Applied
Exercise
Physiology

Applied Exercise Physiology

RICHARD A. BERGER, Ph.D.

Professor of Exercise Physiology
Biokinetics Research Laboratory
Department of Physical Education
Temple University, Philadelphia

1982

LEA & FEBIGER   *Philadelphia*

Lea & Febiger
600 Washington Square
Philadelphia, PA   19106
U.S.A.

Library of Congress Cataloging in Publication Data

Berger, Richard A.
  Applied exercise physiology.

  Includes index.
  1. Exercise—Physiological aspects.   I. Title.
[DNLM: 1. Exertion.   2. Physiology.   WE 103 B496a]
QP301.B416   612'.04   81-2322
ISBN 0-8121-0773-X   AACR2

PRINTED IN THE UNITED STATES OF AMERICA

Print No.   3   2   1

In memory of
Theodore M. Feschuk,
colleague and friend

Preface

The physiologic systems of the body interact to accomplish a variety of tasks. Their interdependence can be likened to a symphony orchestra whose different musical instruments represent various organ systems and whose conductor represents the higher brain center. Some musical compositions and arrangements require all the instruments to blend together; other compositions require one or two instruments to predominate before acquiescing to others. At all times, the precise and melodious interactions are regulated by the conductor.

The emphasis in this book is on specific "instruments" of the body and their unique involvement in certain "musical scores." The organic systems of the body, analogous to the musical instruments, are the skeletal muscles, the nervous system, the cardiovascular system, and the respiratory system. The particular musical scores correspond to different kinds of physical work and exercise. The initiator of the performance is the higher brain center, which coordinates and controls the organic systems involved in exercise. And, just as musical conductors must know the capabilities of the instruments in their orchestras, so must athletes know the capacity of their organ systems for work.

The purpose of this textbook, however, is geared not specifically to the individual athlete but to his or her mentors and to those professionals providing health services. The populations of special concern are physical educators, athletic coaches, physical therapists, recreational therapists, and medical doctors. To provide information about the physiologic systems primarily involved in work and how they can be modified by training, I have followed a specific presentation. The organic systems, which are largely affected by exercise and work, are presented in terms of their structure and function both at rest and during work. The content is substantially elementary so that the student does not need any extensive prior knowledge of physiology, although a general course in anatomy and physiology would greatly help the student to understand the total interdependence of all the organic systems, even those not directly involved during work.

The organic systems of primary concern are the skeletal muscles, the heart and circulatory system, and the nervous and respiratory systems. A chapter is devoted to each system to focus the students' attention on the unique characteristics of each. But, at the same time, chapter content must overlap somewhat for the purpose of showing the interdependence among systems. At the end of the chapters, principles for improving or modifying work performance are presented. These principles are gleaned from research in physiology and, more specifically, from exercise physiology.

The concluding chapter brings all the systems together to focus on their interrelatedness in sports and work. A model of physical performance is presented to assist those individuals interested in dissecting gross physical activity into more easily understood components. Subsequently, greater efficiency and precision in evaluation and assessment of performance become possible.

Philadelphia, Pa.   Richard A. Berger

Contents

CHAPTER 1

Structure, Function, and Force in Skeletal Muscle During Work and Exercise

All movement occurs by the pulling of muscle on bones. The ability to apply a large force in a short time, or a sustained force over a long duration, is possible because of the muscle's capacity to vary energy expenditure according to demand, A working muscle may increase its energy output by 50 times that of the resting level. But to continue this high output, the increased oxygen used by the muscle tissue must be balanced by a corresponding increase in the removal of heat and carbon dioxide from the body. The purpose of the various ways the body responds to work or exercise is to maintain a chemical and physical balance within the muscle cells. The organs of special importance for maintaining cellular equilibrium are the lungs, which supply oxygen and remove carbon dioxide; the heart, which pumps the oxygenated blood and nutrients throughout the body; and the blood vessels, which convey the blood to all the tissues. But the forces required to make all these organs function are provided by muscle tissue. Three types of muscle tissue are in the body: smooth, cardiac, and skeletal. These tissues differ in function (physiologically), structure (histologically), location (anatomically), and innervation (neurologically). This chapter is primarily concerned with skeletal muscle in work and exercise.

GROSS STRUCTURE AND FUNCTION OF SKELETAL MUSCLE

Approximately 40 to 45% of the total body weight consists of skeletal muscle. The cell of muscle tissue is called a muscle fiber and is cylindrical with a diameter of 10 to 100 μ (μ is a micron, which is .001 mm. long) and a length of up to 30 cm. or more. Each fiber is covered by a thin, tough, elastic sheath, called the sarcolemma. Below the sarcolemma are many nuclei. A nucleus is the central mass of protoplasm contained in all cells and is composed of complex proteins that regulate the metabolism and function of the cell. The sarcolemma is closely associated with the cell's cytoplasm, which is the protoplasm outside the cell nucleus. Directly above this sheath is a connective tissue that covers the sarcolemma and is called endomysium (Fig. 1–1). A large number of muscle fibers bound together into bundles, called fasciculi, is enclosed by another connective tissue called perimysium. These bundles, in turn, are grouped together and covered by epimysium. The latter grouping identifies a specific muscle, such as the biceps or deltoid.

Within the sarcoplasm of the cell is a number of thin strands called myofibrils. These strands number from several hundred

1

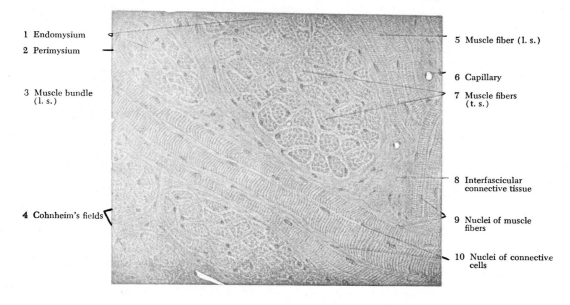

1 Endomysium

2 Perimysium

3 Muscle bundle
(l. s.)

4 Cohnheim's fields

5 Muscle fiber (l. s.)

6 Capillary

7 Muscle fibers
(t. s.)

8 Interfascicular
connective tissue

9 Nuclei of muscle
fibers

10 Nuclei of connective
cells

Fig. 1–1.   The muscle fiber and its component parts. (From Gray's Anatomy of the Human Body. 29th Edition. Revised and edited by Charles M. Goss. Philadelphia, Lea & Febiger, 1973.)

to several thousand in a single fiber. They are about 1 to 2 μ in diameter and run through the length of the fiber. About 80% of the fiber volume is occupied by myofibrils. The myofibrils are the contractile elements in the muscle fiber.

Myofibrils

Myofibrils, when observed under an electron microscope, appear cross striated owing to a consistent pattern of alternating light and dark bands. These bands are comprised of two kinds of protein filaments: a thin filament called actin and a thicker filament called myosin. The overlapping of the two filaments produces the dark band, and the actin filaments alone create the light band. This pattern can be seen in Figure 1–2 where a skeletal muscle is dissected in schematic fashion down to the myofibrils. Note that the dark bands are identified by the term anisotropic, or A; the light bands are identified by the term isotropic, or I. At the center of each I band is a denser portion known as the Z line. The area between two Z lines is called a sarcomere. The center of a resting sarcomere, which is also the center of the A band, reveals a less dense area referred to as the H zone. The varying light and dark bands occur because of the longitudinal arrangement of two different filament sizes. The thicker filaments are in the A band, and the thinner filaments occupy the I band and part of the A band. The overlapping of both filaments results in a dark band, whereas the light band only contains the thinner filaments. These filaments are actually protein rods; the thicker filaments are myosin and the thinner filaments are actin. The cross-sectional view of a myofibril in Figure 1–3 shows the relationship between each thick myosin filament and six thin actin filaments, which form a hexagon. However, the six actin filaments are also shared by other myosin filaments to form other hexagons throughout the myofibril.

Sarcoplasm

The protoplasm of muscle fibers is called sarcoplasm. All living matter, in fact, is

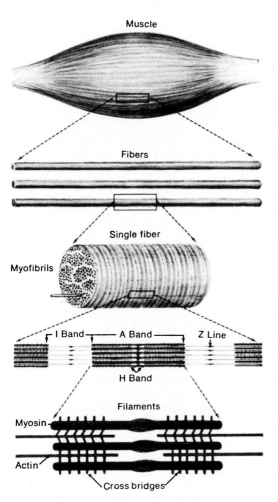

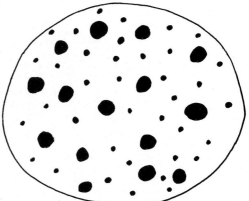

Fig. 1–3.   Cross section of myofibril showing the hexagonal relationship between myosin and actin filaments. (From Guyton, A.C.: Basic Human Physiology: Normal Function and Mechanisms of Disease. Philadelphia, W. B. Saunders Co., 1971.)

Fig. 1–2.   Skeletal muscle dissected schematically. (From Schottelius, B.A., and Schottelius, D.D.: Textbook of Physiology. 18th Edition. St. Louis, The C. V. Mosby Co., 1978.)

made of protoplasm. It is organized into microscopic particles (cells) that form the structure of the human form. Each of these cells possesses a unique structure that is related to its functions in the body. However, the common characteristics of protoplasm for all cells are:

1. Organization into units of specific shape and size.

2. Ability to maintain or increase protoplasm and to transform energy from one expression to another by various chemical activities.

3. Movement.

4. Response to stimuli from outside.

5. Growth by an increase in size and number.

6. Ability to reproduce.

7. Adaptation to changes in the external environment.

The protoplasm of muscle cells, sarcoplasm, contains a variety of structures to perform the specific function of muscle. Muscle cells contain a large number of myofibrils, which are necessary for contraction. In addition, muscle cells contain large quantities of mitochondria in which the chemical reactions occur to produce adenosine triphosphate (ATP), the energy source for all contractions. Other essential substances in the sarcoplasm are potassium, magnesium, phosphate, and protein enzymes.

Sarcoplasmic Reticulum and the T-Tubule System

Substances are transported in and out of the cell to maintain life and function. Two structural systems permit this transference:

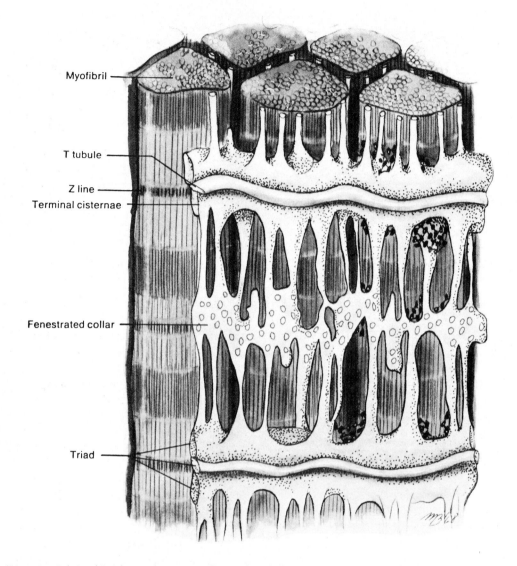

Myofibril

T tubule

Z line

Terminal cisternae

Fenestrated collar

Triad

Fig. 1–4.   Relationship of sarcoplasmic reticulum and T-tubule system to individual skeletal muscle fibrils. (From Schottelius, B.A., and Schottelius, D.D.: Textbook of Physiology. 18th Edition. St. Louis, The C. V. Mosby Co., 1978.)

the transverse tubule system and the sarcoplasmic reticulum. The transverse tubule system, or T system, is a deep infolding of the sarcolemma into the interior of the muscle fiber. Substances are conveyed through this system to the sarcoplasmic reticulum, whose tubules lie parallel to the myofibrils and fuse to form sacs that surround the myofibrils (Fig. 1–4). The nutrients that supply energy for contraction are conveyed from the fluid outside the cell, through the tubules, and into the myofibrils. After the cell uses these nutrients by a series of chemical reactions, the by-products are released from the myofibrils through the sarcoplasmic reticulum and T tubules into the fluid surrounding the cell. The tubules of the sarcoplasmic reticulum and T system also transmit electrical current from the membrane of the muscle fiber into the interior of the myofibril to initiate muscle contraction.

Contractile Mechanism

When the length of a muscle fiber shortens, the length of the A band remains constant, but the I band shortens because the thin filaments of actin proteins slide inward toward each other (Fig. 1–5). During a maximum contraction, the Z line may touch the A band and the filaments may actually fold slightly on contact within the H zone. The sliding of the actin and myosin filaments in a myofibril is explained by the interdigitation or ratchet theory of contraction. The theory states that the protoplasmic projections that outwardly extend from the shank of the myosin filaments and are in contact with the actin filaments move inwardly toward the center of the A band and, at the same time, cause the actin filaments to move with them (Fig. 1–6). This theory has been strongly supported by the observation through an electron microscope of intact sarcomeres. An expansion of this original theory attempts to explain the movement of the projections or cross-bridges of the

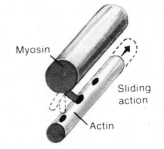

Fig. 1–6. Cross bridges of a myosin filament interdigitating with an actin filament to cause shortening of muscle contraction. (From Schottelius, B.A., and Schottelius, D.D.: Textbook of Physiology. 18th Edition. St. Louis, The C. V. Mosby Co., 1978.)

myosin filaments. Hypothetically, adenosine triphosphate (ATP), which produces energy when broken down, is bound to the cross-bridges of the myosin filaments in the resting state. The negative charge of the ATP is repelled by the same charge of the actin filaments. As a consequence, the actin and myosin filaments remain separated from each other. However, this situation changes when the membrane of the muscle fiber receives an excitatory wave, which is transmitted by the sarcoplasmic reticulum and

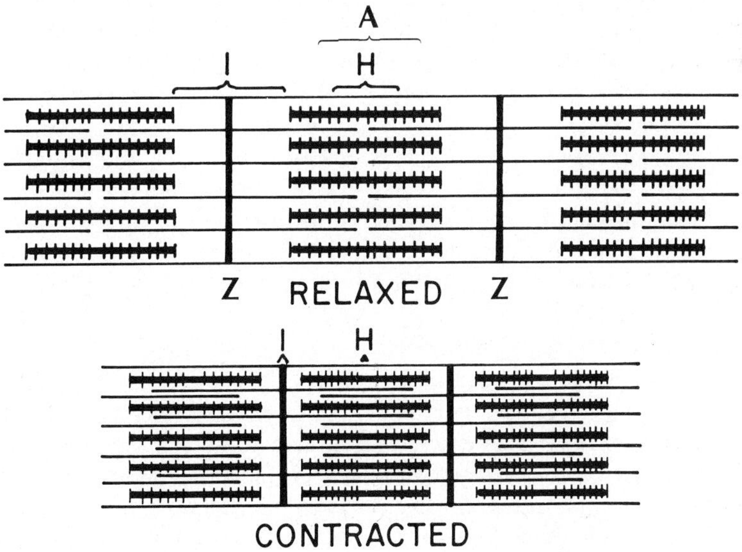

Fig. 1–5. Sliding of the actin filaments during contraction of skeletal and cardiac muscle.

the T tubules into the interior of the myofibril. When this activity occurs, calcium ions are released from the sarcoplasmic reticulum and bind with the ATP on the cross-bridges to neutralize their negative charge. The myosin then attaches to actin and, because the shank of the myosin filaments remains negatively charged, the bridges are attracted and bend in its direction. When the cross-bridges fold in toward the shank, the ATP on the cross-bridges comes in contact with an enzyme (a chemical that accelerates a reaction but does not change itself) on the shank. The contact causes ATP to break down to adenosine diphosphate (ADP) with a release of energy. Consequently, the myosin cross-bridges become negative again and break contact with the actin filament. Almost immediately afterward, energy from other sources causes the ADP to form again into ATP. If an excitatory wave continues to release calcium ions, the cycle is repeated again and again. The cross-bridges of a myosin filament may not function simultaneously in their pulling effect on the actin filaments. While some cross-bridges are pulling, others may have just completed their work and are assuming the resting position in preparation for another activation. The continuous and asynchronous activity of the cross-bridges with actin results in a smooth muscle contraction.

Tendons

Almost all striated muscles are fastened to bones by tendons. A tendon is a connective tissue that is quite dense and is composed of a white fibrous substance. The fibers run the length of the tendon and are grouped into small bundles called fasciculi. These bundles combine to form larger bundles that are held together by a connective tissue referred to as peritendineum. Between these bundles are the tendon cells. The tendons are supplied with blood vessels, lymph vessels, and nerves. Fibers of the tendon are attached to the sarcolemma of the muscle fibers. Because of its great strength, the tendon is less likely to tear than is a muscle or even a bone.

Blood Supply to the Muscles

During severe exercise, the blood flow to skeletal muscles may increase by up to 20 times that of the resting flow. For this increase to occur, all muscle capillaries (smallest blood vessels in which exchange takes place between blood and tissues) are opened. (Only 10% are open during rest.) But the flow is unsteady because of the muscle contraction. Flow increases between contractions and decreases during the contraction phase because of the varying pressure on the blood vessels. After the contractions cease, blood flow remains high for a minute or two and then gradually diminishes.

The great increase in blood flow to working muscles is the consequence of a localized effect on the arterioles (blood vessels leading to capillaries) of the muscles. Apparently, the reduction of oxygen in the muscle tissues and in the surrounding fluids stimulates in some way the dilation of the arterioles in the perimysium. Simultaneously, other vasodilatory (blood vessel dilation) substances are released during contraction. An elevation of arterial pressure, an effect that usually occurs in exercise, also causes an increase in blood flow.

Blood flow to the muscles is also regulated by nerves. Even before vasodilatation is controlled locally, the initiation of muscle activity by the motor cortex of the brain simultaneously excites the vasodilator nerve fibers to the active muscles, and vasodilatation occurs. Thus, extra blood flow is available at the onset of muscular activity.

Nerve Supply to the Muscles

Each muscle fiber is innervated individually but many are innervated by one nerve cell or neuron. The sheath of a nerve fiber, called neurilemma (see Fig. 3–2), appears to be continuous with the sheath of a muscle fiber or sarcolemma (Fig. 1–7). At the muscle fiber, the terminal ending of a nerve branch is embedded in sarcoplasm under the

A

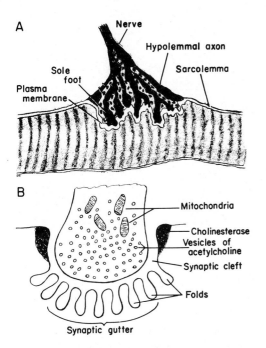

Fig. 1–7.   *A,* The neuromuscular junction and *B,* the sole feet adjacent to the membrane of the muscle fiber. (From Guyton, A.C.: Basic Human Physiology: Normal Function and Mechanisms of Disease. Philadelphia, W. B. Saunders Co., 1971.)

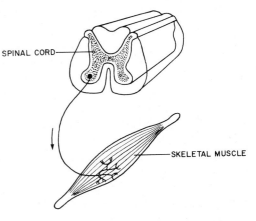

Fig. 1–8.   Motor unit with its motor neuron and muscle fibers. (From Elson, L.: It's Your Body. New York, McGraw-Hill, Inc., 1975. Used with permission of McGraw-Hill Book Co.)

sarcolemma. Single fibers may be stimulated by more than one motor neuron. However, the majority of muscle fibers are stimulated by only one nerve fiber. Each of the nerve cell bodies located in the ventral (front part of the body) horns of the spinal cord sends out a nerve fiber, or axon, which travels from the spinal cord to the muscle it activates. The axon divides into either several or more than 150 branches. Each branch terminates at a single muscle fiber.

The Motor Unit

The axon of the neuron and all the muscle fibers it innervates are called a motor unit (Fig. 1–8). Muscle fibers in the same motor unit do not lie next to each other but are scattered throughout the whole muscle. And, because they are supplied by nerve branches of varying lengths, the muscle fibers contract asynchronously over a considerable area of the entire muscle when a

motor nerve is stimulated. Even motor units to the same muscle (biceps, triceps) are excited asynchronously because they fire at different times.

Transmission of Impulses Along Muscle Fibers

A muscle must be stimulated before its potential energy can be released to cause a contraction. Stimulation of the muscle fibers is provided by the electrochemical impulse that travels along the motor nerves to the muscle. At the junction between a nerve fiber and a muscle fiber, called the neuromuscular junction or end-plate, the electrochemical impulses from the nerve fiber cause a release of a chemical called acetylcholine (see Fig. 1–7). The end-plate invaginates into the muscle fiber but does not penetrate the muscle membrane. The place of invagination is called the synaptic gutter. Many nerve branches of the end-plate, called sole feet, lie adjacent to the fiber membrane (see Fig. 1–7B). Mitochondria and small vesicles containing acetylcholine are contained in the sole feet. Nerve impulses cause the release of acetylcholine from these vesicles into the synaptic cleft between the sole feet and muscle fiber membrane. Within about 2 msec. after acetylcholine is released and enters the synaptic cleft, the enzyme, cholinesterase, which is stored around the rim of the synaptic gutter, destroys the acetylcholine. The excitation of the muscle fiber is thus halted so that the fiber can "recharge itself" in preparation for the next impulse.

The electrical potential between the inside and the outside of a muscle fiber or nerve fiber, called an action potential, is responsible for the electrical flow. When the sarcolemma of the muscle fiber or the neurilemma of the nerve fiber, both thin membranes surrounding their fibers, allow positive and negative ions to pass through them, an electrical impulse travels along these membranes. The impulses are transmitted via the T tubules and sarcoplasmic reticulum into the muscle fibers, where calcium ions are then released to initiate a contraction of the myofibrils.

The electrolytic chemicals that create the action potential across the sarcolemma and neurilemma are sodium, potassium, and nondiffusible negatively charged ions. During rest, the greater number of positively charged sodium ions on the outside of the muscle and nerve cells relative to the smaller amount of positively charged potassium ions on the inside plus the larger amounts of negatively charged ions on the inside result in an action potential or membrane potential of about 85 millivolts. When a stimulus changes the permeability of the membrane, electrochemical impulses travel along the fibers by the movement of sodium ions into the fiber and of potassium ions out of the cell. After a fraction of a second, the membrane is no longer permeable and the balance of positive and negative ions assumes its former resting condition. The process of impulse transmission occurs in two stages called depolarization and repolarization, and applies to both muscle and nervous tissue. These two stages are illustrated in Figure 1–9.

The resting condition of the cell is shown by Figure 1–9A, where relatively more positive ions are shown on the outside than on

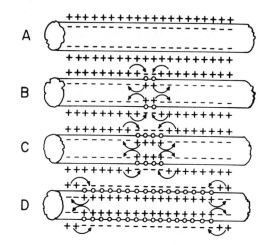

Fig. 1–9.   Impulse transmission along a conductive fiber.

the inside of the membrane. When the cell is excited at its midpoint, as shown by Figure 1–9B, the increase in membrane permeability allows sodium to pass in and potassium to pass out. The current flow is called the depolarization stage, and is illustrated by Figures 1–9C and 1–9D. Immediately after the impulse passes, the positive and negative ions reverse and reach a normal resting potential again. This latter stage is called repolarization. During repolarization, impulses cannot be transmitted along the membranes.

The velocity of impulses traveling along muscle and nerve cells varies. Impulses travel at the rate of about 5 m per sec. in muscle but vary in nerve fibers according to fiber diameter. In small nerve fibers, velocity may be as low as 0.5 m per sec., but can reach 130 m per sec. in the largest fibers.

MUSCULAR CONTRACTIONS

When a muscle fiber contracts, the actin and myosin filaments of the myofibrils slide in toward each other (see Figs. 1–5 and 1–6). Although the fibers respond this way in a contraction, the whole muscle may or may not change its length. The terms used to identify the three kinds of muscular contractions are: concentric, isometric, and eccentric. These contractions occur simultaneously and in sequence to accomplish work and to counteract the effects of gravity on the body.

Concentric Muscular Contraction

A contraction that results in the shortening of a muscle is called a concentric contraction. A concentric contraction occurs when the elbow is flexed by the biceps or extended by the triceps. Movement happens when the origin and insertion of the muscle are brought closer together by the contraction. Occasionally, this kind of contraction is referred to as isotonic, dynamic, or phasic.

There are basically two kinds of concentric contractions, and they differ in the amount of muscle fibers that contract throughout a joint range. During an isodynamic contraction, the number of muscle fibers involved remains about the same from the beginning to the end of the movement. During an allodynamic contraction, the number of contracting fibers is greater at one point in the joint range and less at all other joint angles. The terms, isodynamic and allodynamic, were derived from the Greek words, "iso," which means "the same" and "allo," which means "not the same." They describe the extent to which the muscle fibers are involved in a dynamic (or concentric) contraction. In a maximum isodynamic contraction, the force in the muscle is 100% of its capacity at all joint angles, whereas in a maximum allodynamic contraction, the force capacity is 100% at one angle and less at all others.

ALLODYNAMIC CONTRACTION. When lifting a barbell vertically against gravity in an allodynamic contraction, the degree of force required by the muscle varies according to the joint angle. There is a point in the movement range where the effort is greatest, and that point is called the "sticking point." Variation in joint leverage as the weight is raised produces this effect. The "sticking point" in this case is primarily owing to the poorest leverage at that joint

angle. Other allodynamic contractions occur when a barbell is lifted in a rotational movement, such as when flexing the elbows. In this case, the "sticking point" depends more on the direction in which the load is moved in relation to the force of gravity, not to leverage.

When lifting a constant load in a vertical direction, a "sticking point" is evident because of the differences in leverage throughout the joint range and because of the variations in muscle length. Leverage is more advantageous at some joint angles than at other angles. When this fact is superimposed on muscle length, where a shortening muscle loses some of its force capacity, the combination of the two produces the "sticking point." Because of the variations in leverage arrangements at the joints, each joint has a different strength pattern. For example, when maximum force is determined and plotted at different joint angles in a movement of the deep knee bend or elbow flexion, the curves look similar to those in Figure 1–10.

When lifting a load in a rotational movement where the joint or axis is stationary and the movement of the load proscribes an arc, there is one point where the force of gravity is at a 90° angle to the rotating arm. Only at that point in the joint range does the muscle exert the greatest force. In other words, the "sticking point" in a rotational movement is always at the joint angle where the force of gravity is at a 90° angle to the rotating arm. The factors of leverage and muscle length, which determine the "sticking point" in a vertical movement, are of minimum concern in the determination of the "sticking point" in a rotational movement. The exertion of a force equal to the actual weight of the object is necessary only when the direction of applied force is in line with the force of gravity.

ISODYNAMIC CONTRACTION. For a muscle to contract isodynamically with the same potential force capacity, whether the force is 100% or 50% at all joint angles, the load lifted must vary precisely so that it is

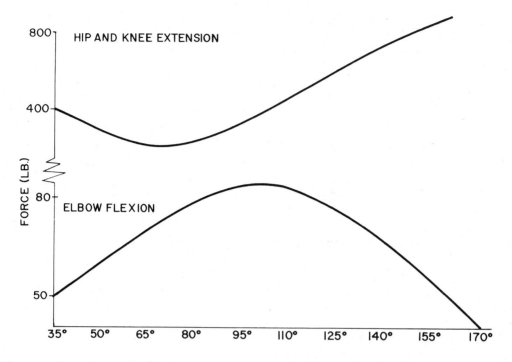

Fig. 1–10.   Strength curves for elbow flexion and hip and knee extension. Curves are not drawn to scale relative to each other.

lightest at the weakest joint angles and heaviest at the strongest angles. An isodynamic contraction is achieved by basically two different kinds of muscle loading: isokinetic loading and accommodating resistance loading.

The equipment providing a constant velocity, or isokinetic movement, falls into two different categories in terms of the method of applying a resistance load to the contracting muscles. The first category includes devices that have a rope wrapped around a pulley within a cylinder. Variations in resistance are provided by varying the contact of the rope around the pulley. Other isokinetic devices provide resistance by electromechanical means. Resistances can be varied so that movements may be fast or slow.

The second category of devices that permits some form of an isodynamic contraction involves a combination of weight plates and leverage. For example, the leverage of a machine is varied so that the resistance load is heaviest at the joint angles with the best leverage and lightest at the joint angles with the poorest leverage. To comprehend this concept, one must understand the formula for a leverage system

$$R \times RA = F \times FA$$

where R is the resistance or load; RA is the length of the resistance arm from R to A; A is the axis; F is the force; and FA is the length of the force arm, from F to A. A situation is illustrated in Figure 1–11 in which the force (F) necessary to lift a load (R) depends on the length of the resistance arm (RA). As the RA becomes longer, more F is needed to raise the same R of 300 lb. The same principle is followed by accommodating resistance machines, which match exercise loads to the different force capacities of skeletal joints throughout a movement range. The machines vary the resistance arm (RA)

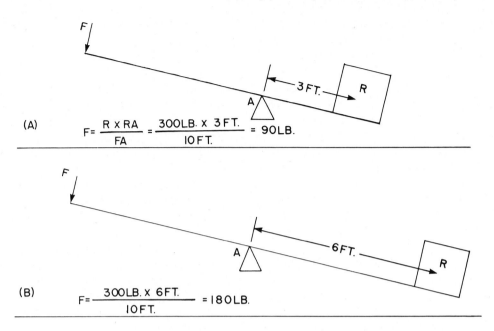

Fig. 1–11.   Lengthening the resistance arm (RA) from 3 ft. (*a*) to 6 ft. (*b*) results in a 100% increase of force (F), from 90 lb. to 180 lb., to raise a 300-lb. resistance (R).

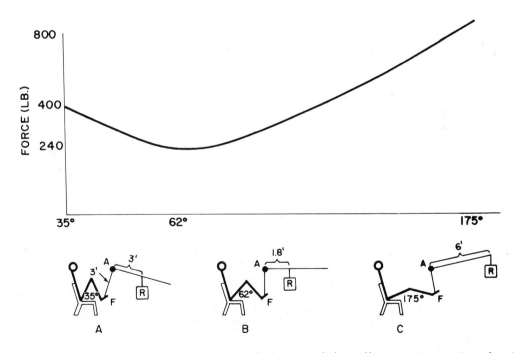

Fig. 1–12.   Changes in resistance (RA) to accommodate the force curve for hip and knee extension.[1] Maximum force is (a) 400 lb. at a knee angle of 35°, (b), 240 lb. at an angle of 62°, and (c), 800 lb. at an angle of 175°. The force arm (FA) and resistance (R) remain the same at 3 ft. and 400 lb. respectively. Varying the RA to 3 ft. at 35°, 1.8 ft. at 62°, and 6 ft. at 175° permits the contracting muscle to exert a similar force throughout the joint ranges. The R is exerting a pull of 400 lb. at a 90° angle to the RA.

while keeping the resistance (R) and the force arm (FA) constant. Force (F) is provided by the contracting muscles.

An example in Figure 1–12 shows how the RA is changed so that a maximum contraction of the leg muscles in the movements of a hip and knee extension is obtained.[1] Three different positions are shown with the knee at 35°, 62°, and 175°. The hip and knee forces needed at each knee angle to match the force curve for a hip and knee extension as shown in Figure 1–12 for a hypothetic individual with a 1-RM of 160 lb. were 270 lb., 160 lb., and 600 lb. at knee angles of 35°, 62°, and 175°, respectively. With the FA and R remaining constant at 3 ft. and 400 lb., the RAs were varied to conform to the appropriate F values. Note how the R shifts back and forth to match or accommodate the F capacity at each knee angle. Moving from a knee angle of 35 to 62°, where strength decreases, the resistance load (R) moves toward the axis (A) to accommodate the weaker position, but, beyond 62°, the resistance load moves away from the axis to accommodate the increased force capacity beyond this angle. RA increases with increased F capacity and decreases with decreased F capacity.

Eccentric Muscular Contraction

Running, throwing, and jumping are the result of concentric contractions. Whenever positive work is done, concentric contractions are responsible. The force of this contraction determines success in athletic performance. However, other kinds of contractions are necessary for coordinated and purposeful movement.

Positioning the body parts so that muscles can effectively shorten by a concentric contraction requires another kind of contraction of the same muscle. Because a muscle must lengthen before it can contract concentrically, there must be a lengthening contraction. A muscle that contracts as it lengthens is experiencing an eccentric contraction. The knee bend exercise, which strongly involves the quadriceps muscle on the front of the thigh, requires that these two kinds of

contractions work together. As the knees flex, the quadriceps group contracts and lengthens at the same time to control the force of gravity on the body. This eccentric contraction places the body in a position that requires a concentric contraction of the same muscle to raise the body to a starting position. All jumping and throwing movements involve both kinds of contractions to a lesser or greater degree. An eccentric contraction is also involved, and prevents joint injury, when jumping to the ground from a high platform. When the feet contact the ground, a reflex action causes the quadriceps and gluteus maximus muscles to contract eccentrically, thereby easing the body's descent. If an eccentric contraction did not occur, the legs would simply collapse and cause injury. Even if the muscles contract concentrically as the feet hit the ground, the tension in the muscles may not be sufficient to support the weight of the falling body. In this case, either the muscle tears and/or the tension is so great on other tissues around the muscle and joint that damage occurs.

Even when both concentric and eccentric contractions occur normally, effective movement is impossible without the third kind of contraction.

Isometric Muscular Contraction

The length of the whole muscle does not change during an isometric contraction; it neither lengthens nor shortens. This kind of contraction maintains the various joints in certain positions against the force of gravity while other joints move under the control of concentric and eccentric contractions. When maintaining a stationary position, the muscles must contract isometrically to support the skeleton. When rising to a standing position, the muscles of the shoulder girdle and trunk contract isometrically to assure a generally vertical posture of the trunk; at the same time, the leg and hip muscles contract concentrically. The same isometric contractions are involved when sitting down, but the leg and hip muscles contract eccentrically. In more complex movements, such as those involved in sports, body posture continually varies so that muscles constantly change their contractions among isometric, concentric, and eccentric responses.

Force Capacity of Concentric, Eccentric, and Isometric Contractions

The tension developed in a muscle during a maximum contraction depends on the type of contraction and on the velocity of shortening. The relationships among the three types of contractions and movement velocities are presented in Figure 1–13. Maximum forces are attained in eccentric contractions and exceed both isometric and concentric contractions by a considerable amount. Almost 50% more force is developed eccentrically than concentrically, and about 25% more than isometrically.

Changes in force occur with movement velocity in both eccentric and concentric contractions. However, the changes follow a different pattern in these two types of contractions. Whereas the concentric pattern of force is highest at slow velocities, the eccentric pattern of force initially rises as velocity increases and then drops with continued velocity.[2] The reasons for differences in force capacity with velocity changes and with the three types of contractions are not known, although the answer probably lies in the physical connections between the actin and myosin filaments. Apparently, the relationship between these filaments, in terms of how they are connected, maintained, and released, holds the clue to the answer.

In many exercises and in work when loads are raised and lowered, it is noticeably easier to lower a load eccentrically than to raise it concentrically. Performing a squat with a heavy barbell resting on the shoulders is a good example of this phenomenon. Lowering the bar eccentrically at a constant velocity is always easier than standing up with the weight at a constant velocity. This effect corresponds to the physiologic responses occurring in the muscles during the work. An eccentric contraction uses less oxygen,[3] a smaller amount of energy,[4,5] and fewer muscle fibers[6] than does a concentric contraction when lifting the same load.

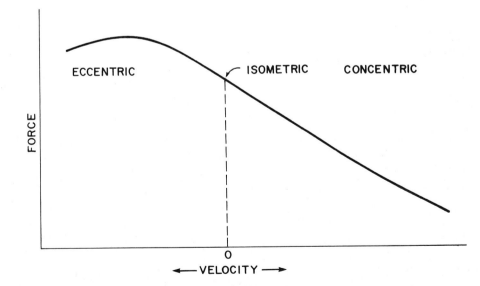

Fig. 1–13. As velocity increases, concentric force decreases. Increasing velocity in eccentric contractions initially increases eccentric force. Further increases in velocity diminish eccentric force, however. (Data from Rodgers, K.L., and Berger, R.A.: Motor-unit involvement and tension during maximum, voluntary concentric, eccentric, and isometric contractions of the elbow flexors. Med. Sci. Sports, 6:253, 1974.)

MOTOR UNIT INVOLVEMENT

The tension developed in a muscle is related to the number of contracting fibers; the more fibers stimulated, the greater the tension. Because all muscle fibers are members of motor units, the number of motor units that fire together determines the tension. Tension is related not only to number of motor units firing, but also to the frequency with which impulses are conveyed by the motor neurons to the fibers. The combination of both number of active motor units and frequency of firing is called motor unit involvement (MUI).

Electrical activity generated by contracting fibers of a muscle can be measured by electrodes either placed on the skin or within the muscle itself.[7] The amount of electrical activity indicates the extent of MUI.[8] A recording of MUI is called an electromyogram or EMG. The relationship between MUI and muscle tension has been studied by examining the EMG. Significant relationships have been discovered between tension and the

extent of MUI.[2] As a muscle contracts with increased tension, the MUI increases proportionately. This relationship is shown in Figure 1–14 where the MUIs corresponding to a concentric and eccentric contraction with different resistance loads are depicted. Note that as force increases, the amount of electrical activity also increases. The two different slopes of the curves show that more motor units are recruited for each unit increase in force with concentric contractions than with eccentric contractions. In addition, the higher concentric curve indicates that, for the same force output, an eccentric contraction requires less motor units than does a concentric contraction. Figure 1–14 represents forces that are generated in nonfatigued muscle. When a muscle becomes fatigued, force obviously diminishes. However, because MUI is a consequence of electrical activity in the muscle and does not reflect the fatigued condition, MUI during a maximum contraction remains essentially the same when force declines with fatigue (Fig. 1–15). If a sub-

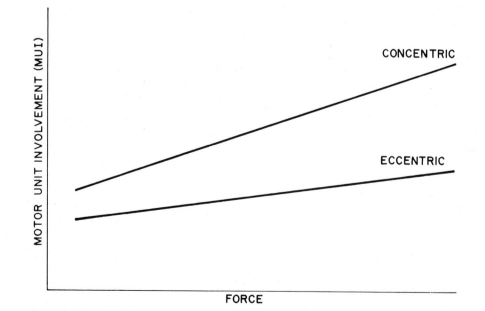

Fig. 1–14.   Motor unit involvement (MUI) of concentric and eccentric contractions at the same muscle forces. (Data from Rodgers, K.L., and Berger, R.A.: Motor-unit involvement and tension during maximum, voluntary concentric, eccentric, and isometric contractions of the elbow flexors. Med. Sci. Sports, 6:253, 1974.)

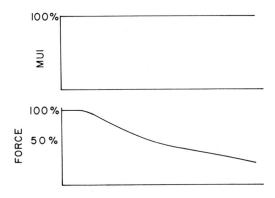

Fig. 1–15. Maximum motor unit involvement (MUI) is maintained as maximum muscle force decreases in fatigue.

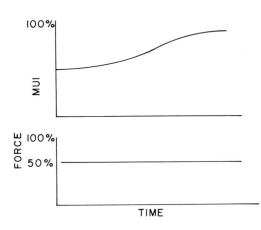

Fig. 1–16. Motor unit involvement (MUI) while maintaining a constant submaximal force. As fatigue occurs, more motor units are required to sustain the force and, therefore, MUI increases to maximum.

maximal load is held until fatigue sets in, the force of contraction remains the same and the MUI increases as more fibers begin to lose their force capacity (Fig. 1–16). As more fibers are brought into play to maintain a given force, the EMG activity is enhanced, reflecting greater MUI.

FACTORS DETERMINING MUSCLE FORCE

The ability to lift a heavy load depends on the force capacity of the muscles and the leverage system through which this force operates. The combination of the two, force and leverage, determines maximum strength. But for strength to improve, force capacity of the muscles must increase because the leverage system of the skeleton is established at birth and cannot be changed. The actual force of a muscle depends on the number of stimulated motor units and their frequency of firing or MUI.

Several factors determine MUI: the length of the muscle at the time of contraction, the velocity with which it contracts, and the extent of neuromuscular control.

Muscle Length

A muscle's length at the time of stimulation to contract determines the amount of force with which it can contract.[9] The relationship between the length of a sarcomere and the tension developed by the muscle fiber is illustrated in Figure 1–17. Sarcomere length is plotted against relative isometric tension for a fiber from the semitendinosus of a frog muscle. When the sarcomere is at a resting length of 2 μ (0.002 mm.) to 2.2 μ (B and C), the isometric tension is maximum. Any length greater (D) or less (A) results in reduction of tension.[9a] The degree of overlap of the myosin actin filaments, corresponding to the sarcomere lengths, is illustrated to the right in Figure 1–17. When the length is at point D, the actin filaments do not overlap with the myosin filaments and the resulting tension is zero. As the sarcomere shortens, filaments overlap and tension increases to about 2.2 μ. At that point, all the actin filaments have overlapped all the cross-bridges of the myosin filaments. As the sarcomeres continue to shorten to less than 2 μ (A), the tension reduces drastically because the increased overlapping interferes with the formation of myosin-actin links.

These results have been confirmed by other experiments with intact muscles in the body. Figure 1–18 shows a curve, similar to that in Figure 1–17, for a whole muscle rather than for an isolated fiber. Although the curves are not identical, their forms are similar. The differences between the curves are probably owing to the larger amount of

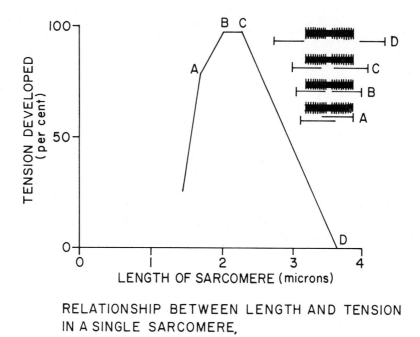

RELATIONSHIP BETWEEN LENGTH AND TENSION
IN A SINGLE SARCOMERE,

Fig. 1–17.   Relationship between length and tension in a single sarcomere. (From Guyton, A.C.: Basic Human Physiology: Normal Function and Mechanisms of Disease. Philadelphia, W. B. Saunders Co., 1971).

elastic connective tissue in the intact muscle and to the sarcomeres in various parts of the intact muscle that do not contract in unison as they do in a single fiber.

Velocity of Shortening

Fewer muscle fibers are involved when a light load is moved rapidly by a concentric

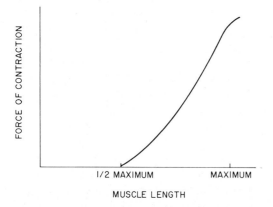

Fig. 1–18.   Relationship between length and maximum tension in an intact muscle. (From Guyton, A.C.: Basic Human Physiology: Normal Function and Mechanisms of Disease. Philadelphia, W. B. Saunders Co., 1971.)

contraction than when a heavier load is moved as rapidly as possible. This statement is understandable because a light load is lifted with less force than is a heavier one. This relationship between muscle force and velocity of shortening has been shown in the laboratory with isolated frog muscle[10–12] and with intact muscle.[1,13] By using an isokinetic device to measure muscle force at different movement velocities, the inverse relationship between force and velocity for knee extension can be demonstrated (Fig. 1–19).

In most sports, the athlete who can move quickly and explosively is more successful. Thus, force improvement at high velocities of movement is apparently more important than improvement at slow velocities. In terms of strength training, some may assume that exercising with light loads and rapid movement is more effective for improving force at fast movements in sport than is exercise with heavy weights, which automatically slow down muscle contraction. However, this assumption has not been supported by research.

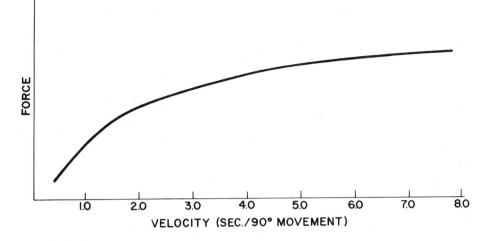

Fig. 1–19.   Relationship between force and velocity of muscle shortening in knee extension. (Data from Berger, R.A., and Higginbotham, R.B.: Prediction of dynamic strength from static strength in hip and knee extension. Am. Correct. Ther. J., 24:23, 1970.)

Muscle Size

The increase in strength from weight training is largely attributable to the increase in the cross-sectional area of the muscle. The greater area is a result of more and larger contractile units within the muscle fibers. And, the increase in contractile units is a consequence of protein build-up resulting from increased protein synthesis stimulated by exercise and work-induced responses in hormones and nervous control of muscle. Although muscle force increases with and is related to muscle size, one should not conclude that a large muscle in one individual has more force capacity than a smaller muscle in another individual. Differences in innate quality of muscle tissue may actually favor the individual with the smaller muscle. If so, the smaller muscle may have more force capacity than the larger muscle. The application of force through the leverage system of the skeleton in terms of the angle at which muscles pull at the joints and at the point of their insertion largely determines strength independent of muscle size.

Neuromuscular Control

An isolated frog muscle, completely disconnected from the animal and prepared for a laboratory experiment, was stimulated electrically to contract under different conditions.[11] In one condition, the muscle was stretched to a predetermined length and, after a pause of several seconds, was stimulated to contract. In another condition, the muscle was again stretched but was immediately given the same electrical stimulus. A comparison of the two forces obtained under the two testing conditions showed that the second stimulus elicited a larger force than did the first. For some unexplained reason, a muscle that is stretched and then immediately contracted has a larger force capacity than a muscle that pauses several seconds after stretching before contracting.

The same phenomenon has been shown in humans. Twenty college students were able to develop a greater force when their muscles were stretched and immediately shortened than when a pause occurred between the stretch and the contraction.[1] Actually, this phenomenon is unconsciously applied in work and exercise. When jumping or throwing, the backswing prior to the forward movement allows more forward force. Athletes, especially, have learned unconsciously not to pause between backswing and forward movement when the primary intent is to increase muscle force. Weight trainers know from experience that lowering a barbell to the starting position and then immediately applying a force to raise it allows more weight to be lifted. Some authorities attribute part of the explanation to special sensory organs in skeletal muscle, known as muscle spindles. These senses respond to stretch and result in the eventual augmentation of muscle force. But augmented force comes to fruition when the muscle contracts immediately after stretching; otherwise, the force is lost. The sequence of the nerve pathway runs from the muscle spindles to the spinal cord and then to the motor nerves of the muscle.

The Golgi tendon organs, located in the tendons of skeletal muscle, affect the force of a contraction because of their protective function. If the tension in a tendon reaches a certain high level, the Golgi organs are stimulated to send impulses back to the spinal cord where contact is made with the motor nerves of the muscle to inhibit their activity. This causes the muscle to lose some of its tension. When these organs become less sensitive to tension as training continues, the forces generated in a muscle increase.

This effect is shown when a maximum isometric force precedes a concentric contraction.[14,15] Figure 1–20 shows the effects of inhibition of the Golgi tendons on the force generated in a muscle when lifting various loads. When inhibition of the tendon organs occurs, the force used to move the different loads is less because the time needed to complete the move is greater than the time needed when inhibition does not occur. For every load, movement time was faster when the tendon organs were not overly stimulated. The movement was extension of the arms while in a supine position (bench press). The structure and function of muscle spindles of Golgi tendon organs are presented in more detail in Chapter 3.

FACTORS DETERMINING STRENGTH

Although the actual force capacity of a muscle depends on its length, the velocity of contraction, its size, and the nature of its neuromuscular control, the ability of an individual to exert a force to an external object or to body weight, such as when jumping, depends on the leverage system of the skeleton through which forces act. Poor leverage may not permit a high application of force to an external weight even though the force capacity of the muscle itself may be high. However, a large external force may be applied if the leverage is favorable, even when muscle force is relatively low. Of course, when leverage is the same for two individuals, the one with the greatest force capacity of the muscles involved will be able to apply the largest force to an external weight. A distinction is made here between the force capacity of a muscle and the force

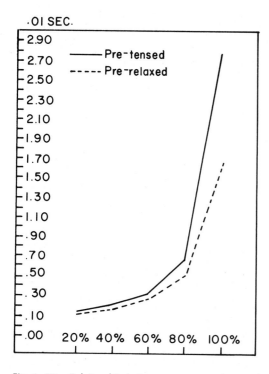

Fig. 1–20. Relationship between movement time and resistance load in pretensed and prerelaxed contractions. Inhibition of muscle force for pretensing by the Golgi tendon organs results in greater (slower) movement time at varying resistance loads. (Data from Berger, R.A., and Mathus, D.L.: Movement time with various resistance loads as a function of pretensed and prerelaxed muscular contraction. Res. Q., 40:456, 1969.)

applied through the leverage system in lifting a load. The latter application of force via the skeletal system is referred to as strength in this text. With this in mind, muscle strength is presented as a function of the leverage system, sex, and age.

Leverage System

To understand how strength is a consequence of leverage, one must first know how leverage is used to apply an external force. Three classes of leverage are in the human body (Fig. 1–21). Note that all classes have an axis (A), resistance (R), force (F), resistance arm (RA) or distance from R to A, and force arm (FA) or distance from F to A. The arrangement of the A, R, F, RA, and FA determines the leverage class.

In the skeletal system, the A represents a joint, the F is provided by a muscle, the R is the resistance or load lifted, the RA is the distance from the resistance to the joint,

usually along a bone, and the FA is the distance from the joint to the point on the bone where the muscle applies F. When the formula for a leverage system $R \times RA = F \times FA$ is balanced, movement occurs.

For example, in a second-class lever of the elbow joint where the muscle (F) is attached 2 in. or .17 ft. from the joint (FA), the resistance arm (RA) is 1 ft. long, and the resistance (R) is 30 lb., the amount of force (F) necessary to lift 30 lb. can be determined by balancing the leverage formula. Transposing the formula so that F is on one side of the equal sign, the formula is:

$$F = \frac{R \times RA}{FA} = \frac{30\,lb. \times 1\,ft.}{.17\,ft.} = 176.47\,lb.$$

In other words, 176.47 lb. of muscle force are needed to lift a 30-lb. resistance in flexion of the elbow. By changing the FA and/or RA, one can readily see by this formula that F would change. If the forearm were 1.25 ft. instead of 1 ft., the F needed to lift 30 lb. would be 220.58 lb. An individual with a long RA relative to the FA would need to apply more muscle force to lift a R than would a person with a shorter RA. A long RA, or short FA, is considered to represent poor leverage; leverage is improved by lengthening the FA or shortening the RA.

Athletes with relatively short forearms and forelegs have a leverage advantage when lifting heavy loads because of their shorter RA. One reason for the power lifter's success in weight-lifting competitions is this leverage advantage. The shorter the RA, the larger the weight that can be lifted. If two individuals have the same force capacity in the biceps muscle (200 lb.) and their muscles are inserted the same distance from the joint (.125 ft.) but one has a longer forearm (1 ft. versus 1.2 ft.), the maximum load or 1-RM (1 repetition maximum) lifted by each is as follows:

Individual A

$$R = \frac{F \times FA}{RA} = \frac{200\,lb \times .125\,ft.}{1\,ft.} = 25\,lb.$$

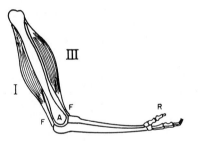

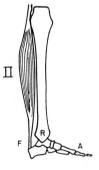

Fig. 1–21. Examples of the three leverage classes in the body: first class (I), second class (II), and third class (III). (From Ricci, B.: Physiological Basis of Human Performance. Philadelphia, Lea & Febiger, 1967.)

Individual B

$$R = \frac{F \times FA}{RA} = \frac{200\,lb. \times .125\,ft.}{1.20\,ft.} = 20.83\,lb.$$

Individual A can lift about 17% more weight than individual B because of the shorter resistance arm.

Sex

Of young children up to 10 to 12 years old, boys are slightly stronger than girls, but the differences are not as significant as they are after these ages. During the adolescent years, as the biologic and structural differences between the sexes become more pronounced and cultural influences encourage males to be physically active and girls to be docile, the strength gap between the sexes widens.[16,17] Many of the physical changes are brought about by the greater hormonal secretions in the male of testosterone, which enhances muscle and bone size. In terms of performances involving strength and power, the physical variations between males and females are reflected in the standing long jump, 50-yard run, shuttle run, and hand grip (Fig. 1–22). Generally, the differences between males and females continue to increase from the ages of 12 to 18. The males continue to improve with age, but the females do not change significantly, except in grip strength.

By the time the average male reaches college age and older, he has almost twice the strength of the average female in the upper

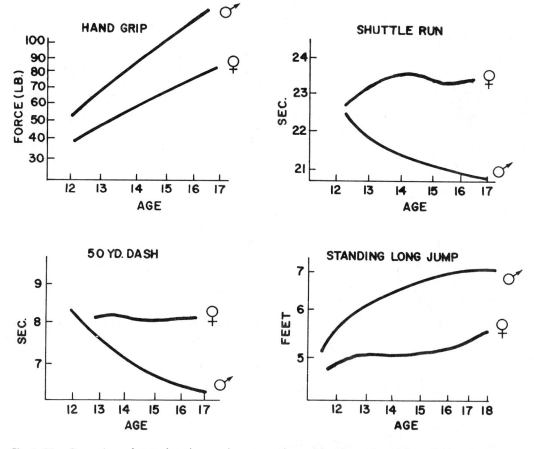

Fig. 1–22. Comparison of strength and power between males and females. (Adapted from Fleishman, E.A.: The Structure and Measurement of Physical Fitness. Englewood Cliffs, Prentice-Hall, 1964.)

Table 1–1.

Absolute and Relative Strength Differences Between Adult Males and Females*

Sample	Sex	Height (in.)	Weight (lb.)	Leg Press Absolute	Leg Press Relative	Grip Absolute	Grip Relative	Bench Press Absolute	Bench Press Relative
College students[20] Study I	F	65.90	127.49	.75	1.00	.61	.80	.57	.51
	M	71.34	170.52						
Military Academy[19] Study II	F	65.91	134.22	.82	.94	.68	.80	.53	.64
	M	69.62	155.45						
Police officers[21] Study III	F	65.30	142.60	.61	.78	.60	.75	.50	.63
	M	69.50	182.40						

*Values indicate the percentage of a male's strength attained by a female for both absolute and relative strength. Relative strength is expressed per pound of body weight.

body and about one-third more in the hips and legs.[18-20] The results of three studies comparing adult males and females are presented in Table 1–1. Only the lifts that were common in all three studies are included. In studies I and II, subjects were college-aged females and males but, in the latter study, the females were significantly larger in body size. The females in study II represented first-year cadets at the United States Military Academy. Study III represented an older population of police officers whose average body sizes were larger than those in the other groups.

When strength is expressed as absolute, males are noticeably stronger than females, based on a compilation of scores from all groups (Fig. 1–23). This gives males an advantage in performances involving a high degree of absolute strength, such as the shotput and discus throw. But, when strength is expressed per unit body weight (the shaded areas), differences between sexes decrease or disappear as shown by

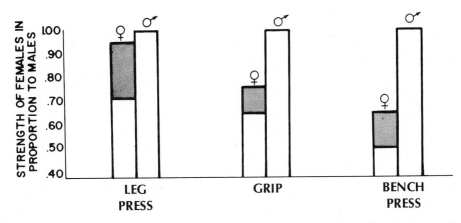

Fig. 1–23. Comparison of absolute and relative strength (st./lb.) between adult males and females based on data from three studies.[18-20] The shaded areas indicate the increased strength of females when strength is expressed according to unit body weight.

the comparison of leg and hip strength in study I.

Part of the difference in performance is owing to the kinds of physical activities in which females and males participate during their youth. Cultural attitudes often encourage males to engage in sports and activities that develop strength and power, such as wrestling and weight training. As a result, they tend to approach their performance potentials more closely than do females who often are discouraged from participating in activities that develop strength. Evidence supports the contention that females are farther than males from their strength potential. This hypothesis is based on the premise that individuals who are farthest from their full potential generally tend to improve more than others when exposed to the same kind of training experience. When college-aged females were trained with weights for 10 weeks, their average relative improvement was greater than the improvement shown by college-aged males.[22] There is no indication that the average female will ever catch up to

the average male in absolute strength. However, with more overload training, the gap between them certainly will narrow.

Age

Physical growth and muscular activity play a large part in determining muscular strength. As a child grows physically from early age to adulthood, force capacity of the muscles rapidly increases. The increase in muscle mass is positively related to force capacity. When physical maturation is reached, an increase in muscle force is only provided by overload training. Unless this training is done, the muscles follow the general downward trend characteristic of other organ systems with advancing age and begin to diminish in force capacity. Overload training continued into adult life often enhances strength significantly beyond the strength experienced during the early stages of adulthood. But, if relatively little overloading is done by the muscle, the steady decline in strength generally follows the curve illustrated in Figure 1–24. These two

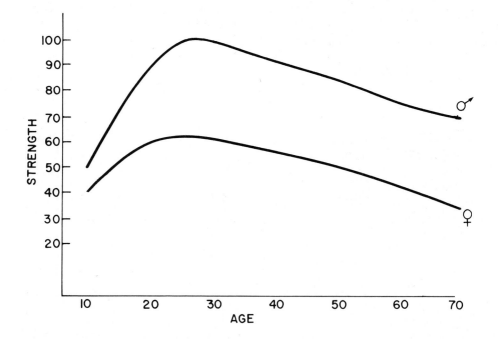

Fig. 1–24. Strength of males and females at various ages. (Data from Fisher, M.B., and Birren, J.E.: Age and strength. J. Appl. Psychol., *31*:490, 1947.)

curves, one for males and one for females, are based on the results of several studies on the average strength of different muscle groups at various ages.[23,24] Maximal strength is reached between the ages of 20 and 30 and gradually declines until, at age 65, strength is about 20% less.

Body Weight

Individuals with heavy body weight tend to have more absolute strength and less relative strength than do those with light body weight. This is illustrated in Figure 1–25 in which mean values for total allodynamic strength are related to body weight. Total strength is the sum of the maximum lifts for curl, upright rowing, standing press, bench press, bend-over rowing, sit-ups, and squat lifts. In the same figure, when total strength is expressed per lb. of body weight, the relationship of strength to body weight reverses, indicating that lighter body weights have more strength per lb. These relationships help to explain why gymnasts tend to be smaller in stature than are football linemen or shot-putters. To perform successfully in gymnastics, a high level of strength is needed per unit body weight to best control the movements of the body in space or suspended from apparatus. However, when heavy opponents must be shoved out of the way, such as in football, a large absolute level of strength and, in turn, body size is an advantage. Generally, in sports where only body weight is the load moved and success depends on speed, agility, and coordination, such as in tumbling, diving, and soccer, body size is usually less than that among athletes who must move or propel such external objects as a shot put or discus.

EFFECTS OF HEAVY RESISTANCE EXERCISE ON MUSCLE, BONE, LIGAMENTS, AND CARTILAGE

The tension in a contracting muscle often reaches several hundred pounds and varies according to muscle mass. The effects of these large forces pulling on bones and on the connective tissues surrounding skeletal joints are reflected in the structural make-up of bones, ligaments, cartilage, and tendons. In all these tissues, structural changes occur

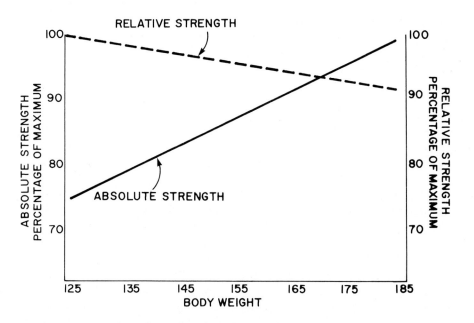

Fig. 1–25.   Relationship between body weight and absolute and relative strengths of college-aged males based on the 1-RM sum of seven lifts. (Data from Berger, R.A.: Prediction of total dynamic strength from chinning and dipping strength. J. Assoc. Phys. Ment. Rehabil., *19*:18, 1965.)

as a result of work and exercise. These adaptations to work are related to changes in the function of skeletal muscle. When muscle tissues increases in force capacity, corresponding alterations in other tissues occur.

Structural and Functional Changes in Muscle From Heavy Work and Exercise

Muscle fibers become larger because of an increase in protein synthesis.[25,26] The result is a multiplication of myofibrils within fibers and a corresponding enlargement of the cross-sectional area of a muscle. Hypertrophy is attributed by most researchers to the increase of myofibrils rather than to an increase in muscle fibers.[27] However, some researchers have suggested that the number of fibers also increases.[28,29] The stimulus for growth is the repeated and continuous contraction of muscle with heavy loads for a period of several weeks. Increases of 3 to 6% have been found in humans who trained with a variety of programs.[30,31]

Muscle hypertrophy may also occur from the stimulus provided when a muscle is stretched. The importance of stretch in hypertrophy, or in retarding atrophy, was shown when a muscle was stretched and secured in a cast.[32] Atrophy occurred at a much slower rate in the stretched muscle than in a muscle cast in a shortened position. For some reason, the tension of stretching reduces the rate of protein breakdown.

Part of the increase in the cross-sectional area of a muscle from exercise is owing to structures other than protein. Work has been reported to induce a proliferation of collagen,[33] which is a fibrous protein of great strength. The collagen fibers in the connective tissue that surrounds the muscle act as a structural framework to which muscle fibers are attached. Because the forces created by the contracting muscle fibers are transmitted to the bone by the connective tissue and tendons, one can understand how muscle hypertrophy is associated with an increase in collagen. In fact, after six days of exercise in rats, a 50% increase occurred in collagen

concentration in the hypertrophied muscle.[33,34]

Effects of Androgens on Hypertrophy

There are several male sex hormones which together are called androgens. They have both androgenic effects and anabolic effects on the body. The androgenic effects are the development of such secondary male characteristics as the enlargement of the external genitalia and accessory sex organs, growth of body hair, and enlargement of the vocal cords, resulting in a deeper voice. The anabolic effects also involve growth, but primarily by increasing protein synthesis in muscle tissue. As a result, girth of skeletal muscle increases. The dominant hormone of the androgen group is testosterone, which is secreted by the male testes and adrenal cortex and, to a much lesser degree, by the female adrenal cortex and ovaries. The difference between females and males in muscle size is primarily owing to testosterone, which is present in larger amounts in males.

The nature of the external work performed by an individual determines whether hypertrophy will occur. Lifting heavy loads is associated with gains in muscle size. Some of these gains can be attributed to the greater increase in testosterone, which is secreted during heavy work. This increase was shown in male swimmers after a heavy workout in water[35] and in college males after weight training.[36] However, significant increases were not noted in females after heavy lifting.

Apparently, the greater amount of testosterone in males is the primary reason for the greater hypertrophy experienced by males than by females after weight training. Studies have shown that, although both sexes respond to training in terms of strength increases and hypertrophy, males exceed females in proportional increases in girth.[22,37] This effect is obvious when the physiques of female gymnasts are compared with those of male gymnasts. In both their training, much emphasis is placed on overloading the musculature, but the effect after years of training is decidedly different.

Effects of Anabolic Steroids on Strength and Hypertrophy

Anabolic steroids, produced synthetically in the laboratory, are chemically and functionally similar to testosterone in their anabolic effects. When taken orally, these steroids have been shown in some studies to increase lean muscle mass and/or body weight, and strength above that attained by weight training alone.[38-42b] Other studies have not shown these results.[43-45] However, in all the studies in which protein supplements were taken in addition to anabolic steroids, a greater improvement in strength occurred.[38-42] These results are supported by interviews with champion shot-putters who cited significant improvements in strength as a result of taking synthetic steroids.[46] Increases in a clean and jerk, from 335 to 365 lb., and in a maximum squat, from 425 to 520 lb., have been reported. Apparently, the use of steroids in sports is advantageous for athletes who move heavy loads, such as shot-putters, discus throwers, football players, and weight lifters. The disadvantages are in the physiologic side effects that result when steroids are taken for prolonged periods of time.[41,47] Some of these adverse effects are reflected in function and structure of the testes, liver, and prostate gland.

Females would probably experience similar improvements in strength from using anabolic steroids, but the consequences in terms of modifying secondary sex characteristics and the other side effects just mentioned may far outweigh any advantages. Ethical problems are also associated with the use of anabolic steroids in athletics. Value judgments are not presented here, not because they are unimportant, but because the content is limited to physiologic function and corresponding structural changes in tissue.

Structural and Functional Changes in Bone, Ligaments, Tendons, and Cartilage from Heavy Work and Exercise

Overload training places stress on the skeletal structure just as it does on the muscles. The large pulling and tugging forces on the bones eventually produce structural changes if the intensity of work is high. Although most studies have used rats to show that high-intensity running or overload increases bone girth and density,[48-51a] some observations and studies with humans have shown similar changes.[52,53] Increases in bone density are largely owing to elevation in mineral content, probably calcium.[50,54-56] Some evidence also shows that bone strength is increased from training[49-51] and that prior training can accelerate the healing process in broken bone.[50] The significant relationships found between bone weight and muscle weight during atrophy[33,57] and under normal conditions,[48] suggest that heavy resistance exercise results in hypertrophy of both muscle and bone. The effects of training on increasing bone density are reflected in the effects of physical inactivity on bone. As a result of inactivity, there is a loss of both the mass and size of bone.[58,59]

Ligaments strengthen joints by extending between the bones that form joints, whereas tendons pull on bones. However, both ligaments and tendons are affected similarly by training because they function together. The information about the effects of training on ligaments and tendons comes largely from research studies that examined rats before and after training. The usual procedure for measuring strength of these tissues is to isolate them and determine their breaking strength. Physical training tends to increase the strength of tendons and ligaments and their attachments to bone so that they can withstand more stress.[60-63] The exact substances responsible for the increase in tensile strength are not known, but evidence points to collagen.[3,60,64,65]

Exercises that stretch the ligaments extensively may reduce the stability of joints and may tend to make them more susceptible to injury. The particular joint of concern among athletes and trainers, and the joint that causes consternation among orthopedic surgeons, is the knee. Evidence shows that performing deep knee bends with weight stretches the ligaments and, thereby, weakens them, reducing joint stability.[66] This conclusion was reached after examining the knee flexibility of competitive weight lifters and other athletes. Weight lifters had more lateral and medial movement of the femur than did the other athletes.

The evidence is not conclusive however, because when ligaments of animals in a related study were stretched to 108% of their length at rest, change in their maximum tensile strength was observed.[67] In fact, most injuries in sports are not a result of damage to the ligament itself, but of its tearing away from the bone.[63]

In addition to the increase of strength in ligaments and tendons from training, there is also a thickening of the cartilage between articulating joints.[60,68] This increase in size comes largely from more intercellular substances rather than from greater cellular components.

MUSCLE STRENGTH AND MOVEMENT VELOCITY

Increased muscle strength has an effect on performances that require quick movements. An individual who improves in strength from 100 to 130 lb. can move 100 lb. faster after the strength increase than he could before the increase. Also, loads of 90, 80, and 70 lb. can be moved faster. However, as the loads become increasingly lighter, until only a body limb is moved, increased movement time (MT) as a result of an improvement in strength becomes less certain. When a maximum strength is based on an isometric contraction and is related to MT of the limb, stronger individuals may move faster.[69,70] However, this is not always the case.[15,71] When maximum strength was based on a concentric contraction in the bench press lift and a relationship was determined between strength and MT with various loads from heavy to light, significant

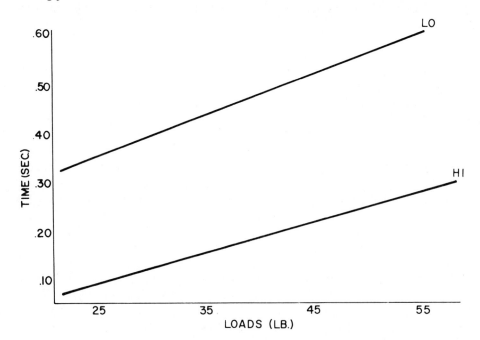

Fig. 1–26.   Movement time with various resistance loads between high-strength and low-strength individuals based on the bench press lift.[72]

associations were found.[72] The movement speeds of high- and low-strength individuals who performed with varying loads are shown in Figure 1–26. With the same loads, individuals of high strength are always faster than those of low strength. In fact, stronger people may move almost twice the loads of weaker persons and at the same velocity.

The advantage of high strength is further indicated when comparisons are made between MTs of strong and weaker individuals when the loads lifted are the same proportions of the 1-RM for both groups (Fig. 1–27). Even when loads are proportionately the same at 20, 40, 60, 80, and 100% of maximum, stronger individuals are faster.[73] When comparisons are made between the two groups on the basis of power, which involves velocity and acceleration, high strength is associated with greater power. In athletic performances requiring quick movements and power, especially with heavy loads involving either body weight and/or an external weight, a high level of strength is certainly an advantage. Apparently, the larger the load to be moved in athletics, the greater the advantage of being strong. This concept is shown by the greater disparity between the high- and low-strength individuals in Figure 1–27 as the loads increased to 80 and 100% of the 1-RM. In summary, not only does an increase in strength permit a faster movement of a given weight but, in addition, there is an increase in the ability to rapidly move a heavy load of the same proportionate percentage of the 1-RM.

Strength and Power Relationships in Performance

When an explosive movement occurs, power is the physical component involved. Power is the amount of work performed in a unit of time. The physicist defines work as the application of force through a distance. For example, when vertically raising a 16-lb. shot put 2 ft., the work done equals 32 ft. lb. The formula for work is:

$$Work = F \times D$$

where F is force (a constant force) and D is the distance through which the force is moved. Then, for this example, Work = F × D = 16 lb. × 2 ft. = 32 ft.-lb.

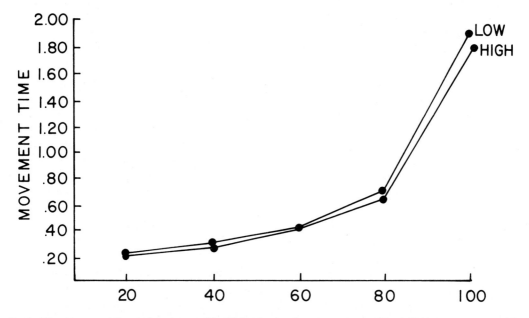

Fig. 1–27. Movement time in bench press lift with loads of various percentages of the 1-RM between young adult males of high and low maximum strength.[72]

As previously defined, power is work done in a unit of time. The formula is:

$$\text{Power} = \frac{\text{Work}}{\text{Time}} \text{ or } \frac{F \times D}{t}$$

When the work in raising the 16-lb. shot put is expressed as power, the amount of time (t) required to complete the work must be known. If the load is moved 2 ft. in .5 sec., the power would be:

$$\text{Power} = \frac{F \times D}{t} = \frac{16\,\text{lb.} \times 2\,\text{ft.}}{.5\,\text{sec.}}$$
$$= 64\,\text{ft.-lbs.}/\text{sec.}$$

The value for F is considered constant in this example. However, in explosive sports, force possesses a factor of acceleration or change in velocity so that $F = M \times A$ (M = mass, A = acceleration). When this aspect is considered, the formula becomes:

$$\text{Power} = \frac{M \times A \times D}{t}$$

The acceleration given to the mass (M) or body weight in running or jumping is provided by the force of muscle contraction. By increasing the force and speed with which the muscles contract, acceleration (A) and time (t) required to complete the work are increased and decreased, respectively. In the power formula, when A is increased and/or t is decreased, power increases. An athlete must have great power to perform certain sports well. Football linemen are large in stature because their size gives them a greater capacity for power, which is essential for blocking or overcoming opponents. So, for a lineman, both quickness (A) and large body weight (M) are essential.

In some sports, the total amount of power generated by a moving body is not as important as the time required to move a specific distance, such as in a 40-yd. dash or a quick move in fencing. For such sports, power relative to body weight or power per lb. of body weight is more essential for maximiz-ing performance. Large muscle mass may be detrimental to athletes who must succeed primarily on running speed and quickness. However, increasing muscle size by over-load training may enhance force to such an extent that acceleration is increased. By the same token, reducing muscle size and body weight with hopes of running faster may not produce the desired result if muscle force is lost in the process.

The decision to maximize acceleration and movement speed (which is relative power) or absolute power depends on the qualities considered most important for ath-letic success. An athlete running sprint races should reduce body weight (M in the power formula) to the point that best maximizes acceleration (A). An athlete who wants to maximize absolute power, such as a defen-sive end in football, should increase muscle mass (M) to the point where the reduction in acceleration (A) offsets or reduces absolute power. But, even though absolute power is essential for success as a football lineman, the sacrifice of some absolute power for more quickness or acceleration may be to the player's advantage. In this event, he would not increase muscle mass to the same extent as he would if absolute power were the only concern. The idea is to find the combination of both absolute power and ac-celeration that best optimizes playing abil-ity. Increasing acceleration invariably in-creases relative power and absolute power.

Other positions in football, such as wide receiver or defensive back, place more em-phasis on relative power than on absolute power. In these positions, the athlete must move rapidly. An offensive back should possess both absolute power to overcome a tackler and relative power to avoid being caught by an intended tackler.

Absolute Strength and Power

Individuals of high absolute strength tend to perform better in tests of absolute power than in tests of relative power. This is under-standable because, in both absolute strength and absolute power tests, force is applied

Table 1–2.

*Relationships Between Absolute 1-RM Strength and Relative Power Among 169 Junior High School Males**

		Relative Power			
	Lift	Standing jump	Shuttle run	50-yd. run	Softball throw
Absolute 1-RM Strength	Squat	.52	.43	.39	.45
	Dead lift	.43	.43	.44	.55
	Curl	.44	.44	.39	—
	Sit-up	.36	.43	.39	.53
	Bench press	.39	.37	.41	.52

*All correlation coefficients are significant (P = .05). Data from Eastwicke and Berger.[75]

largely to such external forces as a barbell or shot put rather than to body weight alone. Nevertheless, in tests of physical fitness where relative power is frequently measured, some component of absolute power is also usually present.[74]

The significance of absolute strength in performances involving relative power among junior high school males is shown in Table 1–2.[75] Absolute strength was the 1-RM values for the weight-training lifts of squat, dead lift, curl, sit-up, and bench press. Note that absolute leg strength is significantly related to the fitness items of relative power. Although the relationships are not high, they do indicate that absolute strength contributes to success in performances of relative power.[75a]

The significant relationships between absolute strength and relative and absolute power emphasize the importance of strength in athletic ability and fitness. Increasing strength by overload training often improves performances in which strength is a significant factor. These performances may require moving an external object of moderate or heavy weight or propelling body weight up or forward.

Relative Strength and Power

Just as tests of relative strength are related to each other (Table 1–3) (although different muscle groups are involved in these relationships), so are tests of relative power.[74] Table 1–4 contains tests that require explosive movements during which only body weight is moved. These tests of relative power involve the hip and leg muscles either alternating in action, such as in running, or moving together, as in the standing jump. The 10-yd. and 50-yd. sprint tests require identical joint actions, but the other two tests vary. The shuttle run requires quick stops and starts and direction reversal whereas the standing jump involves jumping forward with both legs at once. The nature of the muscle contractions also varies among the tests because the jump test is done in one

Table 1–3.

Relationship Between Tests of Relative Strength

	Dipping	Rope climb	Push-up
Chinning	.57	.72	.58
Push-up	.56	.48	
Rope climb	.58		

Data from Fleishman.[76]

Table 1–4.

Relationships Between Tests of Relative Power

	Standing jump	10-yd. sprint	50-yd. sprint
Shuttle run	.69	.67	.80
50-yd. sprint	.58	.69	
10-yd. sprint	.58		

Data from Fleishman.[76]

Table 1–5.

Relationships Among Tests of Relative Strength and Relative Power

		Relative Power			
		10-yd. sprint	Standing long jump	50-yd. sprint	Shuttle run
Relative Strength	Chining	.40	.43	.53	.52
	Push-up	.31	.34	.38	.34
	Rope climb	.43	.46	.58	.52
	Dipping	.37	.41	.52	.46

*All coefficients significant at the .05 level or less. Data from Fleishman.[76]

explosive movement whereas the other three tests are done with repeated and alternating contractions. Even when these differences in joint actions and muscle involvement are considered, all tests still measure the same basic performance component, which is relative power.

The ability to repeatedly move body weight in moderately slow movements, the measure of relative strength, relates significantly to performances of relative power. Higher relationships are found when the relative strength and relative power tests involve both the upper limbs or lower limbs. These results indicate that relative power may be increased as a consequence of improving the force capacity of muscle (Table 1–5).

OVERLOAD PRINCIPLE AND MUSCLE FORCE

To increase force capacity of a muscle, relatively heavy loads must be lifted. Loads may be in any form—barbells, dumbbells, body weight, isokinetic devices, steel or rubber cables, or the action of one muscle against another muscle. Muscles respond to the overload per se, not to the nature of the overload.

Barbells and Dumbbells

Overloading with barbells and dumbbells is done by increasing the exercise load, the number of times the load is lifted (repetitions), or the number of times a particular exercise is repeated (sets). Before proceeding to the specific application of the overload principle, one must understand how weight training has evolved to its present form. The overload principle for increasing strength is certainly not new. Even before Christ, Milo of Crotona in 500 B.C. overloaded by carrying a bull calf on his back every day until the calf reached maturity. He was undefeated as an Olympic wrestler for many years. Through the ages, man has overloaded by carrying heavy objects or by training with heavy weapons. At the turn of the century, circus strong men were in vogue. They achieved tremendous strength by lifting heavy loads for few repetitions. Researchers did not begin to substantiate in published papers until the 1930s that strength is enhanced by overloading with heavy loads in a progressive manner. More recently, researchers compared different kinds of weight-training programs to determine whether one was more effective than another for improving strength. The earliest studies compared the effects of training with heavy loads with the effects of training with light loads. The results of these studies showed that training with heavy loads for a few repetitions (usually the 10-RM load) was more effective in improving strength than was training with light loads for higher repetitions.[77–79]

Later research was confined to training with heavy loads, which permitted repetitions of 10 with various proportions of the 10-RM load. One study compared training with 25% of the 10-RM load for the first set, 50% of the load for the second set, 75% of the load for the third set, and 100% of the 10-RM load for the fourth set to a program

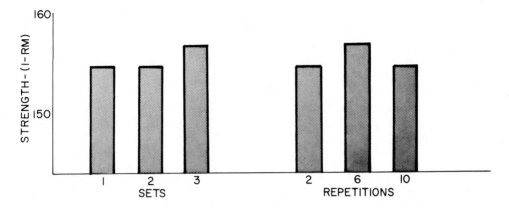

Fig. 1–28. The effects of varying sets and repetitions on strength improvement. Three sets and six repetitions were most effective for increasing strength. (Data from Berger, R.A.: Effect of varied weight training programs on strength. Res. Q., *33*:168, 1962.)

that involved the same number of sets, repetitions, and loads, but a reversed order of proportions of the 10-RM. No significant differences were found between the two programs. Later research compared different numbers of repetitions per set and different numbers of sets to determine which were most effective for improving strength.[80] Repetitions of 2, 6, and 10 per set, and sets of 1, 2, and 3 were compared (Fig. 1–28). The results showed that six repetitions and three sets achieved maximum strength most closely. Another study showed that the optimal number of repetitions to execute when

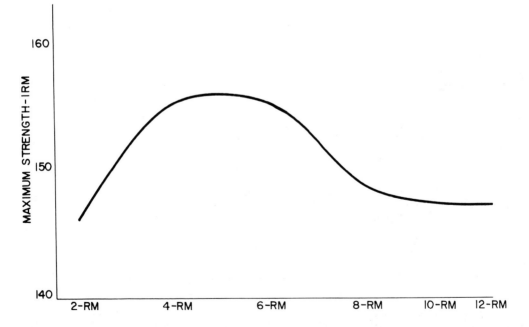

Fig. 1–29. Relationship between training loads and strength improvement after 12 weeks of training, 3 times weekly, and 1 set each session on the bench press. (Data from Berger, R.A.: Optimum repetitions for the development of strength. Res. Q., *33*:334, 1962.)

performing only one set is closest to the 6-RM[81] (Fig. 1–29). Apparently, training for three sets with the 6-RM is better than training for fewer sets with different exercise loads for increasing strength.

Usually, overloading involves both adding weight and increasing repetitions. For example, a lifter may begin with a 5-RM load (a load permitting only 5 repetitions using maximum effort) and will attempt to lift it more times during succeeding training sessions. When 10 repetitions are possible, the weight of the bar is increased by about 5%. Overloading by sets may also be combined with overloading by weight and repetitions simply by adding more sets of each exercise.

Body Weight

In some exercises, body weight alone may be heavy enough to overload the muscles. Overloading with body weight is usually done by repetitions and sets, but is sometimes done by adding more weight to the body. If more than 10 repetitions are possible, however, the effect on improving strength may not be optimal. In this case,

additional weight may be attached to the body in the form of barbell plates. If this is not possible repetitions of up to 20 continue to overload for increasing strength but are not as effective as fewer repetitions and heavier weight. Higher repetitions tend to effect more changes in the endurance capacity of the muscles, but have a diminishing effect on force capacity.

Overloading may be provided to the muscles by changing the position of the body in relation to the pull of gravity. For example, modifying the body position for the push-up exercise so that the feet are elevated on a chair or doing sit-ups on an inclined board instead of on a level surface increases overloading.

The limitations of body weight as an overload for improving strength are related to age. Certain calisthenic exercises, such as push-ups or sit-ups where only body weight is lifted, provide enough resistance for a young child to improve strength. The same exercises for a well-conditioned young adult male, who can do more than 30 push-ups and 100 sit-ups, do not provide enough overload

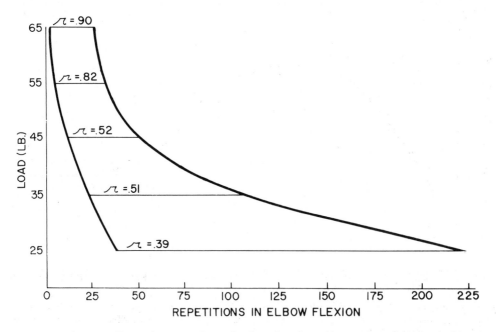

Fig. 1–30.   Correlation coefficients between 1-RM curl and number of repetitions performed with loads of 25, 35, 45, 55, and 65 lb. and corresponding ranges of repetitions for each load. Based on college males.[81a]

for maximizing strength improvement. This situation is indicated in Figure 1–30, in which the relationships between maximum strength and number of repetitions performed with loads of 25, 35, 45, 55, and 65 lb. are presented. As repetitions are done with lighter loads, the ability to perform shifts toward muscular endurance and away from absolute strength. These relationships point out the importance of heavy loads (relative to each individual) in training to increase primarily strength. More than 25 repetitions largely affect muscle endurance. There are relatively few exercises in which body weight is heavy enough to optimally improve strength in young adult males. Therefore, barbells and other kinds of overload equipment are frequently used in strength training.

One Muscle Resisting Another

Overloading can be done by forcing one muscle to resist the movement of another.

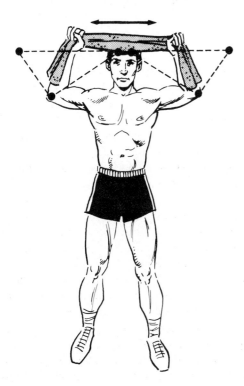

Fig. 1–31. Example of overloading by one muscle resisting the movement of another muscle.

An example of this form of overloading is shown by the exercise in Figure 1–31. A towel is held taut in the position shown. Movement occurs at the elbow joints; one arm extends by a concentric contraction while the other arm flexes by an eccentric contraction of the same muscle. The elbows remain in the same relative position throughout the exercise and the towel is kept taut. If the movement is done moderately slowly and with a constant velocity, the concentric contractions are isodynamic (same motor unit involvement), and the results are similar to those obtained by overloading with isokinetic devices.

Isokinetic Devices

Isokinetic devices are unique because each repetition in a set may be done with a maximum concentric contraction for any number of repetitions. This cannot be done when a constant load is used in training because the muscle force does not approach maximum until nearly the end of a series of repetitions. When lifting a 10-RM load for 10 repetitions, only the ninth and tenth repetitions are maximum or close to maximum.

The best way to overload with isokinetic devices has been studied.[72] The purpose of the study was to determine which combination of repetitions, either 5, 10, or 15, and which time per each repetition, either 1, 2.5, or 4 sec., were better for increasing muscle force as measured at different movement velocities. The subjects were 130 high school students who trained 3 times weekly for 9 weeks. The results of the study are presented in Figure 1–32. Mean values increase as velocities of movement slow down because of the inverse relationship between velocity and muscle force (see Fig. 1–19). The only significant difference (based on statistical probability) between the 3 groups that trained at movement velocities of 1 sec./rep., 2.5 sec./rep., and 4 sec./rep. was between the strength average of the 4 sec./rep. group and the strength average of the other two groups when muscle force was measured at the slow movement of 7 sec./

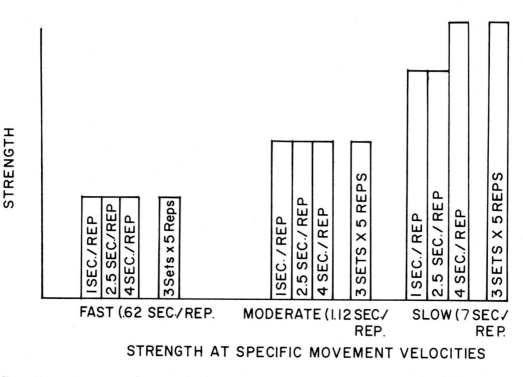

STRENGTH

FAST (.62 SEC./REP.   MODERATE (1.12 SEC./ REP.   SLOW (7 SEC./ REP.

STRENGTH AT SPECIFIC MOVEMENT VELOCITIES

Fig. 1–32.   Maximum strength measured with an isokinetic device at three different movement velocities (.62 sec./rep., 1.12 sec./rep., and 7 sec./rep.) for groups that trained isokinetically for nine weeks at velocities of either 1 sec./rep., 2.5 sec./rep., or 4 sec./rep., or that trained allodynamically for three sets of five repetitions each. The bars of the same height are not significantly different from each other.[101]

rep. Because no differences in strength improvement were found among the 3 treatments when force was measured at the other 2 velocities, that is, .62 sec./rep. and 1.12 sec./rep., isodynamic training at a slow velocity of 4 sec./rep. was determined just as effective for improving force at fast and moderate movement velocities as was training at faster velocities. When comparisons were made among the 3 treatments of repetitions (5, 10, and 15), no significant differences were found in strength improvement at any of the measuring velocities, that is, .62 sec./rep., 1.12 sec./rep., or 7 sec./rep. Apparently, the intensity of each contraction in training has a greater effect on strength improvement than does the frequency of contractions.

Accommodating Resistance

Exercise machines that vary weight resistance to accommodate the force curves of skeletal joints are used to overload in the same way as are barbells and dumbbells. That is, overloading is accomplished by increasing exercise loads, repetitions, and sets. Whereas the maximum contraction is at the weakest joint angle with "free weights," such as barbells, the maximum stress with accommodating resistance is theoretically throughout the joint angle. In reality, however, this rarely happens for several reasons. First, no accommodating resistance machine can vary the exercise loads with enough precision to exactly match every individual force curve. These machines, at best, are calibrated to accommodate individuals with average force curves but, because everyone is not average, all individuals are not accurately accommodated. Second, unless movement velocity is constant and moderately slow, the contraction force is not the same throughout the joint angle (assuming, of course, that accommodating is accurate). This force variation is shown in Figure 1–19, where muscle force varies with movement velocity, that is, the faster the move, the less the contraction force and vice versa. Because accommodating resistance machines do not accurately achieve a maximum force throughout a joint movement, there often is a "sticking point" just as there is with barbells. But usually the "sticking point" with accommodating loads is above that found when the exercise loads are barbells. Consequently, the 1-RM values for most individuals are higher when they are measured with accommodating resistance machines.

ISOMETRIC, ALLODYNAMIC, AND ISODYNAMIC TRAINING

In most sport activities, success depends on how quickly the muscles contract concentrically to propel the body forward or vertically. As a result, one might expect that concentric training is more effective than isometric training for improving athletic performance. Research comparing the two types of contractions indicates that power is more effectively improved by concentric contractions than by isometric contractions in overload training.[82–84a] However, both are similarly effective for increasing strength.[85–87a] Although concentric training is more effective for improving athletic performance, it is not known whether allodynamic and isodynamic training have different effects on physical performance.

Comparisons have been made between the training effects of allodynamic contractions and isodynamic contractions on strength improvement. Allodynamic contractions, which occur when training with a barbell, have been compared to isodynamic training using either an isokinetic device or an accommodating resistance machine. When the effects of training between barbells and accommodating resistance machines are compared, the basic comparison is actually between the two different kinds of muscular contractions that are elicited by the equipment. The allodynamic contraction

is greatest at only one joint angle whereas the contraction achieved with an accommodating resistance machine results in the greatest force occurring at more positions in the joint range. If an accommodating load is accelerated (change in velocity), the effect of momentum on the load results in the application of a maximum force through a joint range that is shorter than that involved with a constant velocity. The relative differences in the joint range over which maximum force is applied when lifting a barbell and an accommodating load are shown in Figure 1–33. The ordinate represents relative muscle force while lifting under three different conditions. In condition A, a constant load is

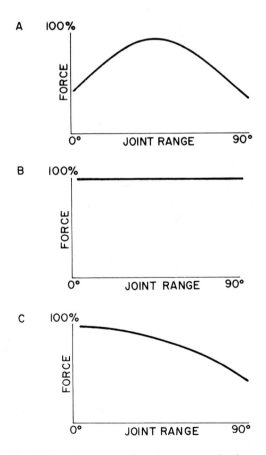

Fig. 1–33. Percentage of maximum muscular force capacity in a joint range when lifting at the same velocity, A, a constant load and B, an accommodating load. C, Moving the same load as that in B, but with maximum acceleration.

lifted; in condition B, an accommodating load is raised with constant and moderate velocity; and, in condition C, the same accommodating load as in B is lifted with maximum acceleration. Condition A results in maximum force over a shorter joint range than that in conditions B and C. Condition C is less than condition B. A contraction with an accommodating machine has both an allodynamic component and an isodynamic component because the system for providing accommodating loads is not often accurate enough to achieve a truly isodynamic contraction and a maximum force at all joint angles. Only an electromechanical isokinetic device has that ability. Nevertheless, training with an accommodating resistance machine probably increases maximum muscle force thoughout a greater range than does training with a constant load. However, this hypothesis has not been examined in research studies because the measures of maximum strength have not been taken at all joint angles.

When the effects of training with a barbell were compared with the effects of training with an accommodating resistance machine, similar improvements in strength were noted. Slightly greater improvements were obtained when the 1-RM was measured with the accommodating resistance machine, but the reverse was true when strength was measured with a constant weight load or barbell.[88] These results reflect the specificity of training because the best improvements are obtained when the criterion involves the same resistance loads and movement patterns that are used in training.[88a] In other words, the best way to improve strength, as measured by lifting a barbell, is to train with a barbell in the same movement. The same reasoning holds true if one wants to increase maximally in strength as measured with an accommodating resistance machine—train with an accommodating load.

Comparisons have been made between the effects of training with loads that produce allodynamic contractions and loads that produce isodynamic contractions

throughout a joint range. The results of studies comparing allodynamic training with a constant exercise load to training that provides an isodynamic contraction by an isokinetic device do not always agree. Patients receiving physical therapy showed greater increases when they trained with an isokinetic device than when their training involved weight training.[89,90] In a study using 169 high school males, comparisons were made between the effects of training allodynamically in knee extension and the effects of training isodynamically with an isokinetic device.[72] Allodynamic training was done with loads permitting five repetitions, using maximum force, for three sets. Isodynamic training was maximum for 5, 10, or 15 repetitions and at movement velocities of either 1, 2.5, or 4 sec. for each repetition. The criterion was muscle strength measured isodynamically at three different movement velocities: .62, 1.12, and 7 sec. per repetition. The results of the comparisons between allodynamic training and isodynamic training at three different numbers of repetitions and three movement velocities, with strength measured at three movement velocities, are shown in Figure 1–32. No significant differences were found between training isodynamically and allodynamically when strength was measured at a fast or moderate velocity. But, when strength was measured at a slow velocity (7 sec./rep.), allodynamic and isodynamic training were significantly more effective than isodynamic training at fast (1 sec./rep.) or moderate velocities (2.5 sec./rep.). When comparisons were made among the same treatments using the criterion of maximum (1-RM) allodynamic strength, there were no significant differences among groups. Apparently, isodynamic training at various movement velocities is as effective for increasing strength, measured allodynamically, as is allodynamic training with a free weight. Based on these results, improvement in the ability to exert a force on a heavy resistance, when movement velocity is slow or moderate, is apparently best achieved by training with high resistance and slow movements. An accelerated movement can be more effectively increased by isodynamic training at fast, moderate, or slow movements or by allodynamic training with heavy loads (5-RM). If the primary concern in strength training is the improvement of both absolute strength and power and relative strength and power, heavy resistance loads are recommended.

Assessment of Strength

When measuring strength, the force of a muscle is measured indirectly through the leverage system of the skeleton. Of course, changes in muscle force as a consequence of training can be measured by comparing strength before and after training. Because the leverage system does not change, any strength differences represent increased force capacity of the muscle. Usually, absolute strength is measured by a maximum effort that involves either a concentric contraction or an isometric contraction. Strength of an eccentric contraction is rarely measured because special equipment is needed, and the significance of the measurement is questionable for assessing or predicting work or athletic ability.

Concentric Contractions

In 1945, a book on weight training for the rehabilitation of skeletal muscles was written by DeLorme.[77] The words, progressive resistance exercise (PRE), were coined at that time and referred to a system of overloading the muscles to improve their force capacity. When applying PRE, the general rehabilitation procedure is to establish the strength of the affected body part and then to prescribe the training loads and the number of times they should be lifted. The term 1-RM (1 repetition maximum) was used to indicate maximum strength in a concentric contraction, and 10-RM (10 repetition maximum) was considered the basis for prescribing the number of repetitions in training. When determining the 1-RM load, which is the amount of weight with which

only 1 lift is possible using maximum muscular force, the load on the muscle is gradually increased after each successful lift. The 10-RM load, or load that permits just 10 repetitions using maximum effort, is determined in the same way. Usually 1 to 2 min. rest is taken between attempts to minimize the effects of fatigue on the final strength values. In training, the 1-RM is periodically determined and used as a gauge of progress. When improvement occurs, approximately 5% is added to the 10-RM training load. In DeLorme's system, training requires the lifter to perform the first series of repetitions, or set, for 10 repetitions with a load of 25% of the 10-RM load. The second, third, and fourth sets are performed for 10 repetitions, each using loads of 50, 75, and 100% of the 10-RM load, respectively. Two minutes between sets are usually taken as a rest period.

The same terminology is used today to indicate maximum strength (1-RM) and training loads (proportions of the 10-RM) in physical rehabilitation. However, in training to improve muscle force and athletic performance, training loads are customarily varied from 1-RM to 10-RM. The immediate concern here is with the determination of 1-RM strength by tests involving allodynamic contractions (where MUI is greatest at one joint angle) and isodynamic contractions (where MUI is similar at all joint angles).

When absolute strength is measured by a concentric contraction, the nature of the resistance load determines at which joint angle maximum strength is measured. If an isokinetic device is used to measure strength, the isodynamic contraction at the angle with the most favorable leverage produces the highest strength score and 1-RM. However, if the resistance is a constant load so that an allodynamic contraction occurs, the 1-RM load is a measure of strength at the weakest joint angle when a load is lifted vertically, such as in a bench press. If the load is lifted in a rotational direction, such as in knee extension, the combining effect of the angle at which gravity pulls on the limb holding the load and of the leverage at the joint determines the joint angle at which maximum strength is measured. As previously indicated, when a load is lifted rotationally, the strength (exercise force) of the joint must equal the load in order for movement to continue only when the force of gravity is at a 90° angle to the limb. The contrast between allodynamic and isodynamic tests is illustrated in Figure 1–10, which shows the strength curve for hip and knee extension. In an allodynamic strength test, where the same load is lifted, the maximum amount of weight lifted depends on strength at 62° of the knee. However, in an isodynamic contraction, where the resistance load is variable to "fit the strength curve," the maximum strength recorded is with the knee at about 180°.

Usually barbells and dumbbells are the loads used to measure the 1-RM in allodynamic strength tests. In weight training, the individual often determines 1-RM values for each of several lifts. Periodically during training, the 1-RM is assessed to ascertain progress. Loads other than weights may be used to measure allodynamic 1-RMs. Body weight can be used to assess strength in tests of chinning or dipping. If only 1 chin-up can be performed, the 1-RM is equal to body weight. When an individual can do more than 1 chin-up, the procedure for determin-

ing the 1-RM chin requires the attachment of external weights, or barbell plates, to body weight. A person weighing 150 lb. who has a 1-RM chin of 180 lb. is capable of performing 1 maximum chin with 30 lb. attached to the body (150 lb. of body weight plus 30 lb. equals a 180-lb. 1-RM).

Barbells

The ability to lift heavy loads with the back muscles is significantly related to the ability to lift with the arm muscles. In fact, all the large muscles of the body are significantly related to each other in their capacity to generate force. This relationship is shown by Table 1–6 in which the 1-RM values of several different lifts in weight training are interrelated. All coefficients are statistically significant and represent common elements of all tests. These relationships are based on a sample of 174 young adult males.[91] Similar relationships were found among 169 junior high school males (see Table 1–2). Apparently, during the process of physical maturation, at least from the ages of 12 years to about 22 years in males, the strength relationships among all muscle groups are relatively consistent.

The best single lifts for predicting total dynamic strength in males, which is the sum of 6 1-RM lifts, are standing press (r = .87) and bench press (r = .84).[91] When a correla-

Table 1–6.

Intercorrelation Coefficients of Seven Dynamic Strength Tests and Total Dynamic Strength*
N = 174

	Total dynamic strength	Curl	Upright rowing	Squat	Sit-up	Military press	Bench press	Back hyper-extension
Back hyperextension	67	.41	.44	.59	.39	.43	.43	1.00
Bench press	.84	.64	.63	.63	.52	.79	1.00	
Military press	.87	.73	.64	.68	.53	1.00		
Sit-up	.67	.48	.48	.48	1.00			
Squat	.82	.57	.62	1.00				
Upright rowing	.81	.68	1.00					
Curl	.81	1.00						
Total dynamic strength	1.00							

*All coefficients are significant beyond the .01 level. Data from Berger.[91]

tion technique in statistics was used to determine the combination of lifts that best predicts total dynamic strength, the standing press and back extension proved most effective (R = .92). The addition of upright rowing increased the prediction slightly (R = .96). These relationships further support the principle that strength of muscles, measured with allodynamic contractions, is general thoughout the musculature. High strength of the back proved indicative of high strength of the muscles at other joints and vice versa. Of course, if an individual trains by overloading exclusively on one joint so as to increase strength, the accuracy of predicting strength of another untrained joint is not high. Gymnasts, who train primarily the upper body and not the legs with heavy resistance exercise, have relatively high strength in their upper body when compared to the strength they have in their legs. Consequently, predicting total strength of gymnasts from the 1-RM values of the upper body is less accurate.

Maximum strength may also be measured allodynamically by using body weight as part of the resistance load. Ability to chin or dip on parallel bars, which involves raising the body by contracting muscles, may be used as excellent predictors of maximum strength (1-RM) of the arms and shoulder region.[92,93,93a]

1-RM Chin and Dip as Predictors of Total Allodynamic Strength. The movements involved in chinning are performed by the muscles that flex the arms and shoulders, rotate the scapula downward, and adduct the shoulder blades. In dipping, the skeletal actions and the muscles involved are different. However, some parts of the chest muscles (pectoralis major) are also active in chinning. The muscles used in dipping extend the arms and shoulders and abduct the shoulder blades. Although the muscles involved in doing a chin and dip have opposite actions, there is a high relationship between them in force capacity. Generally, individuals with high 1-RM chin have high 1-RM dip,

and vice versa (r = .90).[94] A fairly high relationship also exists between upper body strength and lower limb and trunk strength.

The relationship of 1-RM chin and dip to total allodynamic strength has been studied.[92] Fifty college-aged males were measured for 1-RM values of 7 weight-training lifts. The lifts measured strength of all the large muscles in both the upper and lower parts of the body. Significantly high relationships were found between total strength and both 1-RM chin and dip (r = .82 and .83, respectively). When both 1-RM values statistically combined to predict total allodynamic strength, the relationship gave a better prediction than when each was considered alone (R = .93). Total strength can be predicted by the following formula:

Total Allodynamic Strength = 1.05 ×
1-RM chin + .74 × 1-RM dip + 322 lb.

These results and predictions are based on individuals who had not overtrained certain muscles at the exclusion of others. If the total strength of gymnasts was predicted from upper body strength of chinning and dipping the predictions would be too high.

Isokinetic Devices

Numerous devices can provide an isokinetic effect, or movement of constant velocity throughout a joint range. These devices vary in accuracy and in ability to maintain a constant velocity of movement. The rope-pulley device, in which resistance is provided by a rope circling around a pulley that is contained within a cylinder, controls velocity of movement by varying the number of times the rope is wrapped around the pulley. More winds increase the resistance and slow down the movement; fewer winds permit faster moves. Other isokinetic devices provide resistance to movement by mechanical and electrical mechanisms. Velocity may be controlled to achieve fast or slow movements. These devices are more accurate in determining maximum strength than the rope-pulley devices and are as accurate, if not more so, than tests that measure strength of allodynamic contractions such as barbells. Of course, these devices measure strength at the strongest joint angles, whereas the 1-RM value in allodynamic strength indicates strength at the weakest joint angle or "sticking point." Some isokinetic devices are connected to a recording unit so that force can be plotted on paper throughout a joint range. This is an advantage over other measures of strength because any relative weaknesses in a joint range can be readily detected. Treatment can then be prescribed to remedy the condition.

Isometric Contractions

The amount of force applied to an external object while the muscles contract isometrically is a measure of strength. Basically two kinds of instruments are commonly used to measure isometric strength: a dynamometer and a tensiometer.[95-98a] Generally, a dynamometer is used to measure such large muscle groups as the legs, hips, and back, whereas a tensiometer measures isolated muscle groups usually at single joints.

Dynamometer Strength Test. Probably the most frequently used measure of isometric strength is the back and leg dynamometer (Fig. 1–34). It was introduced in 1925 and became part of a battery of tests that measured general athletic ability.[99] It is used to measure back strength or leg strength. A taut spring is pulled during the test. The instrument can measure up to 2,500 lb. Certain testing techniques are followed to ensure standardization of test scores and to prevent possible muscle injury.

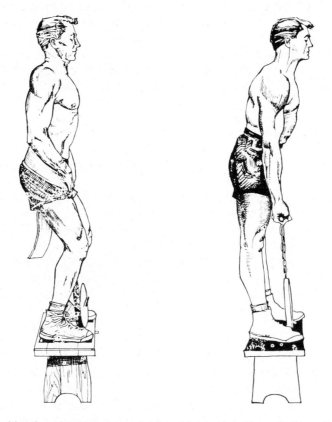

Fig. 1–34. Back and leg dynamometer measures back and leg strength. (From Mathews, D.K.: Measurement in Physical Education. 3rd Edition. Philadelphia, W. B. Saunders Co., 1968.)

Tensiometer Strength Test. A tensiometer measures the tension in a cable (Fig. 1–35). It was originally used in a military convalescent hospital during World War II to measure human strength and was later improved by Clarke.[95] The instrument was initially designed to measure tension of aircraft control cables. Tension is measured in a cable by a force that is applied to a riser and is then converted into pounds. An individual is positioned for a specific test before exerting maximum force. While pulling on a steel cable about one-sixteenth in. in diameter, the tension applied to the cable is recorded on the tensiometer.

Much research has been done with the tensiometer among males and females from the upper elementary grades to the college level.[96,100,100a] The strength-test batteries and norms for each sex are described in a manual.[96] Twenty-five cable-tension tests were administered to 576 subjects from elementary through college age to determine the relationships among the strength scores of different muscle groups.[101] Almost all the test scores related significantly to each other, indicating some generality in strength among different muscles. When a determination was made of the muscles that best predict or estimate total body strength, the muscles of the shoulder region appeared most significant, particularly the muscles that extend the upper arm at the shoulder. These muscles are used in such exercises as chinning and rope climbing. The other muscle groups that contributed to the prediction of total strength were involved in knee extension, trunk extension, trunk flexion, hip extension, shoulder flexion, and ankle plantar flexion. The best combinations of these strength tests varied somewhat according to grade level, but the best three or four predictors for each grade were able to estimate total strength with high accuracy (R = .94 to .98). Similar findings were reported for allodynamic strength tests because relatively few muscle groups can predict, with a high degree of accuracy, total strength.[91]

Measures of Relative Strength

There is a significant relationship between relative strength of different muscle groups. Generally, individuals with high relative strength of the upper body also possess similar qualities in the lower body. This finding is shown by the relationships between different tasks or tests that primarily measure relative strength. Table 1–3 presents the correlation coefficients between all combinations of tests of relative strength. All coefficients are significant and represent elements common to all tests.

Although a higher relationship is generally found between tasks that involve the same muscle groups, nevertheless significant relationships are usually found between tasks of relative strength in which the muscles used are antagonistic. Apparently, both the extent of muscle force and the degree of favorable leverage in the skeletal system are consistent between different muscles and bone joints.

PRINCIPLES FOR TRAINING

1. The force capacity of a muscle is increased by properly overloading so that a

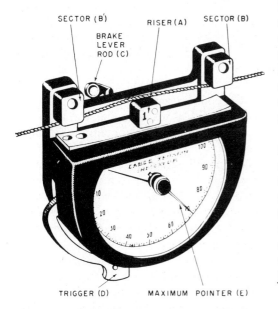

SECTOR (B′) RISER (A) SECTOR (B)
BRAKE LEVER ROD (C)
TRIGGER (D) MAXIMUM POINTER (E)

Fig. 1–35. Tensiometer. (From Mathews, D.K.: Measurement in Physical Education. 3rd Edition. Philadelphia, W. B. Saunders Co., 1968.)

maximum or near maximum force is elicited. Continuous stress of this kind can be applied in several ways: (1) increasing exercise load, (2) increasing number of times a load is lifted (repetitions), (3) increasing number of times, or sets, a series of repetitions is performed, and (4) increasing number of training days per week.

2. Basic principles of strength training apply to most individuals in terms of numbers of repetitions, loads, and training frequency. These principles apply to training loads involving barbells, body weight, or any other weight resistance. The principles are presented, along with the research studies supporting each.

a. To maximize the force capacity of a muscle by allodynamic training, a load should be moved concentrically for 3 to 10 repetitions (3-RM to 10-RM loads).[81]

b. Three sets are more effective than fewer sets for maximizing muscle force in allodynamic training.[80] More than three sets are effective only when the muscles recuperate between training sessions.

c. Every set need not be performed with maximum muscle force to achieve an optimal improvement in strength.[102]

d. No particular sequence of varying loads in a training session, i.e., using light loads at the beginning of a specific exercise, and heavier loads for later sets, or vice versa,[103] is more effective than another sequence in allodynamic training.

e. Training a muscle allodynamically for three sets of five repetitions each is as effective for increasing force capacity as is training isodynamically (concentrically with a load that accommodates the strength capacity throughout a joint range) at a shortening velocity of 4 sec. per repetition for 15 repetitions.

f. Training isodynamically at velocities of 1 sec. per repetition and 2.5 sec. per repetition are just as effective for increasing force capacity as is training at 4 sec. per repetition. However, this applies only when force is measured at fast (.62 sec./rep.) and moderate (1.18 sec./rep.) velocities of shortening.

3. The greater the stretch of a muscle, the larger the initial force of contraction. If the only concern in training is to increase the force capacity of a stretched muscle, training is greatly simplified. But, for some skilled movements, greatly stretching a muscle may hinder execution, e.g., a one-handed shot in basketball or a full squat just prior to a high jump. However, in such sports as shot-putting, discus throwing, bat swinging, or baseball pitching, a long stretch is important. To effectively apply this principle, one must understand the mechanical principles involved in a particular skill movement of a sport. If an extreme stretch does not detract from a skill and if a high force contributes to success, it is advantageous to stretch the muscles.

4. The ability to exert a large force in a fast movement is essential for success in most athletic sports. Success in athletic performance often depends on the amount of force generated in muscles during a quick movement. Running, jumping, and throwing a ball are some activities that require a high force for success. Overload training improves the ability to exert force at all velocities of movement if training involves heavy resistance. If light resistance and fast movements are used, force capacity may only increase at high velocities of movement.[72]

5. A muscle that is stretched rapidly and moved concentrically immediately after can contract with more force than can a muscle that is just stretched and contracted. Many sports require quick movements that are taken in a direction opposite to the movement that accomplishes the specific and desired task. A wind-up in pitching or throwing the arms backward just prior to a forward movement when jumping are examples of this principle. One explanation for this phenomenon involves the behavior of the muscle spindles within all skeletal muscles. When these sensory organs are stretched, impulses are sent to the spinal cord, which, in turn, activates more motor units to the working muscle. Muscle force is augmented

when the contraction occurs immediately after the stretch. Any pause in the backswing obviates this effect. An explanation of the structure and function of muscle spindles is presented in detail in Chapter 3.

REFERENCES

1. Berger, R.A., and Higginbotham, R.B.: Prediction of dynamic strength from static strength in hip and knee extension. Am. Correct. Ther. J., *24:*23, 1970.
2. Rodgers, K.L., and Berger, R.A.: Motor-unit involvement and tension during maxiumum, voluntary concentric, eccentric, and isometric contractions of the elbow flexors. Med. Sci. Sports, *6:*253, 1974.
3. Knuttgen, H.G., and Klausen, K.: Oxygen debt in short term exercise with concentric and eccentric muscle contractions. J. Appl. Physiol., *30:*632, 1971.
4. Curtin, N.A., Svensson, S.M., and Davies, R.E.: Force development and the braking mechanism in stretching activated muscle is not limited by the energy from ATP splitting. Fed. Proc., *29:*714, 1970.
5. Infante, O.A., Klaupiks, D., and Davies, R.E.: Adenosine triphosphate: changes in muscles doing negative work. Science, *144:*1577, 1964.
6. Knuttgen, H.G., Petersen, F.B., and Klausen, K.: Oxygen uptake and heart rate responses to exercise performed with concentric and eccentric contractions. Med. Sci. Sports, *30:*1, 1971.
7. de Vries, H.A.: Efficiency of electrical activity as a physiological measure of the functional state of muscle tissue. Am. J. Phys. Med., *47:*10, 1968.
8. Lippold, O.C.J.: The relation between integrated action potentials in a human muscle and its isometric tension. J. Physiol., *117:*492, 1952.
9. Hutter, O.F., and Trautwein, W.: Neuromuscular facilitation by stretch of motor nerve-endings. J. Physiol., *137*:610, 1956.
9a. Guyton, A.C.: Basic Human Physiology: Normal Function and Mechanisms of Disease. Philadelphia, W. B. Saunders, 1971.
10. Aubert, X.: Le mecanisme contractile in vivo: aspects mecaniques et thermiques. J. Physiol., *48:*105, 1956.
11. Cavagna, G.A., Saibene, F.P., and Margaria, R.: Effect of negative work on the amount of positive work performed by an isolated muscle. J. Appl. Physiol., *20:*157, 1965.
12. Hill, A.V.: The beat of shortening and the dynamic constants of muscle. Proc. R. Soc., *126:*136, 1938.
13. Logan, G.A.: Differential applications of resistance and resulting strength measured at varying degrees of knee extension. Unpublished doctoral dissertation, University of Southern California, 1960.
14. Berger, R.A., and Mathus, D.L.: Movement time with various resistance loads as a function of pretensed and pre-relaxed muscular contraction. Res. Q., *40:*456, 1969.
15. Smith, L.E., and Whitley, J.D.: Relation between muscular force of a limb, under different starting conditions and speed of movement. Res. Q., *34:*489, 1963.
16. Cheek, D.B., et al.: Skeletal muscle cell mass and growth: the concept of the deoxyribonucleic acid unit. Pediatr. Res., *5:*312, 1971.
17. Edington, D.W., and Edgerton, V.R.: The Biology of Physical Activity. Boston, Houghton Mifflin Co., 1976.
18. Becker, B.J.: Construction of a muscular strength test for college women. Microcarded Doctoral Dissertation, University of Oregon, 1967.
19. Stauffer, R.W.: Comparison of USMA men and women on selected physical performance measures. . . project summertime, Dept. of Physical Education, United States Military Academy, 1976.
20. Wilmore, J.H.: Alterations in strength, body composition, and anthropometric measurements consequent to a 10-week weight training program. Med. Sci. Sports, *6:*133, 1974.
21. Bartell Associates, Inc.: The study of police women competency in the performance of sector police work in the City of Philadelphia. State College, Pennsylvania, 1978.
22. Brown, C., and Wilmore, J.: The effects of maximal resistance training on the strength and body composition of women athletes. Med. Sci. Sports, *6:*174, 1974.
23. Fisher, M.B., and Birren, J.E.: Age and strength. J. Appl. Psychol., *31:*490, 1947.
24. Hettinger, T.: Physiology of Strength. Springfield, Charles C Thomas, 1961.
25. Penman, K.A.: Ultrastructural changes in human striated muscle using three methods of training. Res. Q., *40:*764, 1969.
26. Penman, K.A.: Human striated muscle ultrastructural changes accompanying increased strength without hypertrophy. Res. Q., *41:*418, 1970.
27. MacCallum, J.B.: On the histogenesis of the striated muscle fiber, and the growth of the human sartorius muscle. Bull. Johns Hopkins Hosp., *9:*208, 1898.
28. Rowe, R.W.D., and Goldspink, G.: Surgically induced hypertrophy in skeletal muscle of the laboratory mouse. Anat. Rec., *161:*69, 1968.
29. Van Linge, B.: The response of muscle to strenuous exercise. J. Bone Joint Surg. [Br.], *44-B:*711, 1962.
30. Hettinger, T., and Muller, E.A.: Muskelleistung und muskel training. Arbeitsphysiologie, *15:*22, 1953.
31. O'Shea, C.: Effects of selected weight training programs on the development of strength and muscle hypertrophy. Res. Q., *37:*95, 1966.
32. Gutmann, E., and Hajek, I.: Differential reaction of muscle to overload incompensatory by hypertrophy and increased phasic activity. Physiol. Bohemoslov., *20:*205, 1971.
33. Goldberg, A.L., et al.: Mechanism of work-induced hypertrophy of skeletal muscle. Med. Sci. Sports, *7:*248, 1975.
34. Schiaffino, S., Bormioli, S.P., and Aloisi, N.: Cell proliferation in rat skeletal muscle during early

stages of compensatory hypertrophy. Virchows Arch. [Cell Pathol.], *11:*268, 1972.

35. Sutton, C., and Tomkins, G.: Mechanisms of steroid resistance. Cell, *2:*221, 1974.

36. Fahey, T.D.: Serum testosterone, body composition and strength of young adults. Med. Sci. Sports, *8:*31, 1976.

37. McMorris, R.O., and Elkins, E.C.: A study of production and evaluation of muscular hypertrophy. Arch. Phys. Med. Rehabil., *35:*420, 1954.

38. Bowers, R.W., and Reardon, J.P.: Effects of methandostenolone (dianabol) on strength development and aerobic capacity. Med. Sci. Sports, *4:*54, 1972.

39. Casner, S.W., and Early, R.G.: Anabolic steroid effects on body composition in normal young men. J. Sports. Med. Phys. Fitness, *11:*98, 1971.

40. Johnson, L., et al.: Anabolic steroid: effects on strength, body weight, oxygen uptake and spermatogenesis upon mature males. Med. Sci. Sports, *4:*43, 1972.

41. O'Shea, J., and Winklor, W.: Biochemical and physical effects of an anabolic steroid in competitive swimmers and weight lifters. Nutr. Rep. Int., *2:*351, 1970.

42. O'Shea, J.: The effect of an anabolic steroid on dynamic strength levels of weight lifters. Nutr. Rep. Int., *4:*363, 1971.

42a. Ward, P.E.: The effects of anabolic steroids used in the training of athletes. Unpublished master's thesis, Chapman College, 1968.

42b. Ward, P.E.: The effect of an anabolic steroid on strength and lean body mass. Med. Sci. Sports, *5:*277, 1973.

43. Fahey, T.D., and Brown, C.H.: The effects of an anabolic steroid on the strength, body composition, and endurance of college males when accompanied by a weight training program. Med. Sci. Sports, *5:*272, 1973.

44. Fowler, W.M., Jr., Gardner, G.W., and Egstrom, G.H.: Effect of an anabolic steroid on physical performance of young men. J. Appl. Physiol., *20:*1038, 1965.

45. Mayhew, J., and Gross, P.: Body composition changes in young women with high resistance weight training. Res. Q., *45:*433, 1974.

46. Golding, L.A.: Personal interviews with championship-level athletes. *In* Ergogenic Aids and Muscular Performance. Edited by W. P. Morgan. New York, Academic Press, 1972.

47. Johnson, F.L.: The association of oral androgenic-anabolic steroids and life threatening disease. Med. Sci. Sports, *7:*284, 1975.

48. Doyle, F., Brown, J., and Lachance, C.: Relation between bone mass and muscle weight. Lancet, *1:*391, 1970.

49. King, D.W., and Pengelly, R.G.: Effect of running on the density of rat tibias. Med. Sci. Sports, *5:*68, 1973.

50. Kuskinen, A., and Heikkinen, E.: Effects of physical training on development and strength of tendons and bones in growing mice. Scand. J. Clin. Lab. Invest., *29:*20, 1973.

51. Saville, C.D., and Smith, R.: Bone density, break-

ing force and leg muscle mass as functions of weight in bipedal rats. Am. J. Phys. Anthropol., *25:*35, 1966.

51a. Zuckerman, J., and Stull, G.A.: Ligamentous separation force in rats as influenced by training, detraining and cage restriction. Med. Sci. Sports, *5:*44, 1973.

52. Kohbrausch, W.: Ueber den einfluss funktioneller beanspruchung auf das langenwachstum von knochen. Muenchener Medizinische Wochenschrift, *71:*513, 1924.

53. Ross, J.A.: Hypertrophy of the little finger. Br. Med. J., *2:*987, 1950.

54. Heaney, R.C.: Radiocalcium metabolism in disuse osteoporosis in man. Am. J. Med., *31:*188, 1962.

55. Rodahl, L., et al.: Fysiologiske forandringer under langvarig sengeleire. Nord. Med., *75:*182, 1966.

56. Smith, E.L., and Babcock, S.W.: Effects of physical activity on bone loss in the aged. Med. Sci. Sports, *5:*68, 1973.

57. Gillespie, J.A.: The nature of bone changes associated with nerve injuries and disuse. J. Bone Joint Surg. [Brt.], *36:*464, 1954.

58. Deitrick, J.R., Whedon, G.D., and Shorr, E.: Effects of immobilization upon various metabolic and physiologic functions of normal men. Am. J. Med., *4:*413, 1948.

59. Mattsson, S.: The reversibility of disuse osteoporosis. Acta Orthop. Scand. [Suppl.], 144, 1972.

60. Ingelmark, B.E., and Elsholm, R.: A study on variations in the thickness of articular cartilage in association with rest and periodical load. Uppsala Läkareförenings Förhandlingar, *53:*61, 1948.

61. Tipton, C.M., Schild, R.J., and Tomanek, R.J.: Influence of physical activity on the strength of knee ligaments in rats. J. Appl. Physiol., *212:*783, 1967.

62. Tipton, C.M., Matthes, R.D., and Maynard, J.A.: Influence of chronic exercise on rat bones. Med. Sci. Sports, *4:*55, 1972.

63. Vudik, A.: Biomechanics and functional adaptation of tendons and joint ligaments. *In* Studies on the Anatomy and Function of Bone and Joints. Edited by F. G. Evans. Heidelberg, Springer-Verlag OHG, 1966.

64. Kuskinen, O., and Heikkinen, E.: Effect of prolonged physical training on the development of connective tissues in growing mice. Proc. Int. Symp. Exerc. Biochem., 2nd, Abstracts, 1973.

65. Tipton, C.M., et al.: Influence of exercise on the strength of the medial collateral knee ligaments of dogs. Am. J. Physiol., *218:*894, 1970.

66. Klein, K.K.: The deep squat exercise as utilized in weight training for athletics and its effect on the ligaments of the knee. J. Assoc. Phys. Ment. Rehabil., *15:*6, 1961.

67. Vudik, A.: Simultaneous mechanical and light microscopic studies of collagen fibers. Zeitschrift fuer Anatomie und Entwicklungsgeschichte, *136:*204, 1972.

68. Holmdahl, D.E., and Ingelmark, B.E.: Der bau

des gelenkknorpels unter verschiedenen funktionellen verhaltnissen. Acta Anat., *6:*113, 1948.

69. Nelson, R.C., and Fahrney, R.A.: Relationship between strength and speed of elbow flexion. Res. Q., *36:*455, 1965.
70. Nelson, R.C., and Jordan, B.S.: Relationship between arm strength and speed in the horizontal adductive arm movement. Am. Correct. Ther. J., *23:*82, 1969.
71. Clarke, H.H., and Glines, D.: Relationships of reaction, movement, and completion times to motor, strength, anthropometric, and maturity measures of 13-year-old boys. Res. Q., *33:*194, 1962.
72. Berger, R.A.: Relationship between maximum muscle force and loads of varying proportions of maximum. Unpublished study. Biokinetics Research Laboratory, Temple University, 1975.
73. Berger, R.A.: Velocity of stretch and force capacity in skeletal muscle. Unpublished study, 1974.
74. Huffman, W.B., and Berger, R.A.: Comparison between absolute and relative leg power as predictors of physical performance. Res. Q., *43:*468, 1972.
75. Eastwicke, R.A., and Berger, R.A.: Absolute muscular strength in athletic performance. Unpublished study. Biokinetics Research Laboratory, Temple University, 1976.
75a. Larson, L.A.: A factor and validity analysis of strength variables and tests with a test combination of chinning, dipping, and vertical jump. Res. Q., *11:*82, 1940.
76. Fleishman, E.A.: The Structure and Measurement of Physical Fitness. Englewood Cliffs, Prentice-Hall, 1964.
77. DeLorme, T.L., and Watkins, A.L.: Progressive resistance exercise: technic and medical application. New York, Appleton-Century Crofts, 1951.
78. McGovern, A.E., and Luscombe, H.B.: Useful modifications of progressive resistance exercise techniques. Arch. Phys. Med. Rehabil., *34:*475, 1953.
79. Mullor, E.A.: The regulation of muscular strength. J. Assoc. Phys. Ment. Rehabil., *11:*22, 1957.
80. Berger, R.A.: Effect of varied weight training programs on strength. Res. Q., *33:*168, 1962.
81. Berger, R.A.: Optimum repetitions for the development of strength. Res. Q., *33:*334, 1962.
81a. Berger, R.A.: Relationship between strength and absolute muscular endurance with various resistance loads. Unpublished study. Biokinetics Research Laboratory, Temple University, 1970.
82. Berger, R.A.: Effect of dynamic and static training on vertical jumping ability. Res. Q., *34:*22, 1963.
83. Berger, R.A., and Henderson, J.M.: Relationship of power to static and dynamic strength. Res. Q., *37:*9, 1966.
84. Berger, R.A., and Blaschke, L.A.: Comparison of relationships between motor ability and static and dynamic strength. Res. Q., *38:*144, 1967.
84a. Meadows, C.: The effects of isotonic and isometric muscle contraction training on speed, force and strength. Unpublished doctoral dissertation, University of Illinois, 1959.
85. Baer, A.D., Gersten, J.W., and Robertson, B.M.: Effect of various exercise programs on isometric tension, endurance, and reaction time in the human. Arch. Phys. Med. Rehabil., *36:*495, 1955.
86. Dennison, J.D., Howell, M.L., and Morford, W.R.: Effect of isometric and isotonic exercise programs upon muscular endurance. Res. Q., *32:*348, 1961.
87. Salter, N.: The effect of muscle strength of maximum isometric and isotonic contractions at different repetition rates. J. Physiol., *130:*109, 1955.
87a. Singh, M., and Karpovich, P.V.: Effect of eccentric training of agonist on antagonistic muscles. J. Appl. Physiol., *23:*742, 1967.
88. Pipes, T.V.: Nautilus vs. isotonic strength training. Unpublished study. Dominican College, 1976.
88a. Gardner, G.W.: Specificity of strength changes of the exercised and nonexercised limb following isometric training. Res. Q., *34:*98, 1963.
89. Moffroid, M., et al.: A study of isokinetic exercise. Phys. Ther., *49:*735, 1969.
90. Thistle, H.G., et al.: Isokinetic contraction: a new concept of resistive exercise. Arch. Phys. Med. Rehabil., *48:*279, 1967.
91. Berger, R.A.: Classification of students on the basis of strength. Res. Q., *34:*514, 1963.
92. Berger, R.A.: Prediction of total dynamic strength from chinning and dipping strength. J. Assoc. Phys. Ment. Rehabil., *19:*18, 1965.
93. Berger, R.A.: Relationship of chinning strength to total dynamic strength. Res. Q., *37:*431, 1966.
93a. Berger, R.A., and Medlin, R.L.: Evaluation of Berger's 1-RM chin test for junior high school males. Res. Q., *40:*460, 1969.
94. Berger, R.A.: Determination of a method to predict 1-RM chin and dip from repetitive chins and dips. Res. Q., *38:*330, 1967.
95. Clarke, H.H.: Muscular Strength and Endurance in Man. Englewood Cliffs, Prentice-Hall, 1966.
96. Clarke, H.H., and Munroe, R.A.: Test Manual: Oregon cable-tension strength batteries for boys and girls from fourth grade through college. Eugene, Microform Publications in Health, P.E. and Recreation, 1970.
97. Hunsicker, P.: Instruments to measure strength. Res. Q., *26:*408, 1955.
98. Lowenberger, A.G.: Construction of a muscular strength test for college men. Microcarded Doctoral Dissertation, University of Oregon, 1967.
98a. Laycoe, R.R., and Martenium, R.G.: Learning and tension as factors in static strength gains produced by static and eccentric training. Res. Q., *42:*279, 1971.
99. Roger, F.R.: Physical Capacity Tests in the Administration of Physical Education. 4th Edition. New York, Bureau of Publications, Teachers College, Columbia University, 1926.
100. Flower, M.L.: Muscular Strength Relationships Among Upper Elementary, Junior High and

Senior High School Girls. Microcarded Doctoral Dissertation, University of Oregon, 1966.

100a. Bilik, E.: Muscular strength relationships among upper elementary, junior high and senior high school boys. Microcarded Doctoral Dissertation, University of Oregon, 1966.

101. Berger, R.A., and Davies, A.H.: The chronic effects of isokinetic and isotonic training on muscle force, endurance, and hypertrophy. Submitted for publication, Res. Q., 1981.

102. Berger, R.A.: Comparison between resistance load and strength improvement. Res. Q., *33*:637, 1962.

103. Berger, R.A.: Comparison of the effect of various weight training loads on strength. Res. Q., *36*:20, 1965.

Energy for Muscular Endurance

Movement in living creatures requires large amounts of energy. This energy is provided by various chemical reactions that occur in and around muscle fibers. The original source of energy is provided by food. After the food is digested in the alimentary tract, it travels by the blood to the various organs to supply them with needed nutrients and energy. In all muscle tissues of the body, the immediate source of energy for contraction is adenosine triphosphate (ATP). But, the metabolic processes that change food to ATP involve a series of intermediary, biochemical reactions. This chapter is concerned with the production of energy by metabolic processes that are affected by nutrition, hormones, and work. The structural and functional changes in muscle as a consequence of work will also be covered.

ENERGY AT WORK

Metabolism is the sum of all the chemical reactions that occur within the body. The chemical reactions involve either the breaking down of molecules, called catabolic reactions, or the building up of molecules, called anabolic reactions. These reactions occur continuously and simultaneously so that virtually all the organic compounds of a cell are broken down and replaced with new molecules in a relatively short period of time. Some molecules are replaced every few minutes, whereas others may not be replaced for days, weeks, or even years.

The molecules that make up cells may form physical parts or structures, such as the cell membrane or the endoplasmic re-ticulum. Other molecules in cells provide chemical energy when broken down. These molecules maintain cellular structure and function. Such energy molecules are derived from food. Before reading further on the topic of metabolism, one should understand the concept of energy.

Energy in the Cell

Energy cannot be described in terms of size, shape, or mass; it is only definable in dynamic terms that express the ability to produce change. In other words, the presence of energy is shown only when change is occurring or, specifically, when work is being done. The amount of work done is a measure of energy. Work is measured by multiplying the forces acting on an object by the distance it is moved (see Chap. 1). In body function, energy is evident by the movement of joints, which is caused by muscle contraction. The extent of the movement and the force with which the muscles contract indicate the amount of energy expended. Just as body movement is a form of energy, so is the movement of individual molecules in the muscle. After all, the molecules of muscle fibers are set into motion by the energy created from the chemical reactions that produce muscle shortening.

Another form of energy, and one that is associated with movement, is heat. The extent of molecular motion that occurs during chemical reactions in the muscle to produce energy is directly related to the quantity of heat released. This relationship enables energy changes from chemical reactions to be measured in the laboratory by the amount of heat released from the body. Chemical energy is unique because it can be stored until needed. When stored, the energy is called potential energy and is locked within the structure of molecules. When the potential energy is released during a chemical reaction, it is called kinetic energy.

The chemical potential energy that is stored in the structure of a molecule can be likened to the potential energy stored in a stretched spring. The energy required to form the chemical ATP (energy source for all life) in the muscles is similar to the work energy required to stretch a spring. When the spring is released, the stored potential energy appears as motion and heat as the spring returns to its original position. The chemical bond that holds ATP atoms together by electric forces of negative electrons and positive protons represents potential energy, as do the forces in a stretched spring. When the chemical bond of phosphate (P) in ATP is broken off, the potential energy becomes kinetic energy; ADP and P are end products. The process involving the formation of ATP and the energy released from ATP will be explained in more detail.

Enzymes in Energy Formation

In the early nineteenth century, chemists noted that the body's cells had the ability to achieve high rates of organic reactions without the presence of high temperatures. This discovery was puzzling to scientists because the same reactions produced in a test tube required temperatures higher than those in the body. Later research identified a class of chemical substances, present in all cells, that produced these results. Specific proteins were found to accelerate the rates of chemical reactions without undergoing any chemical change themselves and without elevating temperature. Because these proteins acted as catalysts to accelerate the forward and reverse directions of a chemical reaction, they were called protein catalysts or enzymes.

During the formation of energy sub-stances in the cells, many enzymes are involved in the numerous chemical reactions that culminate in ATP energy. Each cell can regulate its own metabolism because it has the ability to control the rate of enzyme synthesis and breakdown. In this way, the products formed in the cell by enzyme activity are kept at a desired level.

Enzymes are highly specific to the molecule upon which they act. Consequently, thousands of different reactions occur within a cell as a result of enzymes. Some enzymes only react with one particular type of molecule, whereas some react with a wide range of different molecules. Enzymes are named by adding the suffix *ase* to the name of the molecules they catalyze or to the type of reaction catalyzed by the enzyme. For example, lactic acid in the working muscle cells is removed by the enzyme lactic dehydrogenase, which breaks down lactic acid by removing its hydrogen atoms.

METABOLISM OF CARBOHYDRATES, FATS, AND PROTEINS

One outcome of metabolism is the formation of ATP, which is a labile chemical compound in the cytoplasm and nucleoplasm of all cells. In essentially all physiologic functions, energy is provided by ATP. A supply of ATP is always available in the cells because the continued oxidation of foodstuffs replenishes the supply used for energy. ATP also provides energy for the transport of substances across cell membranes, e.g., glucose, and for the synthesis of other chemical compounds necessary to the cells.

Energy from Carbohydrates

At least 99% of all carbohydrates consumed by the body form ATP in the cells. But, before ATP is created, carbohydrates are first digested in the alimentary tract and changed to glucose, fructose, and galactose. These sugars pass from the intestines into the blood, which carries them to the liver. In the liver, these sugars are changed almost completely into glucose. Some of the glucose is stored in the liver as glycogen and to a lesser extent, fat. The remaining glucose is transported by the blood into the tissue cells, where it is either stored as glycogen in the muscle or changed to fat in the liver and stored in adipose tissue.

In most tissues of the body, except the liver, glucose cannot diffuse out of the cell. As a result, an exhausted working muscle cannot draw glucose from resting muscle. Glucose can be used immediately for energy in all cells or it can be stored in the form of glycogen. Liver and muscle cells can store relatively more glycogen than can other cells. In fact, the liver can store up to 8% of its weight in glycogen, and muscle can store up to 1%. The liver's high-storage capacity for glycogen is appropriate for its role in maintaining the glucose level of the blood and in providing additional glucose to the muscles during heavy work or exercise. The following chemical pathways for the formation of energy are presented in an abbreviated form, primarily as an introduction to the topic. The changing of glucose into ATP energy (the end-products are water and carbon dioxide) involves 19 chemical reactions in a cell. A different enzyme is involved in each reaction.

Glycogenolysis

When the glucose supply in the muscles is low, the stored glycogen is transformed back into glucose. This chemical process is called glycogenolysis. The glucose molecule is split away from glycogen by the activation of primarily two enzymes (phosphorylase and phosphofructokinase). These enzymes are inactive during rest, but when the muscles contract, certain chemical reactions activate them. Other regulators of glycogenolysis are hormonal in nature and are presented later in this chapter.

Glycolysis

Various chemical steps lead to the formation of ATP. The first step, called glycolysis, involves the breakdown of glucose into pyruvic acid. ATP is created during the pro-

cess. Only about 5% of all the ATP formed comes from this process. Oxygen is not needed for glycolysis.

Pyruvic Acid Conversion

The next step after glycolysis involves the changing of pyruvic acid into acetylcoenzyme A or acetyl-CoA. Oxygen is not needed for this chemical change. But, after this step, oxygen is needed to fully realize the ATP potential of glucose. All chemical reactions beyond acetyl-CoA that require oxygen occur within the mitochondria of the cells where all the necessary enzymes are present. Glycolysis and pyruvic acid conversion occur in the sarcoplasm of the cell, which is located outside the mitochondria.

Krebs' Cycle

The Krebs' cycle (also called the citric acid cycle or tricarboxylic acid cycle) begins with acetyl-CoA and goes through a sequence of 10 chemical reactions, resulting in carbon dioxide and hydrogen atoms. Oxygen is needed for all these chemical reactions. The main purpose of the cycle is to form hydrogen atoms, which are oxidized to liberate large quantities of ATP.

Oxidation of Hydrogen

Glycolysis and the Krebs' cycle provide only about 10% of the total amount of ATP formed. The subsequent oxidation of hydrogen atoms produces the remaining 90%. In fact, the main function of glycolysis and the Krebs' cycle is to make hydrogen available from the glucose molecule in a form that allows oxidation. A series of enzymatically catalyzed reactions result in the oxidation of hydrogen by (1) changing hydrogen atoms into hydrogen ions (H^+) and (2) changing the dissolved oxygen of the fluids into hydroxyl ions. These two products combine to form water, the final end product. During the sequence of these oxidative reactions, large amounts of energy are released to form ATP.

About 56% of the energy formed during the breakdown of glucose is used for oxidative processes and is released as heat. About 44% of the ATP formed either is stored as potential energy or is partially or completely used during work, depending on the severity of the work.

Energy from Fats and Proteins

In the American diet, about 40 to 45% of the calories are derived from fats. Approximately the same percentage of calories are obtained from carbohydrates. But, 30 to 35% of ingested carbohydrates are stored as fat and used later for energy. Therefore, as much as two thirds to three quarters of all energy of the body may be supplied by fat. During aerobic exercise, the use of fat as an energy source may exceed the use of carbohydrates. Prolonged aerobic (with O_2) work of 3 hr. uses fat to supply about 70% of the energy. Work involving primarily anaerobic (without O_2) metabolism uses carbohydrates (CH) as the major source of energy. Protein as an energy source is greatly limited and only occurs to an appreciable extent when the calorie supply is inadequate. However, any excess protein intake is converted either to fat directly, or to glucose first and then stored in the body as fat.

Both fat and protein, when used for energy, must first go through a series of chemical reactions before they can enter into the Krebs' cycle to follow the same pathways as glucose. Because protein plays a minor role in providing energy for muscle contraction under normal circumstances, only fat is discussed as an energy source.

The first step in the conversion of fat to energy is called hydrolysis, which is a chemical reaction changing fat into primarily fatty acids. By a chemical process called beta oxidation, fatty acids are degraded into acetyl-CoA, which then enters into the Krebs' cycle and eventually becomes oxidized for energy in the muscle. The extent to which fat is used as an energy source during rest and exercise will be presented later in more detail.

Energy Release from ATP

When ATP is broken down and energy is released, ADP (adenosine diphosphate) and phosphate (P) are formed.

$$ATP \rightarrow ADP + P + energy$$

For movement to continue, there must be an alternating breakdown of ATP to obtain energy and a building up again of ADP and P to form ATP (a reversing direction in the formula). The energy to regenerate ADP and P to form ATP comes from creatine phosphate (CP), which contains more high-energy phosphate bonds than does ATP. Although CP does not act like ATP as a coupling agent between foods and energy, it can transfer energy interchangeably with ATP. When ATP is abundant in the cell, some of its energy is used to synthesize CP, thus building up a rich source of energy. When ATP is used up, the energy in the CP is transferred back to synthesize ATP from ADP and P. The interchangeable relationship between ADP and CP is illustrated by the following equation:

$$CP + ADP \rightleftharpoons ATP + C \text{ (creatine)}$$

The energy for the resynthesis of CP comes from the oxidation of hydrogen atoms, which are made available by glycolysis and the Krebs' cycle.

METABOLISM IN WORK

The chemical reactions occurring in metabolism during rest and work vary depending on the amount of oxygen available to meet the energy needs of muscle tissue. When oxygen is plentiful, the potential energy in foods is released in sufficient quantities to meet the necessary energy demands. But, when the body cannot provide the necessary energy because of lack of oxygen, the chemical reactions leading to the full utilization of the potential energy in all tissues cannot run their full course.

The metabolism associated with these conditions is commonly referred to in terms of the presence (aerobic) or the absence (anaerobic) of oxygen during the chemical reactions that result in the formation of energy.

Aerobic Metabolism

The chemical pathway for metabolism, when carbohydrate is the energy food and oxygen is plentiful, is presented in a simplified form:

$$\text{Glycogen} \rightarrow \text{Glucose} \rightarrow \text{Pyruvic acid} \rightarrow \text{Acetyl-CoA} \rightarrow \text{Krebs' cycle} +$$
$$O_2 \rightarrow CO_2 + H_2O + \text{ATP}$$

When fat is the energy source, the formula is as follows:

$$\text{Fat} \rightarrow \text{Fatty acids} \rightarrow \text{Acetyl-CoA} \rightarrow \text{Krebs' cycle} + O_2 \rightarrow CO_2 + H_2O + \text{ATP}$$

Note that the two formulas become the same after acetyl-CoA is formed.

The reactions can complete their course only when adequate amounts of oxygen are present in the Krebs' cycle. Physical activity is usually moderate and, therefore, oxygen is plentiful. Even in moderate work, such as jogging slowly, the oxygen supply may be sufficient for aerobic metabolism to take place.

Anaerobic Metabolism

When the energy demands exceed the capability of muscle cells to use oxygen, the end product of glycolysis, pyruvic acid, increases to such an extent that the acidity of the blood and cells impairs performance. The ability to sustain a high level of activity for a short time without adequate oxygen supply indicates that some ATP energy is formed without the presence of oxygen. The process by which ATP is formed without oxygen is called anaerobic metabolism.

Anaerobic metabolism occurs when running 600 yd. with maximum effort. The intake of oxygen by the cells is not sufficient to oxidize all the pyruvic acid formed. After the relatively small amounts of oxygen stored in the muscle myoglobin, in the blood, and in the tissue fluids have been used, the ATP energy for muscle contraction is produced without oxygen. But, this kind of energy production can only continue for several minutes before exhaustion occurs. Energy for the strenuous work is provided by the stored ATP and CP and by the glycolytic breakdown of glucose to pyruvic acid. But, of the total energy in the glucose molecule, only a little more than 5% is used to form ATP without the presence of oxygen.

The increased acidity of the blood is mainly caused by the formation of lactic acid from pyruvic acid and hydrogen atoms. Without the presence of oxygen, lactic acid continues to increase until muscle contractions cease.

Lactic Acid in Work. There is some indication that the formation of lactic acid is more of a limiting factor in muscular endurance than is the availability of energy from ATP and CP stores and from glycolytic sources.[1,2] After exercise, lactic acid is removed at different rates, depending on what is done during the recovery time. If activity is moderate immediately after exhaustive exercise, recovery occurs at a faster rate than when a rest is taken. In fact, research evidence indicates that a workload of 60 to 70% of $\dot{V}O_2$ max (the maximum amount of oxygen absorbed) removes lactic acid at a faster rate than does any other load.[3]

Lactic acid is not lost. Some diffuses into the interstitial fluid and the circulating blood and is either changed to glycogen in the liver or oxidized for energy in the heart. During recovery, about 85% of the lactic acid is resynthesized to glycogen in the muscle,[4] and 15% is oxidized to CO_2 and H_2O in the production of ATP. The presence of oxygen changes the lactic acid into pyruvic acid, which can then be utilized in the Krebs' cycle to provide more oxidation energy. If the ATP stores are filled, the excess pyruvic acid is converted back into glucose.

Anaerobic and aerobic metabolism do not follow entirely different chemical pathways. In fact, the pathways for both are the same through the glycolytic pathway. But, the aerobic pathways take over beyond the glycolytic pathway.

Oxygen Debt. During rest, especially after anaerobic work, the body takes in large quantities of oxygen for several minutes or more. Additional oxygen is needed to reconvert lactic acid into pyruvate and glucose and to build up the ATP and CP stores to their resting levels. In addition, oxygen is needed to replace that which is normally stored in the body during rest, such as in the muscle myoglobin, in the blood, and in the tissue fluids. The oxygen demands during exercise are not limited to the specific muscle groups moving or propelling the body. But, the increased activity of the respiratory muscles and of the heart in delivering oxygenated blood requires large amounts of oxygen. The oxygen absorbed by the body tissues that is above the quantity needed to maintain the resting level is called oxygen debt.

Even after light exercise, when work is performed aerobically, the heart and respiratory rates remain elevated, indicating some oxygen debt. But, in these cases, the debt is primarily owing to the slight oxygen deficit that occurs at the beginning of exercise. There is a period of time at the start of exercise when the circulatory and respiratory adjustments lag behind. As a result, oxygen is not immediately utilized by the working muscles in sufficient quantities. The limited stores of oxygen that are in the muscle myoglobin, in the blood, and in the tissue fluids before exercise are not adequate to meet these initial demands. However, as activity continues, a catching-up

effect maintains or diminishes the initial oxygen deficit.

Cellular Changes and Metabolic Efficiency During Work

Performance level in endurance sports depends on the capacity of the heart and respiratory systems to pump oxygenated blood to the working muscles and on the ability of the working muscles to extract oxygen from the blood. An increase in the ability of the body to absorb more oxygen during exercise is brought about by an increase in the amount of blood pumped by the heart and by the biochemical adaptations that take place in muscle cells, increasing their capacity to extract more oxygen from the blood. At the cellular level, changes that take place as a result of training improve the ability of muscle tissue to produce energy during work. These changes are summarized in Table 2–1.

Exercise increases the myoglobin content of skeletal muscle.[5,6] Because myoglobin increases the rate of oxygen transport through a fluid layer,[7,8] it is possible that myoglobin may also facilitate oxygen utilization in

Table 2–1.

Cellular Changes in Skeletal Tissue from Endurance Training

Cell Component	Trained	Untrained
Myoglobin	Higher	Lower
Mitochondria		
1. Number	Higher	Lower
2. Composition	Higher	Lower
Oxidation of:		
1. Pyruvate	Higher	Lower
2. Fat	Higher	Lower
3. Carbohydate	Higher	Lower
Activity of mitochondrial enzymes	Higher	Lower
Muscle glycogen	Higher	Lower

muscle by increasing oxygen flow through the cytoplasm of the cell into the mitochondria. An increase in myoglobin is associated with an increase in mitochondria.[9-11] Exercise also increases the size of mitochondria and probably their number.[12] The total effect improves the capacity of mitochondria to generate ATP. In fact, approximately 50% of the increase in oxygen consumption by the body from training is owing to the increase in myoglobin and mitochondria.

The amount of fat used by muscle for energy also changes as a consequence of training. Physically trained individuals oxidize more fat and less carbohydrate during submaximal exercise than do untrained individuals.[13] This finding suggests that endurance exercise results in a greater release of fatty acids from adipose tissue.[14,15] Because glycogen is spared in the trained individual, the condition of hypoglycemia (low blood glucose), which may limit endurance during a prolonged race, is less likely to occur because the uptake of blood glucose by the muscle during exercise is decreased. The reasons for the proportionately greater amount of fat used as an energy source as a result of improved cardiovascular fitness may lie in some of the control mechanisms that regulate carbohydrate catabolism. One of these mechanisms is the rate of fatty acid oxidation which, when high, inhibits glycolysis and pyruvate oxidation.[16] Fat is oxidized as long as the concentration of fatty acids in the muscles is substantial.

Endurance training increases the capacity of muscle cells to oxidize pyruvic acid, carbohydrates, and fatty acids and to form ATP via oxidative phosphorylation, largely by the rise in activity levels of the mitochondrial enzymes.[10] These enzymes are involved in the Krebs' cycle, in fatty acid catabolism, and in changes in mitochondrial composition. When their activity level increases, the ability to continue an aerobic activity is enhanced, resulting in increased work capacity. The specific biochemical changes occurring from exercise are presented in detail by Holloszy.[17]

Comparison Between Trained and Untrained Individuals

Individuals trained for endurance work, such as long-distance runners, can absorb much more oxygen than can untrained individuals. The trained may have maximum values of oxygen uptake ($\dot{V}O_2$ max), expressed in ml. (milliliters) per kg. (kilogram) of body weight per min. of 75 ml./kg./min., whereas the untrained may have $\dot{V}O_2$ max values of 42 ml./kg./min. The reasons for these $\dot{V}O_2$ max differences are related to the cellular changes previously presented and are reflected in the rate of glycogen depletion in working muscle, the fat utilization in exercise, the blood flow to muscle, and the blood lactate level (Table 2-2).

Glycogen and Fat Depletion in Trained and Untrained Individuals. During submaximal exercise, trained individuals have the same rate of glycogen depletion from the muscle as do untrained individuals when both work at the same relative $\dot{V}O_2$ max. For example, research reported by Saltin demonstrated that when both trained and untrained individuals worked at 68 to 69% of $\dot{V}O_2$ max (same relative work) for 275 to 291 min., approximately the same amount of glycogen was used and about the same quantity of energy was yielded.[13] But, almost 60% more absolute work was done by the trained persons. Therefore, the additional energy must have come from another energy source. This other source was fat. In the research cited, more than twice as much energy in the trained individual was provided by fat. In fact, of the total energy used in work, 58% was supplied by fat in the trained persons, and only 41% was supplied by fat in the untrained persons.

When both the trained and untrained individual do the same amount of work in the same time interval (e.g., 50% $\dot{V}O_2$ max, trained; 80% $\dot{V}O_2$ max, untrained), less glycogen and fat are used by the trained individual. Consequently, the trained person uses less ATP and CP. Even at the same

Table 2–2.

Comparison Between Trained and Untrained Individuals in Exercise Response

Exercise Response to Aerobic Training	Trained	Untrained
$\dot{V}O_2$ max	Higher	Lower
Muscle glycogen	Higher	Lower
Rate of glycogen depletion 1. At same relative work. 2. At same absolute work.	Same Lower	Same Higher
Oxygen uptake 1. At same relative work. 2. At same absolute work.	Higher Same	Lower Same
Muscle and blood lactate 1. At same absolute work. 2. At same relative work (except maximum) 3. At same O_2 uptake. 4. In maximum work.	Lower Lower Lower Higher	Higher Higher Higher Lower
Respiratory quotient 1. At same relative work.	Lower	Higher
Decrease in muscle CP plus ATP 1. At same absolute work.	Lower	Higher
Blood flow/kg. of working muscle 1. At same absolute submaximal work.	Lower	Higher

work loads, trained individuals use a greater proportion of fat for energy than do untrained individuals. This fact was shown by the R.Q. (respiratory quotient), which was lower for the trained persons at both absolute and relative work loads.

When energy is demanded during exercise, carbohydrate[18] and pyruvic acid[19] are oxidized more readily by the trained person than by the untrained person. Underlying the increased capacity of muscle to oxidize fat, carbohydrate, and pyruvic acid is the rise in the levels of activity of the mitochondrial enzymes.[18] Approximately 50% of aerobic capacity, as measured by $\dot{V}O_2$ max, is based on the ability of the heart, the circulatory system, and the respiratory system to move oxygenated blood to the working muscles. The other 50% of aerobic capacity is based on the ability of the muscle cells to extract oxygen from the blood.

Blood Flow to the Working Muscles. This 50% contribution to aerobic capacity of the cells is largely owing to the biochemical activity of the mitochondrial enzymes. In the past, practically all the aerobic capacity was assumed to be attributable to the amount of blood flow to the muscles. More recent research evidence indicates otherwise. Studies have shown that, after muscles are trained, blood flow per kg. of muscle mass is actually less than blood flow per kg. before training, when doing the same amount of submaximal work.[20] However, during maximum work, total blood flow through the working muscle is increased.[21] Because the amount of oxygen taken from the blood is improved by training, even though blood flow per kg. of mass is less when doing the same work, oxygen is extracted to a much larger extent by the cells.

Blood Lactate in Trained and Untrained Individuals. Blood lactate is lower in trained individuals than in untrained individuals at the same absolute work load and oxygen uptake[22] and at the same relative work load, except when work is maximum.[23] At maximum oxygen consumption, blood lactate is highest in the trained individual. Lack of oxygen, which is the stimulus for anaerobic glycolysis, is apparently not the reason for the increased production of lactic acid in the muscle and blood. Even when oxygen is plentiful, lactic acid accumulates.[22] The lactic acid build-up has been attributed to the imbalance between glycolysis and the rate of pyruvate utilization.[24] The biochemical adaptations from exercise, which occur in the muscle cells, are primarily responsible for the functional relationship between glycolysis and pyruvate utilization. The result is that the trained individual accumulates less lactic acid in the muscle and blood than does the untrained individual while working at the same physiologic intensity or stress (same relative $\dot{V}O_2$ max).

Glycogen Storage and Work Capacity

The amount of glycogen stored in the muscles, liver, and body fluid at the beginning of exercise determines how well an individual performs either during prolonged endurance training, such as running, or in intermittent work, such as soccer.[25] The relative proportions of glycogen stored at these three sites are approximately 29% in the liver, 67% in skeletal muscle, and 4% in the body fluid. The importance of glycogen storage in exercise was shown by Saltin,[26] who compared the soccer performance of five players with normal amounts of glycogen in their thigh muscles with the performance of four players with only half the normal glycogen content. The five players with the normal amount of glycogen covered more distance and ran at maximal speeds for a longer time than did the other four players.

The performance differences were apparently brought about by the greater amount of glycogen expended by the five players with the normal content of glycogen because at the completion of the game, the glycogen stores were practically depleted for all players.

After glycogen is no longer available for work in the muscle, fats are always present as an inexhaustible source of energy. But, because more oxygen is needed by fats than by glycogen to yield the same amount of energy, the work effort is greatly reduced. In fact, the intensity of the work must be less than about 50% of maximal oxygen consumption ($\dot{V}O_2$ max) for exercise to continue. In a long distance race or in prolonged and continued sport activity, performance is greatly impaired when fats are practically the only energy source.

Even when an athlete consumes carbohydrates during the contest, usually in liquid form, the capacity of the digestive system to make new glucose available to the muscle probably meets only 20 to 30% of the total needs for energy. Nevertheless, some carbohydrate intake during a race retards glycogen depletion.

The amount of glycogen stored in the muscle just before an endurance contest determines how well an athlete performs. It is possible to increase the glycogen stored in a muscle by 100% or more through a process referred to as supercompensation.[25] The process begins by depleting the muscle of glycogen through exercise. The idea is to stimulate a greater synthesis of glycogen by the muscle so that the amount of glycogen later stored is beyond that which was expected. There is an overcompensation or supercompensation of glycogen stored. The only way to completely deplete muscle glycogen is through exercise; glycogen cannot leave the muscle fiber once it is inside.

To supercompensate after a muscle is depleted of glycogen by exercise, a diet rich in carbohydrates is followed for the next three days, just before competition. A further increase in glycogen is possible if, after exhaustive exercise and glycogen depletion, a low-carbohydrate diet is followed for the next three days, followed by three days of a rich carbohydrate diet just before competition. For example, a marathon runner preparing for an important event seven to eight days hence first depletes glycogen stores by a hard workout. A diet low in carbohydrates is consumed for the next three days. Greater depletion occurs when exercise is continued during the days of low carbohydrate intake. Care must be taken to ensure that a minimum of 60 g. of carbohydrates are consumed during each of these three days. Otherwise, the function of the nervous system and red blood cells may be impaired. A high carbohydrate diet is consumed and physical activity is minimized for the next three days, just before competition. The increase of 100% or more in glycogen storage improves performance.

Metabolic Processes Involved in Work of Different Intensities and Durations

Energy for work is provided by both anaerobic and aerobic metabolism. The de-gree to which energy is obtained by anaerobic or aerobic processes depends on the intensity and duration of exercise. Continuous exercise of long duration can only be done by low-intensity muscle contractions and, therefore, is performed by energy provided aerobically. In high-intensity work of short duration, most of the energy comes from anaerobic metabolism. Unlike aerobic metabolism, during which the ATP energy comes from the complete oxidation of foodstuffs, anaerobic metabolism provides two sources of ATP energy for movement. These energy sources are related to the severity of work.

Production of ATP Energy in Work of Different Intensities. There are basically three sources of ATP during work. When work is explosive and lasts for only several seconds, the main source of energy comes from the ATP and CP stored within the muscle. However, some of the energy is supplied by the second source, which is the breakdown of glucose to pyruvic acid or glycolysis. In work that goes beyond about 8 to 10 sec. but does not exceed about 2 min. there is a shift

Table 2–3.

Relative Contribution of Anaerobic and Aerobic Processes to Total Energy Output During Maximal Exercise of Different Durations*

Work Time, Maximal Exercise	Relative Contribution (%)		Primary Energy Source	% $\dot{V}O_2$ Max
	Anaerobic Processes	Aerobic Processes		
10 seconds	83	17	ATP-CP	100
1 minute	60	40	glycolysis	100
2 minutes	40	60	glycolysis and oxygen	100
5 minutes	20	80	glycolysis and oxygen	100
10 minutes	9	91	oxygen	95–100
30 minutes	3	97	oxygen	80–95
60 minutes	1	99	oxygen	80–90

*These values are estimates based on the findings of several research studies.[7,13,26,27]

in the importance of stored ATP-CP and glycolysis as the energy source. Because only relatively small amounts of ATP-CP can be stored in muscle, it is greatly depleted after about 10 sec. Consequently, glycolysis provides most of the ATP energy for work that lasts up to 2 min. But, because the work is strenuous for 2 min. and oxygen cannot be delivered to the muscles in sufficient quantities, lactic acid builds up to the point where performance level cannot be maintained or exhaustion occurs. In maximum work lasting over 2 to 3 min., the third source of ATP production plays a larger part in providing energy, although the other two sources still operate but at a diminishing rate. This third source is the aerobic aspect of metabolism during which ATP energy is produced by the presence of oxygen. Work of 60 min. or longer receives almost 100% of its energy from aerobic metabolism (Table 2–3).

HORMONAL REGULATION OF METABOLISM

Energy metabolism is affected by hormones that are secreted by the endocrine system. The glands of the endocrine system secrete their hormones directly into the blood, which transports them throughout the body. At specific sites in the body, hormones control and integrate bodily functions involved in reproduction, organic metabolism, and energy balance.

The endocrine system consists of the glands of internal secretion. These glands are the hypophysis, the thyroid, the parathyroids, the suprarenals, the islet cells of the pancreas, and part of the stomach, duodenum, ovaries, and testes (Fig. 2–1). A hormone is a chemical substance produced by a specific organ or tissue. It comes from a Greek word meaning "to stir up or set in motion." Endocrine glands differ from such other glands as the sweat, salivary, and gastrointestinal because they do not discharge their secretions into ducts that lead to the specific site of their action or use. The endocrine glands convey their hormones to specific organs by way of the blood. For

example, the secretion of epinephrine by the adrenal medulla gland has specific effects on the heart, arteries, and adipose tissue, but little effect on other organs.

Some of the endocrine glands with the largest effect on metabolic action are presented in this chapter. Although one of the primary concerns in this chapter is the production of energy by metabolic processes, to which the hormones of the endocrine glands greatly contribute, the overall significance of the endocrine system, beyond its direct role in regulating metabolism, is also discussed. Consequently, the reader can glean a better understanding of how the endocrine glands have both an immediate effect and an indirect effect on tissue metabolism at rest and during work. Hormones, when not specifically modifying metabolism, better adapt the physiologic systems to meet varying metabolic needs. The short-term and long-term effects of work and exercise on these glands are emphasized where known. Before proceeding, one must understand the interrelationships between the nervous and endocrine systems in regulating metabolism.

Interrelationships Between Nervous and Endocrine Systems

Both the nervous and the endocrine systems are regulatory because their primary role is to maintain homeostasis of the body's internal environment. The nervous system is concerned with rapid adjustments, whereas the endocrine system is concerned with slower metabolic adjustments. These two systems cannot be separated because their function in maintaing a relatively stable condition involves regulating and integrating the activities of all tissues and organs.

A good example of the coordinating activity between the two systems is the function of the hypothalamus, located at the base of the brain. The hypothalamus is part of the autonomic nervous system, which regulates the activity of cardiac muscle, smooth muscle, and glands via motor nerves to these

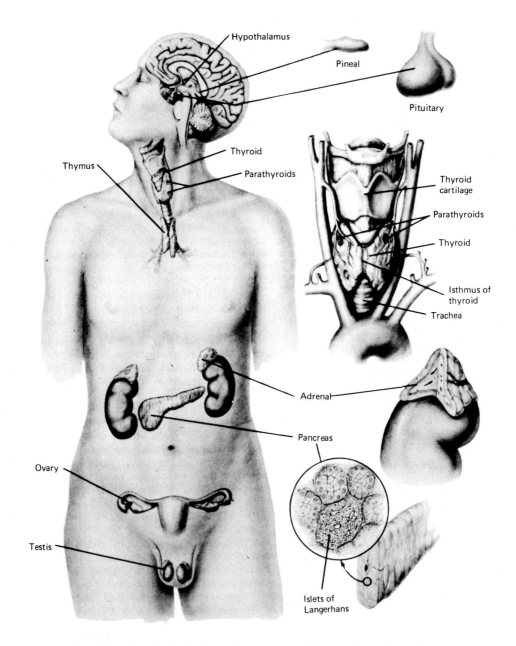

Fig. 2–1.   Location of the endocrine glands. (From Solomon, E.P., and Davis, P.W.: Understanding Human Anatomy and Physiology. New York, McGraw-Hill, Inc., 1978. Used with permission of McGraw-Hill Book Co.)

organs (see Chap. 3). Although the primary functions of the hypothalamus are the nervous control of blood pressure, blood flow to skeletal muscles, temperature regulation, food intake, water intake, and adjustment to such stresses as fear, cold, and anger, it also regulates some of the endocrine glands by either direct or indirect neural stimulation.

Common Effects of Hormonal Activity

Hormones never initiate a process, but they do alter the rates at which specific cellular processes proceed. These alterations in rate either accelerate or decelerate cellular activity. Most hormones act on tissue cells by either influencing the rate of transport of a substance across a cell membrane or affecting the enzymes within the cells.

Hormones alter the enzyme activity within cells in several ways. They may either stimulate an increase in the quantity of certain enzymes in the cell or repress the synthesis of these enzymes. Hormones can also increase enzymatic activity without synthesis. In some cases, certain hormones induce both the synthesis of more enzyme molecules and an increase in enzyme activity. There is an advantage in this dual effect because the activation of molecules already present permits a response in only a few minutes while, at the same time, the synthesis of new enzyme molecules, which takes hours or days, offers the advantage of a long-term adaptation. Thus, the response may be prolonged.

Whereas some hormones may only act directly on the enzymes of the cell, others affect the cell membrane to either facilitate or inhibit the transport of substances into the cell. For example, glucose enters most cells by the action of the hormone, insulin, which increases the rate of glucose transport across cell membranes. Other hormones inhibit glucose transport.

Hormones may have secondary effects on the cells. Insulin, when present in the blood in large quantities, has a primary effect on cell membranes that increases the intake of glucose from the blood. As a result, many chemical reactions involving glucose are activated within the cells as a secondary effect. There are other situations in which the secondary effects do not occur within the cells, but affect the entire body. When blood insulin is deficient, blood glucose rises because glucose is not transported in sufficient quantities into the cells. As a result, large quantities of glucose are secreted in the urine as a secondary effect. This occurs in some cases of diabetes. Because virtually all hormones are continually secreted at some rate in the body, cells are always exposed to the simultaneous effects of many hormones. These interacting effects create difficulties when one tries to determine which hormones play the dominant role in regulating activity under a variety of work conditions.

HORMONES AND PHYSICAL WORK. Some of the most important hormones involved in maintaining homeostasis of the body's cells during exercise and work are presented in Table 2–4. The sites or places in the body where the hormones are secreted, the target areas that are primarily affected by these secretions, the stimuli that initiate hormonal activity, the sites that control the degree of secretions, and the responses often made as a consequence of these hormones are also presented in the table.

CORTISOL AND PHYSICAL ACTIVITY. The main purpose of cortisol is the metabolism of carbohydrates, fats, and proteins. This hormone, secreted by the adrenal cortex, effects in tissues specific chemical changes that result in an increase in blood glucose. Muscle and adipose tissues are primarily affected by cortisol and undergo the transformation that leads eventually to increased blood glucose. Cortisol catabolizes (breaks down) protein in muscle, and the amino acids separated out are changed into glucose in the liver. The increased glucose is either stored as glycogen in the liver or released into the blood where it is conveyed to the working muscles for energy. Glucose is also made more available to the muscles by the effect of cortisol on adipose tissue. This increased availability is brought

Table 2–4.
Hormones in Physical Activity

Hormone	Secretion Site	Target Area	Stimulus	Controlling Site	Response
Cortisol	Adrenal cortex	Liver, adipose tissue, skeletal muscle	Stress: physical and/or psychologic	Hypothalamus-pituitary system	Increase in blood sugar
Androgens	Male: testes Female: ovaries	Reproductive organs, tissues of secondary sexual characteristics, skeletal muscle and bone	Unknown, but probably related to some inherent automaticity	Hypothalamus-pituitary system	Increase in muscle and bone size
Growth hormone	Pituitary	Adipose tissue, cell membranes, bones	Low blood sugar	Hypothalamus	Increase in free fatty acids for energy
Aldosterone	Adrenal cortex	Kidney	Low blood pressure	Wall of renal artery leading into kidney	Increase in blood pressure
Thyroxine	Thyroid	Essentially all tissues	Circulating thyroxine in the blood	Hypothalamus-pituitary system	Increase in basal metabolic rate
Insulin	Pancreas	Most body cells (except brain tissue)	Elevated blood sugar	Pancreas	Glucose increases in muscle and adipose tissue; decreases in blood plasma
Catecholamines: Epinephrine	Adrenal medulla	Heart, blood vessels	Stress: physical and/or psychologic	Sympathetic nervous system	Increases blood glucose, fatty acids, and blood pressure
Norepinephrine	Nerve endings of sympathetic nervous system	Adipose tissue, heart, blood vessels			

about by the chemical removal of free fatty acids from adipose tissue. These fatty acids travel in the blood to the muscles where they are transported into the cells and converted to glucose for energy.

Although cortisol is continuously secreted in varying quantities, an exceptionally large amount enters the blood as a consequence of all forms of stress. These forms may be either physical, such as injury to a muscle or joint, or psychological, such as preparation for athletic competition. Other stressful situations include prolonged heavy exercise, decreased oxygen supply, prolonged exposure to cold, fright, pain, and infection. In fact, the term, "stress," is often defined as any event that increases cortisol secretion. In addition to cortisol, there is always a nervous response to the same stresses by the activation of the sympathetic nervous system. Traditionally, in physiology, stimulation of the nervous system had always been considered the first overall response to stress. Cortisol was recognized later as contributing to the response.

The adrenal gland is stimulated to secrete cortisol by the action of another hormone that is secreted by the pituitary gland. The initial stimuli for activating the pituitary gland come from the hypothalamus, which receives sensory input from a variety of sources. When the body anticipates a stressful situation or when the actual stressor affects the organism, the hypothalamus is stimulated. These stimuli have a psychic origin, a physical origin, or both, as previously indicated.

During acute exercise, cortisol in the blood plasma increases when moderate to heavy work loads are involved. Work is considered the stressor, and the response of increased cortisol secretion prepares the body for action. Endurance of working muscles increases as a consequence of enhanced cortisol secretion from work stress. Apparently, the increase in blood glucose by the action of cortisol makes the energy source more available to muscle, thereby increasing contractile capacity. But, this effect only occurs when relatively heavy work loads are involved.[28,29] Light to moderate work effort may not be stressful enough to elicit an increase in plasma cortisol.[30,31]

The effect of different work loads on cortisol secretion, an indicator of stress, and the relationship between physical performance and the availability of plasma cortisol, as discussed previously, are a consequence of acute effects of work. But, the long-term effects, or chronic effects, of exercise on cortisol secretion show that several adaptations in structure and function occur. Research studies reported that the adrenal gland hypertrophies as a result of chronic stress and exercise.[32,33] But, there is not complete agreement as to whether the secretory response of cortisol varies as a consequence. Several studies reported that plasma cortisol secretion after acute exercise was lower among trained animals than among untrained animals.[34,34a] Similar results were found with trained human subjects.[35,36] In fact, a study by Henderson[35] showed that differences in cortisol secretion were not only observed between trained and untrained individuals after work, but also between trained and untrained individuals after submergence in cold water. Other studies have shown no difference in cortisol response between trained and untrained individuals.[14,37]

The general consensus is that, in time, light to moderate exercise in training may produce either an increase, decrease, or no change in plasma cortisol, depending on the degree of psychologic and/or physiologic stress from exercise. However, when training involves moderate to exhaustive work, less plasma cortisol appears in the trained individual at rest and in submaximal work. However, in exhaustive work, the cortisol level is about the same for both trained and untrained individuals.

ALDOSTERONE AND PHYSICAL ACTIVITY. During exercise, when blood flow is increased to meet the metabolic needs of the body, several hormones help to maintain flow by increasing blood pressure. One such hormone is aldosterone, which is secreted by the adrenal cortex when blood pressure begins to fall. When aldosterone reaches the kidneys, it decreases the amount of sodium excreted in the urine and, thus, increases sodium concentration in the blood. As a result, more fluid passes from the extracellular spaces into the blood, thereby increasing blood volume and, in turn, blood pressure.

The chain of events that precedes the secretion of aldosterone by the adrenal cortex originates in the wall of the renal artery, which leads into the kidneys. When blood pressure falls, an enzyme (renin) is secreted into the blood by a group of cells located in the wall of the renal artery. This enzyme acts on a specific blood protein (angiotensin I) that eventually is affected by a different blood enzyme and changed to another substance (angiotensin II). Angiotensin II acts directly on the adrenal cortex to release aldosterone. The hormone then stimulates the kidneys to increase blood volume.

ANDROGENS AND PHYSICAL ACTIVITY. Androgens produce masculine sexual characteristics. Primarily two hormones produce these effects, testosterone and androstenedione, and they are responsible for the hair distribution characteristics of the sexes and for the complete development of accessory sex organs. These hormones are secreted mainly by the testes in the male, the ovaries in the female, and to a small extent, by the adrenal gland. In adult men, the secretion of testosterone is 50 to 100 times more than that in the adult female, whereas the secretion of androstenedione in the male is about one half of the secretion in the female.[38] Because testosterone is about five times more powerful than androstenedione, and because it is much more prevalent in the male than in the female, its effects are most evident in the male.

There are several effects of testosterone on body structure and performance. Lean body mass, or muscle size, is enhanced by testosterone, which causes muscle tissue to increase amino acid uptake. The chemical building blocks for protein in the muscle are provided by this increase. Increased muscle mass results in increased force and power. Consequently, males often excel females in athletic performances and in certain occupations that require strength and power for success. In addition to increasing muscle size, testosterone also affects bone size. The hormone effects a thickening of bones by producing a larger protein matrix and by retaining more calcium in the bones. Larger bone size offers more areas on the skeleton for muscle growth.

Athletic performance increases when synthetic anabolic steroids, which have the same chemical properties as testosterone, are consumed. The effects are obvious in strength and power events if a high protein diet is also taken. These effects are presented in more detail in Chapter 1.

Stimulation for the secretion of the masculinizing sex hormones, or androgens, is provided by the anterior pituitary gland, which releases two hormones [follicle-stimulating hormone (FSH) and luteinizing hormone (LH)] into the blood. The blood then carries these hormones to the testes or ovaries. The control of pituitary hormones is provided by the hypothalamus and its hormone-releasing factors. The primary sensory input that controls these releasing factors is not known, but, regardless of the triggering event, the secretion of releasing factors for FSH and LH probably proceed at a normal rate during adult life.

CATECHOLAMINES AND PHYSICAL ACTIVITY. The catecholamines, epinephrine and norepinephrine (also called adrenalin and noradrenalin, respectively), are hormones secreted by the nerve endings of the sympathetic nervous system. These nerve endings are located on the heart, the blood vessels, and the adrenal medulla. The nerve endings on the heart and blood vessels secrete approximately 20% epinephrine and 80% norepinephrine. The reverse is true for nerve endings on the adrenal medulla.

Catecholamines primarily affect the metabolism of fats and carbohydrates and the cardiovascular function.

Adipose tissue is broken down into free fatty acids by the catecholamines circulating in the blood. The greater availability of fatty acids in the blood provides an additional source of energy for the cells, thus sparing blood glucose. At the same time, the catecholamines activate the breakdown of glycogen in the liver so that more glucose can be released into the blood and to the working muscles. A similar effect occurs in skeletal muscle when epinephrine and, perhaps, norepinephrine, hasten the breakdown of glycogen into glucose for readily available energy.[8]

The response of the heart and blood vessels during exercise is modified by the blood-circulating catecholamines, but the greatest effect on these tissues, in terms of activity, is provided by the norepinephrine secreted by the nerve endings of the autonomic nervous system that are located on the heart and blood vessels. Catecholamines increase heart rate, increase force of contraction, and produce vasoconstriction of the blood vessels. The increased blood pressure that results speeds the flow of blood to the working muscles.

As exercise increases in intensity, catecholamines in the blood also increase. But, as a consequence of long-term training, the body can absorb more oxygen. Therefore, performing the same absolute work after training as was performed before training results in reduced levels of plasma norepinephrine. Training may reduce sympathetic stimulation during exercise.[8,39]

The initiation for increased catecholamine secretion is provided by a variety of stimuli, such as physical pain and stress and even emotional stress. The emotional excitement experienced just before athletic competition stimulates catecholamine activity and prepares the body for work. The exact stimulus for increased catecholamine secretion during exercise is not known, but it is not believed to be glucose. It has been suggested that, during exercise, the central nervous system activates motor units to skeletal muscle and sympathetic fibers simultaneously so that they both function together.[40]

GROWTH HORMONE AND PHYSICAL ACTIVITY. This hormone is secreted by the pituitary gland and controls normal growth and metabolism. The releasing factor for growth hormone comes from the hypothalamus, which is apparently stimulated by a decrease in plasma glucose. Growth hormone (1) increases the breakdown of adipose tissue and, thereby, releases more fatty acid into the blood, (2) increases blood glucose, and (3) increases protein synthesis in muscle. When blood glucose is low, growth hormone enters the blood from the pituitary gland and produces effects that elevate glucose. With the breakdown of adipose tissue to fatty acids and the corresponding increase of blood fatty acids, more energy potential is provided to the cells. This fatty acid moves into the cell, where it is converted to energy and used by the cell. At the same time, growth hormone inhibits the entry of glucose from the blood into cells by having an effect on the membrane mechanism for glucose entry. As a result, blood glucose levels rise without seriously affecting the energy requirements of the cells.

Growth hormone also regulates protein synthesis. It does this by primarily increasing the transport of amino acids, the building blocks of protein synthesis, across cell membranes. Although exercise affects the levels of growth hormone, it is not clear as to how these effects relate to level of performance or training effects.

Exercise affects growth hormone during the time of work but does not do so in accordance with work intensity. The highest growth hormone values are reached during moderate work; the lowest values during exhaustive work. But, as a consequence of training during moderate work to exhaustion, growth hormone is maintained at a higher level until exhaustion is approached.[41] Apparently, training supplies more fatty acids as an energy source during work, thus sparing glucose and increasing work endurance.

THYROXINE AND PHYSICAL ACTIVITY. The thyroid gland, located in the neck, secretes a hormone called thyroxine, which has an effect on many functions in the body. The release of this hormone is brought about by the stimulation of the hypothalamus which, in turn, stimulates a pituitary hormone. This pituitary hormone stimulates the production and secretion of thyroxine from the thyroid gland. The ultimate control of secretion depends on the concentration of thyroxine in the blood circulating through the hypothalamus and pituitary gland. If the concentration is high, the pituitary secretes little thyroxine; if concentration is low, secretion increases.

Although thyroxine affects a variety of enzymatic activities in the body and probably plays an important part in some physiologic and biochemical responses to exercise, the exact mechanisms involved and the effect of exercise on thyroxine activity are not known. Some indications of the importance of thyroxine in work and of the relationships between exercise and this hormone have been shown by several studies. Exercise enhances the utilization, or turnover rate, of thyroxine.[42] Apparently, exercise stimulates the thyroid gland to secrete more thyroxine. However, this effect seems to occur only as a consequence of exercise because there is no evidence that athletes are ordinarily hyperthyroid.

During the search for the implications of thyroxine in exercise, several researchers have surmised that the hormone is needed for the normal release of fatty acids during exercise. They base this conclusion partly on the fact that free fatty acids released from adipose tissue are decreased in dogs whose thyroid gland does not function during exercise.[43]

Some relationships have been discovered between thyroxine and training effects on cardiac function. Both training[44] and thyroxine administration[45] produce hypertrophy of the heart. Other studies have shown that thyroxine has a controlling influence on cardiac contractions[46] and that it enhances cardiac tension[47] and the rate of tension development.[48] Whether thyroxine clearly mediates these responses is not known.

INSULIN AND PHYSICAL ACTIVITY. Insulin is a protein hormone secreted by the pancreas gland, located just below the stomach. The control of secretion is provided primarily by the concentration of blood glucose passing through the pancreas. A high concentration stimulates secretion, and a low concentration inhibits secretion. Other types of input information to the pancreas influence secretion, such as the plasma concentration of certain amino acids and certain digestive hormones, but much of the control comes from plasma glucose.

The most important function of insulin is the facilitation of the entry of blood glucose into certain cells, especially muscle and adipose tissue cells. When glucose concentration increases in the cells, all the chemical reactions in which glucose participates are enhanced, such as glucose oxidation, fat synthesis, and glycogen synthesis. Protein synthesis also occurs, but in a different way. Insulin stimulates the membrane transport of amino acids, particularly into muscle cells where more protein is formed. But, when insulin secretion is excessive, blood glucose depletes to such an extent that the main source of fuel for brain metabolism and for the central nervous system becomes inadequate and poses a potential danger to life. A large drop in blood insulin, which inhibits glucose uptake by the cells, increases plasma glucose. Much of the glucose is then lost to the urine.

Of course, if insulin is not present in the blood in adequate amounts, not enough glucose enters the cells. As a result, glycogen, protein, and fat break down more rapidly. The breakdown of fats into free fatty acids and their release into the blood increase the availability of fat as an energy source for all cells. The increased quantities of fat in the blood facilitate cellular uptake and the utilization of fat for fuel. But, when fat is primarily used for energy, the increased quantities of oxygen needed for oxidation and energy formation, compared with the quantities needed when glucose is used as a fuel, diminish performance in work of long duration.

Insulin is an important regulatory hormone for glucose metabolism in exercise. During exercise, the demand for glucose by the muscles is met by a corresponding increase in glucose released by the liver. Although large amounts of glucose are taken from the blood by the cells and equally large quantities are released by the liver, the plasma glucose concentration in the blood that travels to the muscles does not change markedly. The presence of insulin in the blood helps to regulate the transfer of glucose across cell membranes. In fact, if a minimal amount of insulin is not present during strenuous exercise, glucose cannot be utilized in adequate amounts to meet the metabolic needs of the working muscles.[49]

Combined Hormonal Activity During Exercise

During exercise, and even before, the endocrine glands are stimulated in varying degrees as a response to physical activity. The extent of the response depends on the strenuousness of the work. All the specific actions of the hormones during exercise are not known. As a result, a total and clear picture of their composite effects is difficult to present; some obvious gaps between theory and fact will appear. Nevertheless, hormonal responses to exercise or work will be presented in this chapter.

Before proceeding, one must understand that many other organ systems, in addition to hormones, are involved in controlling and regulating responses to work stress. These other systems interact with hormonal influences to accomplish physical activity. In fact, some research has shown that hormones play a minor role in the control of physiologic functions in exercise when compared with the roles of other systems;[50] other research indicates that hormonal control is significant.[28,32]

Even before exercise begins there is an anticipation of stress, especially if the activity involves athletic competition. The hormonal response to such a situation is initiated in the higher brain center, from which thought signals are conveyed to the hypothalamic-pituitary system and eventually to the adrenal cortex, where cortisol is released. At the same time, the sympathetic nervous system is stimulated to release primarily epinephrine from the adrenal medulla and norepinephrine at the blood vessels, heart, and adipose tissue. The combination increases blood glucose and the production of glucose in the liver; decreases protein synthesis in the working muscles; and increases sweat gland activity, heart rate, force of the heart beat, and blood pressure.

When actual exercise begins, the secretion of cortisol continues if the work is strenuous, and the catecholamines are released in larger amounts. This process results in still more blood glucose owing to the greater production of glucose in the liver and to the breakdown of glycogen to glucose also in the liver. Because of the increased amount of epinephrine in the blood that flows through the working skeletal muscles, the blood vessels vasodilate. At the same time, the secretion of norepinephrine at the nerve endings on the blood vessels causes constriction of the vessels in organs and tissues not directly involved in the work. The vasodilation in the working muscles caused by epinephrine, the oxygen need in the muscle which stimulates vasodilation, and the vasoconstrictive effect of norepinephrine at other body sites maximize blood flow to working muscles. The catecholamines also increase heart rate and force of contraction. The combination of vasoconstriction and heart activity increases blood pressure.

After some adaptation to the work stress takes place, cortisol secretion probably drops. Epinephrine and norepinephrine continue to be secreted and to exert their influence on the cardiovascular system. If work is at a relatively high level, blood glucose may drop. If so, the pituitary gland is stimulated to release growth hormone, which acts on adipose tissue by mobilizing free fatty acids. These acids can then be used for energy by the cells. When exercise lasts for a prolonged time, at least over 2 min., the combination of cortisol, epinephrine, and growth hormone stimulates an increase in the rate of fatty acid mobilization. More of the total energy is then provided by fat and less is provided by glucose as a result. As a result, some of the glycogen stores can be saved until needed later.

ENERGY COST OF WORK

A large portion of energy in foods becomes heat before it can be transferred to the functional systems of the body. About 25% of all food energy is finally used by the systems, but much of this energy also becomes heat after it is used. Because of the strong relationship between energy production and heat, the quantity of energy released from the different foods, or expended by the body functions, is expressed by a unit of heat. This unit is the small calorie (with a small "c"), and reflects the quantity of heat required to raise the temperature of 1 g. of water 1°C. In practice, the large calorie (spelled with a capital "C") is used and is equivalent to 1,000 calories. Because essentially all the energy expended by the body is derived from the reaction of oxygen with foods, the amount of oxygen used to perform a specific work is a measure of both energy cost and heat produced from that work. The energy used for work, or the sum of the chemical reactions in the body, is expressed in terms of rate of oxygen consumption or, more commonly, as metabolic rate.

Measurement of Energy Cost

As was just mentioned, the metabolic rate can be calculated with a high degree of accuracy from the rate of oxygen utilization. A metabolic rate measured in this way is called indirect calorimetry. Direct calorimetry measures actual energy output by the body heat produced. During direct calorimetry, the heat of an individual's metabolic processes is measured in a special, enclosed chamber where all the heat in the air and walls of the chamber is used to calculate the total energy output. This method is seldom used in exercise physiology because the equipment and chamber are expensive and difficult to use.

There are two methods of indirect calorimetry: the closed-circuit and the open-circuit methods. The closed-circuit method requires the individual to breathe into a face mask. The face mask connects to an oxygen chamber from which inspired air is taken and to which expired air is released. Before the expired air reaches the oxygen chamber, it passes through a canister containing soda lime. The soda lime chemically combines with the carbon dioxide, thereby removing it from the air. As the oxygen is used by the body, it gradually depletes in the chamber. The amount of oxygen in the chamber is continually recorded over a known time interval so that rate of oxygen utilization can be determined.

Although this method is relatively simple, it may be in error by as much as 10%. In addition, the amount of carbon dioxide produced is not obtained and, therefore, the foodstuff that is used for energy cannot be determined. The relationship between carbon dioxide and oxygen in the determination of the kinds of foodstuff used for energy (respiratory quotient) will be discussed further.

A more accurate method of calorimetry is the open-circuit method during which the atmospheric air is inspired directly and then expired into a container in which the air is collected. The time during which gas collects is carefully monitored. Samples of the expired air are taken from the container to determine the percentage of oxygen and carbon dioxide gases present in a known volume of air. By knowing the concentration of O_2 and CO_2 in the atmosphere, which are constant at 20.93 and 0.03% respectively, and the percentage concentrations of O_2 and CO_2 in the expired air, one can calculate the amount of energy expended. The O_2 consumed is obtained by subtracting the volume of O_2 remaining in the expired air from the volume of O_2 in the inspired air for the same volume of air. The volume of CO_2 produced can be computed in the same way. When both the CO_2 produced and the O_2 consumed are known, the foodstuffs used for the energy supply can be ascertained by the respiratory quotient (R.Q.).

Respiratory Quotient

The amount of energy liberated from food depends on the food's content of carbohydrates, fats, and proteins. Each gram of the three foods releases a different amount of energy, as measured by heat, when oxidized. Carbohydrate releases 4.1 calories per gram; fat, 9.3 calories; and protein, 4.35 calories. But, these values are obtained by different amounts of oxygen. More oxygen is needed to completely oxidize 1 g. of fat or protein than is needed to oxidize 1 g. of carbohydrate. Stated another way, for each liter of oxygen metabolized with glucose, 5.01 calories of energy are released; for each liter metabolized with fat, 4.70 calories are released; and for each liter metabolized with protein, 4.60 calories are released. This fact should be kept in mind when heavy work or exercise is performed and when the heart and respiratory systems are greatly taxed to supply oxygen to the muscles. In such conditions, the greatest yield in energy comes from carbohydrates. Thus, carbohydrate is considered the "energy food."

To determine which foodstuff is supplying energy, the ratio between oxygen consumed by the body and carbon dioxide produced is used. This ratio can be determined because the number of oxygen molecules used for the oxidative process varies in a known way according to the foodstuff oxidized. For example, when one molecule of glucose is oxidized, the number of liberated molecules of carbon dioxide equals the number of oxidative molecules required for the oxidative process. Therefore, the ratio of carbon dioxide output to oxygen usage is 1.00 when glucose is oxidized. The formula is:

$$R.Q. = \frac{\text{Vol. } CO_2 \text{ produced}}{\text{Vol. } O_2 \text{ consumed}} = 1.00$$

The ratio of carbon dioxide output to oxygen usage falls to about 0.71 for fat and 0.80 for protein.

Consequently, if one achieves a steady state while running, and the metabolic rate is such that the oxygen consumed is equal to the carbon dioxide produced, the R.Q. of 1.00 indicates that carbohydrate is providing the energy. An R.Q. between 0.70 and 1.00 indicates that a mixture of fat and carbohydrate is being burned. Because protein plays a small part in energy metabolism under normal circumstances, it is considered a negligible factor in the interpretation of an R.Q. value.

Work and Exercise in the Energy Balance of the Body

The breakdown of organic molecules provides the source of energy, in the form of ATP, for the performance of work. In animal cells, most of the energy is expended as heat, and only a small amount is used for work. Energy used for work is evident in the movement of external objects, such as the lifting of a barbell by the skeletal muscles. Energy also does work within the body to permit the proper functioning of internal organs.

The term used to indicate total energy expenditure, as expressed per unit time, is metabolic rate. When metabolic rate equals the amount of energy consumed by the body in food, no change in body weight occurs. But, if there is an imbalance between food intake and energy expended, the body either gains or loses weight, depending on the direction of the balance. Most often in modern society, energy intake exceeds output, and the balance is stored as fat. The factors that determine metabolic rate also determine body weight because they affect energy expended.

Factors that Determine Metabolic Rate

During rest, most energy is expended by such internal organs as the heart, liver, kidneys, and brain. The amount of this energy used depends on physical size, age, and sex. In a growing child, the resting metabolic rate, relative to size, is rather large because a large amount of energy is used for the formation of new tissue, such as muscle and bone. The reverse is true during advanced age when the metabolic rate is smallest. The resting metabolic rate is usually less for a female than for a male, even when body weight is considered. However, the female's metabolic rate increases considerably during pregnancy and lactation.

Such factors affecting metabolic rate are small when one compares the effects on metabolic rate of muscular activity owing to work or exercise. During heavy exercise, metabolic rates more than double. This increase indicates the significance of exercise in "burning up" excess calories. Nevertheless, the amount of food intake is the dominant factor in controlling energy balance or body weight, especially in modern society which uses less than half of its energy input for external work.

Control of Food Intake

The physical structures primarily concerned with food intake are specific groups of nerve cells in the hypothalamus. The hypothalamus is located in the brain stem, the unconscious portion of the central nervous system. When various areas of these nerve clusters are stimulated, they effect either the sensation of hunger or satiety. These hypothalamic centers involved in the control of food intake act only as integrating centers that process afferent input and control efferent output. They function dependently, responding to the body's need for food.

The exact nature of the sensory receptors that inform the hypothalamus that the body needs more energy, and that thereby increase appetite, is not known. Some early theories have been greatly weakened. One hypothesis suggested that hunger was associated with contractions of an empty stomach and that distending the stomach could lessen hunger. Consequently, afferent pathways from the stomach and other areas of the gastrointestinal tract were believed to send signals to the hypothalamus, thus initiating the desire to seek food. However, experiments have shown that complete denervation of the upper gastrointestinal tract, which prevents afferent nerves from sending signals to the hypothalamus, does not interfere with a normal maintenance of energy balance. Apparently, other afferent pathways to the hypothalamus control appetite over a long period, even though gastrointestinal signals may play a modifying role in regulation.

Several theories have been postulated about the mechanisms responsible for regulating energy balance by affecting appetite via the hypothalamus. One theory is based on the belief that glucose receptors on the hypothalamus are stimulated by the concentration of blood glucose. After eating, when blood glucose is high, the sensory receptors in the hypothalamus signal satiety and inhibit eating. The reverse response occurs after a period of fast. Another theory holds that a substance released from fat deposits has a controlling effect on hunger. Large amounts of adipose tissue would release proportionately large quantitites of this substance to inhibit appetite whereas small amounts of fat would release lesser amounts to stimulate hunger. This substance would reach the hypothalamus via the blood to either inhibit or stimulate the appetite. A third theory suggests that the rise in body temperature induced by eating is the signal that inhibits appetite. This theory has received some support because people in colder climates eat more than those in warmer climates. None of these mechanisms is considered as the sole regulator, but all are involved to some degree.

Some psychologic and sociologic factors also regulate food intake. It is probably safe to say that obese individuals are more affected by these factors than are normal individuals. Complex emotional factors are associated with the desire for food. These factors are not biologically motivated, but may have some effect on the hypothalamus. Often, these same factors dispose an obese individual to docility and limit the physical expenditure of energy. The total effect further shifts the energy balance toward food intake.

In summary, the factors that influence the hypothalamus centers in controlling food intake are:

1. Plasma glucose
2. Total body adipose tissue
3. Body temperature
4. Extent of gastrointestinal distention
5. Psychologic and social elements

Considering the complexity of the control mechanisms that regulate appetite, it is amazing how energy balance remains relatively constant over a long time period. This constancy is shown by the effects of only a slight imbalance of food intake over a period of years. If only one piece of bread a day is eaten above a maintenance caloric level, about 44 lb. of additional body weight will accumulate in 5 years.

Work Intensity and Food Intake. Even though energy balance is influenced by the energy needs of the body's tissues, there is not a direct relationship between the extent of physical activity and caloric intake. This finding was shown by Mayer, who studied the calorie intakes and body weights of large numbers of workers who labored at different levels of physical activity in the same factory.[51] The results of this study are shown in Figure 2–2. Individuals who had the most sedentary jobs consumed almost as many calories as those with jobs demanding heavy work and more than those with jobs demanding light, medium, or heavy work. The corresponding body weights for each work level indicate that the individuals with sedentary jobs were obese whereas all the other workers had similar body weights. These results suggest that physical inactivity may increase appetite. At the other levels of activity, there was a more direct relationship between work output and caloric intake. These relationships were generally supported by a study using rats as subjects.[51] The sedentary rats ate more than the rats that exercised for almost 2 hr. Rats that exercised from 2 to 5 hr. or more had greater food intake than did the sedentary rats.

Physical Activity in Controlling Energy Balance

When the amount of energy consumed in food is greater than the amount expended, overweight or obesity occurs. The notion that all obese individuals eat more than individuals of normal weight is a misconception. This statement is not necessarily true, even though the obese eat more than they "burn up" in calories. The caloric intake and physical activity of two groups of high school girls, one obese group and one normal-weight group, were compared.[51] The study showed that, generally, the obese girls ate less and participated less in physical activities than did the normal girls. Another study demonstrated that obese children are generally less active than nonobese children when participating in tennis, volleyball, or swimming.[51] Similar results were found when adult males and females, who were either obese or nonobese, were compared.[52] Obese individuals, on the average, were much less active than nonobese individuals in their daily lives.

Thus, some obesity is largely caused by inactivity rather than by overeating. The ex-

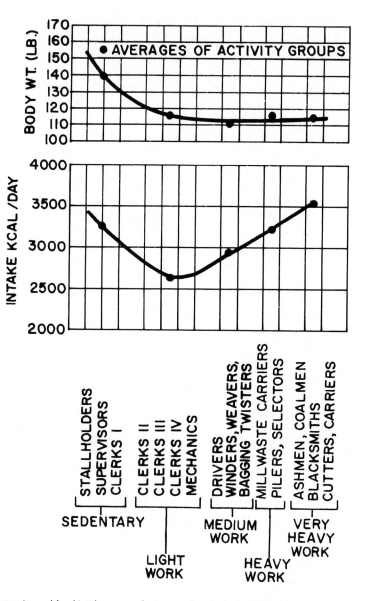

Fig. 2–2. Work intensity and food intake among factory workers in India. (From Mayer, J., Roy, P., and Mitra, K.P.: Am. J. Clin. Nutr., 4:169, 1956.)

tent to which obesity results from inactivity is not clear and certainly varies from person to person. Nevertheless, physical activity may contribute substantially to controlling energy balance.

NUTRITION AND EXERCISE

An inadequate intake of carbohydrates results in early fatigue because energy avail-able for work cannot meet bodily needs. When too much food energy is consumed, the excess is stored as fat. In both condi-tions, physical performance is adversely affected and health is impaired.

Nutritional needs other than energy must be met. Some of the results of an inadequate diet often are not visible to the eye but, in time, are reflected in a decrement of physical performance. This decrement occurs because food is required not only to provide energy, but also to build new tissue and to chemically regulate metabolic functions.

Even when food intake is balanced to meet all the bodily needs, the level of physical activity affects the use of various nutrients. Strenuous exercise creates certain metabolic needs that are different from the needs found during rest. In addition to the acute metabolic effects of exercise, long-term training produces certain changes in tissue structure and in substances used for energy that are beneficial for improving physical performance.

Nutrients in Food

The nutrients in food are classified six ways: water, minerals, vitamins, proteins, fats, and carbohydrates.

WATER. An adequate supply of water is essential for all energy production in the body, for temperature control in rest and exercise, for the transportation of nutrients to the cells, and for the elimination of the by-products of cell metabolism. The importance of adequate water intake during exercise and under extreme environmental temperatures is presented in Chapter 5.

MINERALS. These nutrients are classified into two groups: those needed by the body in large amounts and those required in small amounts. The first group includes sodium, potassium, calcium, phosphorus, magnesium, sulfur, and various chlorides. Some of these will be discussed because they relate to physical work capacity.

Sodium, potassium, and chlorine are present in the body as electrically charged particles called ions. They function together to control and regulate the rate of fluid exchange within the body. In this function they regulate the flow of nutrients into the cells and of waste products out of the cells. During work or exercise, they maintain a proper balance of fluids so that the body can cool by evaporation of sweat and the cells can simultaneously maintain homeostasis. In addition

to achieving fluid balance, these electrolytes are essential for keeping the proper electrical gradients around nerve and muscle membranes. In this way, they make possible depolarization and repolarization, events that occur in the transmission of impulses along nervous and muscular membranes and in the return of these membranes to a polarized state.

Calcium, phosphorus, and magnesium are minerals bound to protein molecules as structural parts in bone. Calcium represents about 40% of the total mineral content in the body. It combines with phosphorus to form bones and teeth. Calcium is also essential for blood clotting, for the transport of fluids across cell membranes, and for muscular contractions. In addition to its role in the formation of bones and teeth, phosphorus is an essential component in the high-energy compounds, ATP and CP.

The second minerals group, required in small amounts, is called trace minerals. Some of these minerals and their roles are: fluorine, essential for healthy dental and bone formation; iodine, a necessary ingredient for the hormone, thyroxin; zinc, needed for normal growth, tissue repair, blood cell formation, and reproductive function; and iron, involved in energy metabolism of all cells because of its concentration in the red pigment of muscles and blood.

Because iron is highly important for endurance and physical performance and because an inadequate amount of iron results in a nutritional deficiency common in this country, it should be given special attention. Male adults who have reached full body stature use only about 10% of the ingested iron, whereas menstruating females absorb about twice that amount. Approximately 85% of the daily absorbed amount is used to produce new hemoglobin, which is a protein substance in blood that creates the red color and carries oxygen. The rest of the absorbed iron either is used for growth or is stored.

During the adolescent years, more iron is needed for the rapid growth of bone and muscle tissue. During this period, more than

85% of male growth and 60% of female growth is in lean body tissues. However, menstruation in females increases their iron needs to about the same as those of males. Adolescent girls are more likely than boys to be iron deficient, although both of their iron needs are similar. Because the overall dietary needs of boys are greater than those of girls the larger food intake by boys is more likely to result in adequate iron consumption.

VITAMINS. Vitamins are organic substances that regulate chemical reactions. Vitamins are necessary for growth and the maintenance of life. Although they are involved in these functions, vitamins do not contribute significantly to body structure, nor do they supply a direct source of energy for body function. As a result, the vitamin needs of an athlete are usually no greater than those of a nonathlete. An athlete, therefore, need not consume more than the quantities of vitamins recommended for a normal diet. In fact, athletes usually eat more food and, therefore, are more likely to consume the vitamins necessary to meet their needs. The B vitamin, thiamine, is an exception because it is required by the body in proportion to the amount of carbohydrates eaten. Because athletes usually ingest large amounts of carbohydrates, they usually need more thiamine.

The next three classes of nutrients—fats, carbohydrates, and proteins—are sources of energy for the body, but have other functions as well.

FATS. In addition to being stored as future energy, fat provides an insulation to extremes in temperature and protects some organs from physical shocks. Fat is stored in the form of triglyceride. Fatty acids are also attached to phosphoric acid (phospholipids), carbohydrates (glycolipids), and proteins (lipoproteins). When combined with cholesterol (another fatty substance), fats are involved in the formation of the membrane structures of all cells. The structural units of the different kinds of fats are fatty acids.

CARBOHYDRATES. Sugars and starches, called carbohydrates, come from plants. The primary basic structural unit of carbohydrates is the simple sugar, glucose. Sugars in such foods as honey, fruits, and milk are all absorbed by the gastrointestinal tract and consequently changed to glucose by the liver. Much of the glucose formed in the liver is passed into the blood, which transports it to body tissues, primarily the brain and muscles. A smaller amount is converted to glycogen and is stored in the muscles and liver. Other tissues in constant need of glucose are the heart, kidneys, and brain. Any slight reduction of plasma glucose to the brain results in dizziness, general feeling of weakness, and hunger.

The amount of glucose in the blood diminishes gradually unless some form of carbohydrate food is ingested periodically during the day. When physical activity is at a high level because of work or athletic training, plasma glucose depletes more rapidly. Consequently, individuals who want to maintain a high level of performance must eat snacks between meals to maintain blood glucose levels. Carbohydrates should provide over 50% of an athlete's total caloric intake.[53]

PROTEINS. The basic structural units of protein are amino acids. There are 23 amino acids that are combined in different ways for a particular kind of animal or plant protein. Proteins are structural parts of cells, hormones, enzymes, and molecules of muscle. Their concentration varies in different tissues. For example, muscle has 20% protein, tendons have 33% protein, and nerve tissue has 10% protein.

The variety of proteins needed by the various body cells requires a source of amino acids. Most amino acids can be manufactured within the cells that use them by the action of cellular enzymes. For this to occur, sugars or fats are utilized in the enzymatic pathways within the cells. Although most amino acids can be formed in this manner, eight cannot be synthesized in the body, but are needed to synthesize other human proteins. These eight amino acids are classified as essential amino acids.

The only common foods that have all the essential amino acids are soybeans and meat. However, when cereals and beans, which both lack a different essential amino acid, are combined, they provide an adequate supply of protein that contains all the essential substances.

Although many athletes consume large quantities of animal protein, their protein needs can be met more cheaply and just as adequately by eating a varied diet of vegetables, grains, and fruits. In fact, some outstanding athletes exist on a vegetarian diet. However, an adequate supply of protein is difficult to ensure on a vegetarian diet unless special care is taken to consume adequate amounts. When just a relatively small amount of animal protein is added to a largely vegetarian diet, the additional amino acids from meat increase the protein efficiency of the vegetable proteins. In fact, the same effect is achieved by adding eggs, cheese, or other dairy products to a strictly vegetarian diet.

Many athletes consume more protein than their bodies can use. Some of the excess is either stored as fat or changed to glucose. Because amino acids cannot be stored by the body, much of the excess is converted to urea and is excreted by the kidney. Athletic activity may not require a significant increase in the need for protein, even though energy expenditure is high. Most of the energy is supplied by fats and carbohydrates and little, if any, by protein. Any increased need for protein can be met by eating more food containing all the nutritional essentials. In this way, more than adequate amounts of protein are available.

Nutrition and Exercise

Because the amounts and kinds of food an individual eats determine body size, endurance, and strength, one must follow a proper diet, especially if success in athletics is a goal. Two requirements must be met in order to be well nourished. These require-

ments relate to the kinds of foods eaten and the energy content, or calories, of the foods. Both must be balanced to optimize performance and to maintain health.

Daily Caloric Requirements for Athletes. The recommended daily dietary allowances, established by the National Academy of Sciences, for moderate activity of various age groups are presented in Table 2–5. The average weights and heights for males and females are also shown. These averages are based on moderate activity; therefore, greater activity requires more calories. The amount of calories needed daily to maintain body weight with moderate activity can be estimated more precisely with the information in Table 2–6. To estimate the number of calories needed each day, multiply body weight by the number of calories the average male or female expends each day per pound of body weight (Table 2–7). For example, a 160-lb., 20-year-old, male athlete must consume 3,040 calories (160 lb. × 19 cal. = 3,040 cal.) to maintain body weight. If daily work exceeds a moderate level, more calories are needed to prevent loss of body weight. The relationship between level of activity and caloric cost is shown in Table 2–6. When activity is increased by strenuous exercise, such as cross-country running,

Table 2–5.

Calorie Requirements for Males and Females in Moderate Activity

	Age (Years)	Weight (Pounds)	Height (Inches)	Calories*
Males	10–12	77	55	2500
	12–14	95	59	2700
	14–18	130	67	3000
	18–22	147	69	2800
Females	10–12	77	56	2250
	12–14	97	61	2300
	14–16	114	62	2400
	16–18	119	63	2300
	18–22	128	64	2000

*Recommended daily dietary allowances established by the National Academy of Sciences.

Table 2–6.

Estimated Energy Cost of Selected Exercises and Sports

Sport or Exercise	Total Calories Expended per Minutes of Activity
Climbing	10.7–13.2
Cycling 5.5 mph	4.5
9.4 mph	7.0
13.1 mph	11.1
Dancing	3.3–7.7
Football	8.9
Golf	5.0
Gymnastics	
Balancing	2.5
Abdominal exercises	3.0
Trunk bending	3.5
Arms swinging, hopping	6.5
Rowing 51 str./min.	4.1
87 str./min.	7.0
97 str./min.	11.2
Running	
Short-distance	13.3–16.6
Cross-country	10.6
Tennis	7.1
Skating (fast)	11.5
Skiing, moderate speed	10.8–15.9
Up-hill, maximum speed	18.6
Squash	10.2
Swimming	
Breaststroke	11.0
Backstroke	11.5
Crawl (55 yd./min.)	14.0
Wrestling	14.2

Table 2–7.

Calories Expended Per Pound Each Day for Males and Females

Age (years)	Calories Per Pound Per Day*	
	Males	Females
10–12	32	29
12–14	24	23
14–18	23	21
18–22	19	19

*Values based on data in Table 2–3.

approximately 320 calories are burned up in 30 min. In about 11 days, approximately 1 lb. of fat will be lost if food intake remains unchanged during that time. Obviously, a heavier individual must eat more calories than a smaller person to maintain body weight. A large football athlete weighing 240 lb. may require 4,560 calories a day (240 lb. × 19 cal. = 4,560 cal.) to prevent weight loss. Both the 160-lb. athlete and the 240-lb. athlete have basically the same bodily requirements for vitamins and minerals. However, the absolute amounts of carbohydrate, protein, and fat consumed are greater for the larger athlete. When these foods are expressed relative to total calories consumed, there is not much difference between the two athletes. Both require a similar percentage of carbohydrate and protein. Athletes should not obtain more than 30 to 35% of their calories from fats.[44]

Sugar Supplements in Performance. Most athletes have a sufficient supply of stored energy to meet the physical demands of the sport. The glycogen stored in the liver (29%) and muscle (66%), and the glucose in the body fluid (5%), can supply up to about 1,500 calories. Because the most strenuous exercise performed for up to 60 min. requires about 900 to 1,000 calories, a limitation in a performance of such a duration is not caused by energy depletion. Running relatively short races, from 100 meters up to 10,000 meters or more, may not be made easier by eating sugar or honey just before the race, even though the energy used may be replaced more readily. But, during strenuous work, when activity is continued beyond 60 min., such as marathon running, the stores of energy may be depleted. In these events, glucose taken during the race partially replenishes the energy stores and may permit better performance. Marathon runners and cross-country skiers usually consume sugar solutions during a race. The sugar should be consumed with water in moderately small quantities throughout the race. Large quantities of sugar consumed at each feeding may cause nausea during the race.

The exact amount of glucose that should be consumed during a race is not known.

Some athletes take a 10% glucose solution whereas others may consume a 40% solution. But, whatever the amount, the athlete should become accustomed to the solution before the competition. In addition to possible nausea, too much glucose inhibits the stomach from emptying water. Excess fluid in the stomach may be uncomfortable and could hinder performance.

Pre-Event Meal

The pre-event meal should be eaten at least 2.5 hr. before the competition to permit sufficient time for digestion. Otherwise, the digestive system's need for blood may compete with the muscle's need during exercise. A light meal consisting of foods that will not upset the athlete during the emotionally exciting period just before the competition is recommended. If the contest involves prolonged and continuous activity, such as a marathon run, saturating the muscles with glucose by supercompensation, as previously discussed, may be most appropriate. But, in any sport event, the meal eaten prior to the contest should be readily digestible. A meal consisting mostly of carbohydrate digests faster than a meal of fat or protein. Also, glycogen becomes depleted in the muscle and liver during exhaustive activities, and a high carbohydrate diet could further increase the energy stores. Carbohydrate can be made available for energy in the body with less energy expended in the metabolic process than occurs during the metabolism of protein or fat. Recovery from strenuous exercise is also usually augmented by a high carbohydrate meal, and the energy expended during the exercise is replenished more rapidly.

Meal Frequency

The number of meals eaten in a day seems to influence body weight by an unknown process involving the way foods are distributed and used. Rats that eat fewer meals per day tend to gain more body weight than rats that consume the same number of calories but through more frequent meals. Other responses, in terms of plasma-free fatty acids and liver glycogen, are affected differently by meal frequency, but studies have not found that one meal frequency is superior to another in terms of physical performance. However, more frequent meals, at least three per day, are recommended.

Making Weight

In certain sporting events, athletes must perform in weight classes. It is common practice among athletes to lose body weight so that they can compete in a lower class. The assumption is that when an athlete loses body weight in fat and/or liquid to qualify for a lighter weight class, the same strength and endurance typical of the higher class are still maintained. Consequently, the athlete has the supposed advantage of competing in a lower weight class but with the strength and endurance equal to those of a higher class. This assumption is not necessarily true. When weight loss involves a combination of food restriction, fluid deprivation, and, often, dehydration, the typical result is a reduction in muscular strength and work performance.[56,57] The physiologic bases for these decreases in work capacity are lower cardiac output and, consequently, higher heart rates,[56,57] smaller stroke volumes,[57] lower oxygen consumption,[58] and impaired thermoregulatory processes.[56,59]

When these changes occur in the young athlete, they can inhibit normal growth and development. To prevent these consequences, the following recommendations have been made by the American College of Sports Medicine:[60]

1. The body composition of each athlete should be assessed several weeks before the competitive season.[61-63] Athletes with less than 5% fat content should obtain medical clearance before competing.

2. The daily caloric requirements should be obtained from a balanced diet and should be based on age, body surface area, growth, and physical activity level. If an athlete consumes less than the minimal caloric requirements, which range from 1,200 to 2,400

calories for high school and college athletes, prior medical approval of this diet should be required.

3. The use of fluid deprivation and dehydration of athletes to lose weight should be discouraged. The use of rubber suits, steam rooms, saunas, laxatives, and diuretics to lose weight are especially prohibited.

ENERGY FROM MUSCLE FIBERS

Endurance training produces in skeletal muscle cells certain biochemical changes that increase their capacity to do work. But, the extent of these changes depends on the kind of training undertaken by the different kinds of skeletal muscle. When exercise is continuous and prolonged, one kind of muscle fiber shows more biochemical changes than does another kind. If exercise is performed in short spurts of near-maximum contractions, interspersed with short rest periods, a different fiber type is affected.

Red and White Muscle Fibers

There are three kinds of muscle fibers: two kinds of red fibers and one kind of white fiber. The concentration of a red-colored protein, myoglobin, in the fibers accounts for the differences in color. Myoglobin is similar to the protein, hemoglobin, which gives blood a red appearance. The characteristic properties of red and white muscle, as shown in Table 2–8, indicate differences

in work performance and in response to physical training. The two types of red fibers and their properties are presented in the table; however, they actually differ in the extent to which they possess these properties. There are slow-twitch and fast-twitch red fibers. The fast-twitch red fibers possess characteristics that result in less respiratory capacity than do the slow-twitch red fibers; however, the fast-twitch red fibers produce more respiratory capacity than do the fast-twitch white fibers. The laboratory technique used to analyze muscle tissue taken by biopsy from endurance-trained muscle does not clearly differentiate among the three kinds of fibers. However, this same technique does allow a more accurate distinction between the white, fast-twitch (FT) fibers and the other fibers, most of which are red, slow-twitch (ST) fibers. Consequently, in the following research studies relating fiber type to performance, the fibers are classified as FT and ST.

Nearly equal quantities of myosin appear in the different fibers, but the myosin ATPase activity (an enzyme that initiates contraction by splitting ATP for energy at the actomyosin cross-bridges) is much higher in the white fibers, which probably accounts for the white fibers' faster release of energy and shorter contraction time. White fibers have larger concentrations of glycolytic enzymes (enzymes that change

Table 2–8.
Properties of Red and White Muscles

	Red Fibers	White Fibers
Contraction time, msec.	75	25
Nerve activity to muscle	Continuous low frequency	Intermittent high frequency
Primary source of ATP	Oxidative phosphorylation	Glycolysis
Glycogen	Low	High
Myosin ATPase activity	Low	High
Capillary blood flow	High	Low
Fatigue	Difficult to fatigue	Easily fatigued
Nerve fiber diameter	Small	Large
Nerve conduction velocity	Low	High
Myoglobin content	High	Low

glycogen into glucose for energy). This characteristic results in a more rapid breakdown of glycogen to glucose and a quicker release of energy from the ATP thus formed. The metabolism of white fibers is primarily glycolytic, which means that most of the ATP energy for contraction is derived from the glucose in the cytoplasm of the cell. But, because the breakdown is so rapid, the glycogen stores are quickly reduced and lactic acid is formed. This process results in the formation of relatively small amounts of ATP. In fact, of the total amount of ATP produced in a cell, only about 5% occurs from glycolytic activity, whereas 95% occurs from oxidative phosphorylation (the process whereby ATP is formed from a combination of oxygen, inorganic phosphate, and ADP) in the mitochondria of the cells. As previously indicated, the sequence of chemical reactions through the end of the glycolytic stage comprises the anaerobic phase of metabolism during which oxygen is not needed for the formation of ATP energy. If sufficient oxygen is present in the cell, the end chemical product of the glycolytic phase, pyruvic acid, can be further changed by enzyme activity in the mitochondria to produce more ATP. This second state is the process of oxidative phosphorylation and is the aerobic phase of metabolism.

The white fibers are easily fatigued because of their increased concentration of lactic acid created by the large breakdown of glycogen and glucose and because they are surrounded by only a few capillaries, thereby limiting the flow of glucose from the blood into the cells to replenish the glycogen stores.

The breakdown of glucose in red fibers is not as rapid as in white fibers, partly owing to the red fiber's slower muscle contractions. The capillaries are more plentiful around the red fibers, thus supplying more glucose and oxygen. In addition, red fibers have more mitochondria and obtain most of their ATP from oxidative phosphorylation. Red muscle is different from white because a large quantity of its total energy is derived

from fatty acids. In fact, in prolonged aerobic work of 1 hr. or more, about 50 to 60% of the energy is supplied by fats.[64]

The white muscle's capacity for oxidative metabolism is approximately one-fifth that of red muscle.[65] Even after prolonged and strenuous training, which causes the capacity for aerobic metabolism to increase twofold, white muscle still has the same proportional capacity for oxidative metabolism—one-fifth that of red fibers.

The different nerve fibers in contact with red and white muscle may account for these biochemical distinctions. Nerve fibers to red muscle have a small diameter and a low conduction velocity, whereas the nerve fibers to white muscles have a larger diameter and a higher conduction velocity. In addition, when nerves are monitored in the body, those that reach the red muscle are almost always active, continually discharging at a low frequency. Nerves to white muscles are mostly relaxed. If the nerve to a fast muscle fiber is transplanted to a slow fiber and a nerve from a slow fiber is transplanted to a fast fiber, the slow fiber speeds up and the fast fiber slows down. Therefore, either the nerve fiber itself or its frequency of simulation causes the biochemical differences between red and white fibers.

Response of ST and FT Muscle to Exercise

Differences between fiber types, largely in velocity of contraction and in capacity to form ATP from glycolytic metabolism and from oxidative phosphorylation, also cause differences in training response. In activities requiring short bursts of energy, such as sprint running, FT fibers are more involved; but, in continuous and prolonged work, such as distance running, the ST fibers are most affected. This relationship was shown by a study in which subjects first exercised continuously until they reached exhaustion in 2 to 3 hr.; later, these subjects exercised at heavy loads 5 to 6 times for 50 to 60 sec. The 50- to 60-sec. blocks of working time were interspersed by rest periods of 10 min.[66] Prolonged exercise first depleted the glycogen stores of the ST fibers and then the glycogen stores of the FT fibers. At complete exhaustion, all the ST fibers and practically all the FT fibers were depleted. But when the muscle was examined after the heavy work bouts of 50 to 60 sec., the FT fibers had utilized their glycogen sources much more rapidly than had the ST fibers.

These results indicate that muscle fibers are selectively recruited. The ST fibers are activated at lower work rates and the FT fibers during intensive work.[27] The FT fibers are also activated after the ST fibers are depleted of their glycogen during prolonged endurance work.[66]

Exercise Capacity and Fiber Type

As just indicated, training with submaximal loads and with long, continued movement has a greater effect on ST fibers than on FT fibers in effecting biochemical adaptations. Likewise, heavy loads and/or rapid muscular activity places more stress on the FT fibers than on the ST fibers to adapt. To improve the ability to run long distances, the ST fibers must be exercised more because their biochemical activity largely limits performance in endurance events. By the same token, a sprinter needs to optimize the biochemical activity in FT fibers to reach a higher performance level. However, some sports require both a high glycolytic and a high endurance capacity, such as middle-distance running. At this distance, the FT fibers need to be stressed to increase their glycolytic capacity, and the ST fibers must be stressed to improve their oxidative capacity. Many middle-distance track athletes have learned from experience that both over-distance and under-distance training are important for improving performance. Over-distance running develops primarily the endurance capacity of ST fibers so that a faster steady pace of running is possible. Under-distance running develops the explosive capacity of FT fibers, which is necessary near the end of a race when the runner sprints to the tape.

The composition of muscle fibers among untrained individuals is approximately 40% ST and 60% FT. However this ratio can vary greatly. Champion athletes in endurance events have a majority of ST fibers whereas weight lifters have about 50% of each.[27] Although large variations occur between individuals, similar fiber compositions are found in the shoulders and the legs of the same individual.

Some differences in the proportion of ST fibers in the legs were shown among four track runners.[67] The percentage of ST fibers increased according to the distance run. The sprinter had 26%, the two middle-distance runners (mile) had 52% and 62%, and the long distance runner (10,000 m.) had 75%. There was also a corresponding relationship between maximum oxygen uptake by these athletes and the percentage of ST muscle. The sprinter had the lowest $\dot{V}O_2$ max with 56 ml./kg./min., the middle-distance runners had 72 and 75 ml./kg./min., and the long-distance runner had 79 ml./kg./min. When oxygen consumption is expressed per unit body weight (kg.), comparisons can be made between individuals of different body weights.

Other studies have shown similar relationships between the proportion of ST fibers and physical performance in athletes. Whereas a previous study has shown that track athletes in different events, such as sprinters and long-distance runners, have varying proportions of ST fibers in the gastrocnemius,[26] a later study reported that there are also differences between world-class distance runners and average-trained, middle-distance runners.[68] And, both of these running groups differ from untrained subjects. On the average, the elite distance runners had 79% ST fibers, the middle-distance runners had 61.8%, and the untrained runners had 57.7%. Thus, the outstanding runners had a greater percentage of ST fibers. In addition, these fibers were, on the average, 29% larger than the FT fibers. No differences were observed between the two fiber types in the middle-distance runners and in untrained men.

Although the relative proportions of ST and FT fibers in various atheletes may differ, it is difficult to determine how much of these differences are caused by genetic factors and exercise training. One reason for this difficulty is that the fiber types in a muscle are so intermingled that they cannot be easily separated and studied biochemically. Another difficulty in studying the effects of exercise on fiber types is the large difference among individuals in the proportion of red and white fibers in the same muscle. It is not known exactly how much of the proportions of red and white fibers are caused by genetic factors or exercise training. However, the evidence leans toward the genetic answer based on research findings. Men who exercised for 1 hr./day, 4 days/week, for 5 months showed no difference in relative proportions of red and white fibers in a thigh muscle, even though both fiber types increased in size.[67] This discovery held true for both young children (11 to 13 yr.) and men.

LOCAL MUSCULAR ENDURANCE

When small muscle groups, such as the arms, are worked to exhaustion, the limiting factors in performance are primarily within the muscle cells themselves rather than in the heart-circulatory-respiratory systems. When a load is lifted repeatedly to exhaustion by flexing the arms, the pain is localized to the biceps, and the stress on the heart and the general blood transporting system is minimal.

Lactic Acid in Limiting Endurance

The specific factor primarily responsible for limiting activity is not known, but the increase in muscle lactate appears to play an important role. Lactate continues to increase in the muscle as work progresses even though the oxygenated blood bathing the cells and the glycogen stores may be plentiful.[69] The consequent decrease in pH (higher acidity) may slow down the biochemical reactions that lead to the production of energy (ATP). Because lactate accumulates even when the oxygen supply seems adequate, some researchers attribute its production not to hypoxic (lack of oxygen) stimulation of anaerobic glycolysis but to an imbalance between glycolysis and the rate of pyruvate utilization.[16]

Glycogen Depletion in Limiting Endurance

The intensity of the contraction largely determines the amount of oxygen flowing into the muscle. When the contractions are about 60% or more of the maximum force capacity of the muscle, blood flow is completely cut off. When the force of contraction is 15 to 20% of a maximum force, oxygen flow is continuous, although somewhat diminished. Light loads, such as 5% maximum force, may permit continuous activity until the energy sources are depleted, which takes at least 50 to 60 min.[15,27] In this kind of long-term work, the limiting factor in performance is primarily glycogen depletion, not lactic acid accumulation.

Muscle Endurance and Cardiovascular Endurance

Endurance activities involving local and small muscle groups often require the muscles to contract with a force that indicates the enlistment of mostly white fibers. This is evident by the relatively short time before contraction reaches a fatigue state because white fibers quickly use energy (ATP), and lactic acid increases accordingly. In such sports as wrestling and boxing muscle activity occurs in short bursts of quick movements, and fatigue occurs rapidly. The implication may be that working primarily white fibers may not be effective for increasing the efficiency of the heart and total circulatory system because work cannot continue for a sufficient time period. But, if different muscle groups are activated simultaneously so that several smaller muscles contract together, or if these muscles contract at varying times but sequentially, the greater involvement of total muscle mass places more stress on the heart and circulatory system over a long time period. Consequently, there is a training effect on the larger oxygen-supplying systems of the body. The circulatory-respiratory system may be continuously stimulated for periods of 10 min. or more by work involving primarily white fibers in local muscle groups when exercise is alternated from one group to another. Weight-training exercises involving loads of 40% of maximum, lifted for 10 repetitions with several seconds of rest between sets, resulted in heart rates in 10 young male adults that rose steadily to 165 after 10 min.[70,71] When the same heart rates were duplicated on a bicycle ergometer by the same 10 young male adults, the recovery period was significantly longer after the weight-training exercises. In fact, after 15 min. of recovery, heart rate was 7% higher after the weight-training exercises than after the bicycle work. This suggests that working primarily white fibers (primarily anaerobically) by weight training has a greater effect on energy sources than does working ST fibers (primarily aerobically) on the bicycle ergometer when work continues for approximately 10 min. Apparently, the increase in anaerobic metabolism as a result of a greater involvement of white fibers during work stressing local muscular endurance produces a larger oxygen debt than does work performed primarily aerobically, even though the heart rates for both conditions are similar.

Training by alternating the local muscle groups (often referred to as circuit training) may be just as effective as training requiring work of the same muscle mass for improving the efficiency of the heart and vascular system and of the respiratory system. However, circuit training is most likely to improve the anaerobic capacity of the muscles, whereas long-distance running improves the aerobic capacity of the muscles.

Absolute and Relative Endurance

The ability of a muscle group to contract over a long period of time depends on the blood flow to the muscle and on the amount of oxygen extracted from the blood by the cells. If the muscle is occluded so that oxygenated blood does not reach the cells, the ability to endure depends on the availability of ATP and CP, on the glycolysis of glucose, and on the extent of lactate accumulation. When a muscle improves in endurance, it maintains the same contraction force as before training, but does so for a longer time. The same load can be raised and lowered more times. When endurance is measured with the same load before and after training, the quality measured is absolute endurance. This quality is improved by the larger quantities of stored ATP, CP, and glycogen in the muscles after training[72] and/or by the greater force capacity of the muscle, if this is a training effect.

An increase in force capacity or strength permits a muscle to apply the same force as applied before training, but with less muscle mass. In fact, fewer motor units are activated and a smaller proportion of the total energy capacity of the muscle is required. Consequently, weight training, or any other form of heavy overload training, improves absolute endurance by increasing strength.[73-75]

Ordinarily, overload training to improve strength also produces histologic and chemical changes within muscle tissue. These changes increase endurance. The increase in myoglobin and in the number of mitochondria in the muscle cells enhances endurance,[76-78] as do the increased energy stores of ATP, CP, and glycogen. In addition, there is a general increase in biochemical activity within the mitochondria, the energy storehouses.

Although endurance training unquestionably improves absolute endurance, no evidence shows that relative endurance is improved. Most studies have shown no improvement;[73,79,80] however, one has shown an increase in endurance with loads of 20, 30, and 35% of maximum.[48] Relative endurance is measured by how long a given proportion of maximum strength can be maintained or by the number of times it can be raised and lowered. For example, if an individual's maximum force is 100 lb. before training and 140 lb. after training, but he performs 30 repetitions with 50% of maximum strength before and after training, relative endurance has not improved. In the first test, the load of 50% was 50 lb.; but, after training, the second test was with a load of 70 lb.

The importance of muscle force and enduring work depends on the size of the work load. When the load is relatively heavy, strength largely determines endurance (Fig. 1–30).[81] But, when the load is relatively light and high repetitions of 50 or more are possible, maximum strength is less important as a factor determining endurance. With light loads, when 100 or more repetitions can be done, strength may be a negligible factor in determining or predicting work endurance.

PRINCIPLES FOR TRAINING

1. To optimize athletic performance, one should eat foods that are balanced in terms of calories and nutrients. Athletes consuming the least calories must be especially careful to maintain a balanced diet because their nutritional needs, which are essentially the same for the heavy athlete, are a little more difficult to achieve when caloric intake is less.

2. The pre-event meal should be eaten at least 2.5 hr. before athletic competition so that the food can be completely digested. In this way, blood needed for exercise is not diverted to digestion. A meal consisting of mostly carbohydrates is suggested because they digest faster than fats or proteins.

3. Sugar supplements during exercise of about 60 min. or less do not improve performance because the calories needed are in sufficient supply at the beginning of activity, assuming that the skeletal muscles have their full complement of stored glycogen at that time. However, in exercise lasting over 60 min., the energy stores at the beginning of exercise may be insufficient to meet all energy needs. In this case, liquid solutions containing from 10 to 40% glucose may be taken during exercise. Athletes should be aware that too much glucose can cause the stomach to retain water, thereby contributing to dehydration.

4. To ensure normal growth and development of the young athlete who participates in wrestling or in sport whose competition is according to body weight classes, certain precautions should be taken:

A. Percent body fat should not be less than 5%. If it is, medical clearance should be obtained before competing.

B. Before dieting to lose weight, the athlete should obtain medical approval of the diet.

C. Fluid deprivation and dehydration to lose weight should be discouraged. The use of rubber suits, steam rooms, saunas, laxatives, and diuretics to lose weight should be prohibited.

5. Athletic events that require a large involvement of both ST and FT fibers for success should involve training activities that stress the muscles for about 1 to 4 min. in maximum work.

6. To increase muscle endurance for long-distance racing, the stress of training should be placed primarily on the ST fibers to increase their oxidative capacity. The training that best accomplishes this is activities involving moderate muscle contractions that are continuous and repeated for at least 5 to 10 min.

7. To increase the ability of muscle to endure and repeatedly contract at high levels of force, the FT fibers must be primarily stressed in training to enhance their glycolytic capacity. Activities that require high forces in muscle contractions are best for increasing endurance of the FT fibers.

8. In intermittent work, such as playing soccer or football, performance is optimum when the glycogen stored in the muscles is in plentiful supply. A relatively high carbohydrate diet and sufficient rest between practice time and the game guarantee an adequate supply of glycogen.

9. Muscular endurance for sports involving intermittent contractions ranging from maximum to submaximum, such as in

wrestling and water polo, is achieved by alternating the stress on FT and ST fibers. One approach applies the work stress in a manner similar to that encountered during competition. Training should focus on all-out runs or swims that are interspersed by moderate work. The time intervals for each should be similar to those encountered in competition.

10. The ability to exercise continuously for a long period of time or to work explosively for short periods is related to the proportion of ST and FT fibers in the working muscles. Individuals with a high proportion of ST fibers (70% or higher) have the greatest potential for success in distance events. Those with 40% or less seem to have an advantage in sprint running.

11. Muscular endurance for sports involving prolonged and repetitive movements with submaximum contractions, such as swimming or long-distance running, is improved by repeatedly lifting loads that provide a stress similar to that provided during competition. The stress should be applied for as long as or longer than the time required during competition.

12. In athletic races of more than 60 min., such as the marathon run, during which the limitation in performance is largely caused by glycogen depletion in the working muscles, running times can be improved by increasing the glycogen stores above normal before the race. When depleting muscle glycogen by diet and work for three days and then increasing carbohydrate intake for the next three days, stored glycogen may increase by 100% or more. However, even when small amounts of carbohydrates are taken, at least 60 g. daily are needed to maintain the adequate function of some important systems of the body, such as the nervous system and red blood cells.

REFERENCES

1. Hultman, E.: Studies on muscle metabolism of glycogen and active phosphate in man with special reference to exercise and diet. Scand. J. Clin. Lab. Invest. [Suppl.], *19:*94, 1969.

2. Karlsson, J.: Lactate and phosphagen concentrations in working muscles of man. Acta Physiol. Scand. [Suppl.], *82:*358, 1971.

3. Rowell, L.B.: Cardiovascular limitations to work capacity. *In* Physiology of Work Capacity and Fatigue. Edited by E. Simonson. Springfield, Charles C Thomas, 1971.

4. Gollnick, P.D., et al.: Glycogen depletion patterns in human skeletal muscle fibers during prolonged work. Pfluegers Arch., *344:*1, 1973.

5. Barnard, R.J., and Peter, J.B.: Effect of exercise on skeletal muscle: III. Cytochrome changes. J. Appl. Physiol., *31:*904, 1971.

6. Pattengale, P.K., and Holloszy, J.O.: Augmentation of skeletal muscle myoglobin by a program of treadmill running. Am. J. Physiol., *213:*783, 1967.

7. Gollnick, P.D., and Hermansen, L.: Biochemical adaptations to exercise: anaerobic metabolism. *In* Exercise and Sport Sciences Reviews. Edited by J. H. Wilmore. New York, Academic Press, 1973.

8. Hemmingsen, E.A.: Enhancement of O_2 transport by myoglobin. Comp. Biochem. Physiol., *10:*239, 1963.

9. Gollnick, P.D., Ianuzzo, C.D., and King, D.W.: Ultrastructural and enzyme changes in muscles with exercise. *In* Muscle Metabolism During Exercise. Edited by B. Pernow and B. Saltin. New York, Plenum Press, 1971.

10. Gollnick, P.D., et al.: Effect of training on enzyme activity and fiber composition of human skeletal muscle. J. Appl. Physiol., *33:*421, 1972.

11. Saltin, B., et al.: Effect of physical conditioning on oxygen uptake, heart rate, and blood lactate concentration by submaximal and maximal exercise in middle-aged and old men. Scand. J. Clin. Lab. Invest., *23:*323, 1969.

12. Barnard, R.J., Edgerton, V.R., and Peter, J.B.: Effect of exercise on skeletal muscle: I. Biochemical and histological properties. J. Appl. Physiol., *28:*762, 1970.

13. Saltin, B.: Metabolic fundamentals in exercise. Med. Sci. Sports, *5:*137, 1973.

14. Hartley, L.H., et al.: Multiple hormonal responses to graded exercise in relation to physical conditioning. J. Appl. Physiol., *33:*602, 1972.

15. Issekutz, B., Jr., et al.: Aerobic work capacity and plasma FFA turnover. J. Appl. Physiol., *20:*293, 1965.

16. Paul, P., Issekutz, B., Jr., and Miller, H.I.: Interrelationship of free fatty acids and glucose metabolism in the dog. Am. J. Physiol., *211:*1313, 1966.

17. Holloszy, J.O.: Biochemical adaptations to exercise: aerobic metabolism. *In* Exercise and Sport Sciences Reviews. Edited by J. H. Wilmore. New York, Academic Press, 1973.

18. Molé, P.A., Oscar, L.B., and Holloszy, J.O.: Increase in levels of palmityl Co A synthetase, carnitine palmityl-transferase, and palmityl Co A dehydrogenase and in the capacity to oxidize fatty acids. J. Clin. Invest., *50:*2323, 1971.

19. Morgan, T.E., et al.: Effect of long-term exercise on human muscle mitochondria. *In* Muscle Metabolism During Exercise. Edited by B. Pernow and B. Saltin. New York, Plenum Press, 1971.

20. Elsner, R.W., and Carlson, L.D.: Post exercise hyperemia in trained and untrained subjects. J. Appl. Physiol., *17:*436, 1962.
21. Varnauskas, E., et al.: Effects of physical training on exercise blood flow and enzymatic activity in skeletal muscle. Cardiovasc. Res., *4:*418, 1970.
22. Ekblom, R., et al.: Effect of training on circulatory response to exercise. J. Appl. Physiol., *24:*518, 1968.
23. Hermansen, L., Hultman, E., and Saltin, B.: Muscle glycogen during prolonged severe exercise. Acta Physiol. Scand., *71:*129, 1967.
24. Jöbsis, F.F., and Stainsby, W.N.: Oxidation of NADH during contractions of circulated mammalian skeletal muscle. Respir. Physiol., *4:*292, 1968.
25. Bergstom, J., et al.: Diet, muscle glycogen and physical performance. Acta Physiol. Scand., *71:*140, 1970.
26. Saltin, B., and Hermansen, L.: Glycogen stores and prolonged severe exercise. *In* Nutrition and Physical Activity. Edited by G. Blix. Upsala, Almquist and Wiksell, 1967.
27. Saltin, B., and Karlsson, J.: Muscle glycogen utilization during work of different intensities. *In* Muscle Metabolism During Exercise. Edited by B. Pernow and B. Saltin. New York, Plenum Press, 1971.
28. Bunyatyan, A., and Erez, V.: Effect of physical exertion on transcortin binding of corticosteroids in the plasma. Probl. Endocrinol., *18:*13, 1972.
29. Davies, C., and Few, J.: Adrenocortical activity in exercise. J. Physiol., *213:*35P, 1971.
30. Korenskaya, E.: Fatigue in physical exercise and the adrenal cortex function. Probl. Endocrinol., *13:*65, 1967.
31. Rose, L., et al.: Plasma cortisol changes following a mile run in conditioned subjects. J. Clin. Endocrinol. Metab., *31:*339, 1970.
32. Buuck, R., and Tharp, G.: Effect of chronic exercise on adrenocortical function and structure in the rat. J. Appl. Physiol., *31:*880, 1971.
33. Selye, H.: The Sress of Life. New York, McGraw-Hill, 1956.
34. Foss, M., Barnard, R., and Tipton, C.: Free 11-hydroxycorticosteroid levels in working dogs as affected by exercise training. Endocrinology, *89:*96, 1971.
34a.Dieter, M.: Glucose metabolism in the rat lymphatic tissues: Effects of actue and chronic exercise. Life Sci., *81:*459, 1969.
35. Henderson, D.J., and Berger, R,A.: Aerobic capacity and adrenocortical response to work and cold water stressors. Proc. Natl. College Phys. Educ. Assoc., 1974.
36. White, J., Ismail, A., and Bottoms, G.: Changes in serum corticosteroids resulting from conditioning. Med. Sci. Sports, *4:*60, 1972.
37. Frenkl, R.: Pituitary-adrenal response to various stressors in trained and untrained organisms. Acta Physiol., *39:*41, 1971.
38. Baulieu, E., and Robel, P.: Catabolism of testosterone and androstenedione. *In* The Androgens of the Testis. Edited by K. B. Eib-Nes. New York, Marcel Dekker, Inc., 1970.
39. Hartley, L.H.: Growth hormone and catecholamine response to exercise in relation to physical training. Med. Sci. Sports, *7:*34, 1975.
40. Hartley, L.H., et al.: Multiple hormonal responses to prolonged exercise in relation to physical training. J. Appl. Physiol., *33:*607, 1972.
41. Jones, L.G., et al.: The effects of muscular leg exercise on neuroendocrine levels. *In* Proc. Army Sci. Conf., II:195, 1970.
42. Irvine, C.H.G.: Effect of exercise on thyroxine degradation in athletes and non-athletes. J. Clin. Endocrinol., *28:*942, 1968.
43. Paul, P.: Uptake and oxidation of substrates in the intact animal during exercise. *In* Muscle Metabolism During Exercise. Edited by B. Pernow and B. Saltin. New York, Plenum Press, 1971.
44. Tipton, C.M., Terjung, R.L., and Barnard, R.J.: Response of thyroidectomized rats to training. Am. J. Physiol., *215:*1137, 1968.
45. Beznak, M.: Cardiovascular effects of thyroxine treatment in normal rats. Can. J. Biochem. and Physiol., *40:*1647, 1962.
46. Taylor, R.R., Covell, J.W., and Ross, J.: Influence of the thyroid state on left ventricular tension-velocity relations in the intact, sedated dog. J. Clin. Invest., *48:*775, 1969.
47. Crews, J., and Aldinger, E.E.: Effect of chronic exercise on myocardial function. Am. Heart J., *74:*536, 1967.
48. Penpargkul, S., and Scheuer, J.: The effect of physical training upon the mechanical and metabolic performance of the rat heart. J. Clin. Invest., *49:*1859, 1970.
49. Vranic, M., Kawamori, R., and Wrenshall, G.A.: The role of insulin and glucagon in regulating glucose turnover in dogs during exercise. Med. Sci. Sports, *7:*27, 1975.
50. Gollnick, P.D., et al.: Exercise-induced glycogenolysis and lipolysis in the rat: hormonal influence. Am. J. Physiol., *219:*729, 1970.
51. Mayer, J.: Overweight and weight control. Englewood Cliffs, Prentice-Hall, Inc., 1968.
52. Chirico, A., and Unkard, A.: Physical activity and human obesity. N. Engl. J. Med., *263:*935, 1960.
53. Smith, N.J.: Food for Sport. Palo Alto, Bull Publishing Co., 1976.
54. Oscai, L.B., and Holloszy, J.O.: Effects of weight changes produced by exercise, food restriction, or overeating on body composition. J. Clin. Invest., *48:*2124, 1969.
55. Bosco, J.S., Terjung, R.L., and Greenleaf, J.E.: Effect of progressive hypohydration on maximal isometric muscular strength. J. Sports Med. Phys. Fitness, *8:*81, 1968.
56. Robinson, S.: The effect of dehydration on performance. *In* Foot Injuries. Washington, National Academy of Sciences, 1970.
57. Saltin, B.: Circulatory response to submaximal and maximal exercise after thermal dehydration. J. Appl. Physiol., *19:*1125, 1964.
58. Taylor, H.L., et al.: Performance capacity and effects of caloric restriction with hard physical work on young men. J. Appl. Physiol., *10:*421, 1957.
59. Bock, W.E., Fox, E.L., and Bowers, R.: The effect of acute dehydration upon cardiorespiratory endurance. J. Sports Med. Phys. Fitness, *7:*62, 1967.
60. Position stand on weight loss in wrestlers. Med. Sci. Sports, *8:*xi, 1976.
61. Clarke, K.S.: Predicting certified weight of young

wrestlers: a field study of the Tcheng-Tipton method. Med. Sci. Sports, *6:*52, 1974.

62. Sinning, W.E.: Body composition assessment of college wrestlers. Med. Sci. Sports, *6:*139, 1974.

63. Tcheng, T.K., and Tipton, C.M.: Iowa wrestling study: anthropometric measurements and the prediction of a "minimal" body weight for high school wrestlers. Med. Sci. Sports, *5:*1, 1973.

64. Christensen, E.H., and Hansen, O.: Arbeitsfähigkeit und ehrnährung. Skandinav. F. Physiol., *81:*160, 1939.

65. Baldwin, K.M., et al.: Respiratory capacity of white, red, and intermediate muscle: adaptive response to exercise. Am. J. Physiol.,*222:*373, 1972.

66. Gollnick, P.D., et al.: Glycogen depletion patterns in human skeletal muscle fibers after exhausting exercise. J. Appl. Physiol., *34:*615, 1973.

67. Gollnick, P.D., et al.: Effect of training on enzyme activity and fiber composition of human skeletal muscle. J. Appl. Physiol., *34:*107, 1973.

68. Costill, D.L., Fink, W.J., and Pollock, M.L.: Muscle fiber composition and enzyme activities of elite distance runners. Med. Sci. Sports, *8:*96, 1976.

69. Havel, R.L., et al.: Turnover rate and oxidation of different free fatty acids in man during exercise. J. Appl. Physiol., *19:*613, 1964.

70. Rodgers, K., and Berger, R.A.: Heart rate response to prolonged and continuous work involving primarily fast twitch fibers. Unpublished study, Biokinetics Laboratory, Temple University, 1972.

71. Berger, R.A.: Comparison between primarily aerobic and anaerobic work at the same heart rate on recovery heart rate. Unpublished study, Biokinetics Research Laboratory, Temple University, 1975.

72. Karlsson, J., Diamant, B., and Saltin, B.: Muscle metabolites during submaximal and maximal exercise in man. Scand. J. Clin. Lab. Invest., *26:*385, 1971.

73. Berger, R.A.: Effect of varied weight training programs on strength. Res. Q., *33:*168, 1962.

74. Shaver, L.G.: Effects of training on relative muscular endurance in ipsilateral and contralateral arms. Med. Sci. Sports, *2:*165, 1970.

75. Stull, G.A., and Clarke, D.H.: High resistance, low repetition training as a determiner of strength and fatiguability. Res. Q., *41:*189, 1970.

76. Lawrie, R.A.: Effect of enforced exercise on myoglobin concentration in muscle. Nature, *171:*1069, 1953.

77. Lawrie, R.A.: The activity of the cytochrome system in muscle and its regulation to myoglobin. Biochem. J., *55:*298, 1953.

78. Paul, M.H., and Sperling, E.: Cyclophorase system XXIII. Correlation of cyclophorase activity and mitochondrial density in striated muscles. Proc. Soc. Exp. Biol. Med., *79:*352, 1952.

79. Berger, R.A.: Force and relative endurance. Unpublished study. Biokinetics Research Laboratory, Temple University, 1976.

80. Clarke, D.H., and Stull, G.A.: Endurance training as a determinant of strength and fatiguability. Res. Q., *41:*19, 1970.

81. Berger, R.A.: Muscle force in endurance. Unpublished study. Biokinetics Research Laboratory, Temple University, 1968.

CHAPTER **3** # Control of Muscular Activity

The human body is continually bombarded with input information from both the outside world and the internal milieu. Information from the outside is provided to the central nervous system by light, sound, temperature, and touch, and the responses to these take various forms. Sometimes a response is involuntary, as occurs when the hand touches a hot flame and pulls away without prior deliberation. Or, the stimulus may come from pressure on the bottom of the feet to activate sensory receptors, which initiate the chain of events leading to a quick, involuntary response by skeletal muscle. Moves of an involuntary nature are called reflex responses. At other times, an individual is aware of the stimuli before a response is made. In these situations, one deliberates over the stimuli and responds in a specific way. Thus, the control of muscular activity in these instances is voluntary.

Stimuli from within the body elicit responses that are not usually brought to consciousness. Hormonal balances are regulated at an unconscious level and fluctuate with emotional state and level of physical activity. Internal organs are usually activated without voluntary assistance from the conscious mind even though their responses may be initiated by external stimuli and brought to the level of consciousness. In practically all responses to stimuli, whether internal or external, the central nervous system acts as purveyor of messages, often back and forth because the response itself provides additional input information that modifies later responses. The basic unit of the nervous system that conveys signals throughout the body is the nerve cell or neuron.

THE NEURON

The neuron is both the structural and functional unit of the nervous system and is highly specialized to generate and conduct electrical impulses. It contains all the life-sustaining cytoplasmic components usually found in other cells but, in addition, has a special kind of covering or membrane for its unique electrical functions. The major parts of a neuron are shown in Figure 3–1. Impulses travel in a neuron from the dendrites to the soma and then along the axon to the small fibrils extending from its end. Generally, dendrites are not more than a few millimeters from the soma or cell body; however, dendrites in parts of the brain stem may extend farther. Somas vary greatly in diameter, from .03 mm. in some cells of the brain to .07 mm. in motor neurons. Axons in neurons show the greatest differences in length, ranging from several micrometers to several feet in some motor and sensory fibers.

Neurons can be divided into three classes according to their function: (1) afferent neurons, (2) efferent neurons, and (3) interneurons. Afferent neurons and efferent neurons are usually located outside the skull and vertebral column whereas interneurons lie inside the central nervous system. Afferent neurons carry information from the sensory receptors, such as the skin and muscles, to the brain and/or spinal cord. The

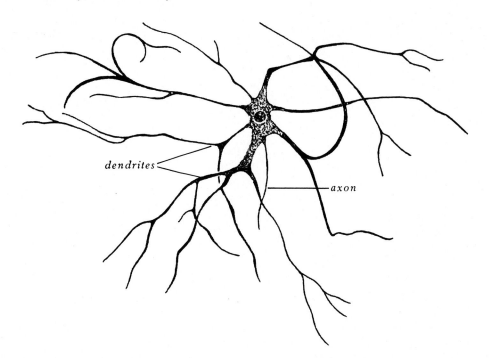

Fig. 3–1.   A motor neuron from the ventral horn of the spinal cord. (From Gray's Anatomy of the Human Body. 29th Edition. Revised and edited by Charles M. Goss. Philadelphia, Lea & Febiger, 1973.)

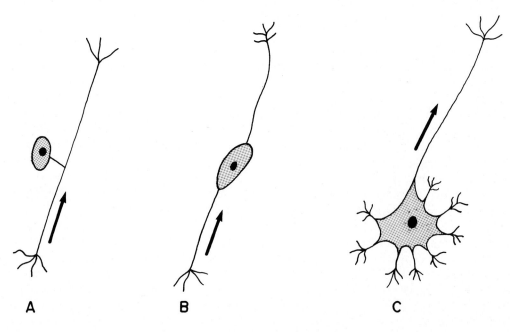

Fig. 3–2.   Types of neurons: *A*, unipolar, *B*, biopolar, and *C*, multipolar.

brain and spinal cord make up the central nervous system. After the information is integrated within the central nervous system, it is transmitted by the efferent neurons to the effector organs, such as muscles or glands. Effector neurons that innervate skeletal muscles are called motor neurons. Interneurons originate and terminate within the central nervous system and make up about 97% of all nerve cells.

There are basically three types of neurons in terms of structural makeup, and they differ in the number of processes leading to the cell body (Fig. 3–2). These neuron types are unipolar (or nonpolar), bipolar, and multipolar. The unipolar neuron is usually a sensory receptor whose dentrite lies in the skin or deep tissue. The dentrite fiber extends to its cell body, which is located directly outside the spinal cord or brain stem. Cell bodies from many other sensory nerves group together to form a ganglion. From here the axon enters the spinal cord or brain stem. The bipolar neuron is also a sensory receptor, but is found only in cranial nerves involved with the special senses of vision, hearing, smelling, and balance. The third type of neuron, the multipolar neuron, has many dentrites and is the most numerous. Multipolar neurons form much of the gray matter of the central nervous system and function as interneurons and motor neurons. A unique feature of multipolar neurons is their ability to integrate (add and subtract) many inputs from other neurons before making the appropriate response. These sophisticated computers number several billion in the central nervous system.

Neurons outside the central nervous system aggregate to form bundles called nerves or nerve trunks. Nerves transmit information between the same areas of the body or carry the same kind of information. Nerve fibers differ in that some are surrounded by a myelinated (liquid or fatty substance) sheath whereas others are not. Figure 3–3 shows a cross section of a typical nerve trunk with several large fibers and more small fibers. The large fibers are myelinated; the small

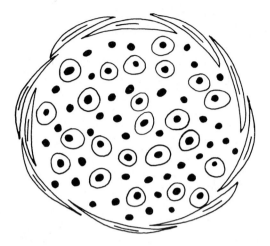

Fig. 3–3.   Cross section of a nerve trunk with myelinated and unmyelinated nerve fibers. (From Guyton, A.C.: Basic Human Physiology: Normal Function and Mechanisms of Disease. Philadelphia, W.B. Saunders Co., 1971.)

fibers are unmyelinated. The average nerve trunk has about twice as many unmyelinated fibers as myelinated fibers. An electrical current or impulse travels along the membrane of the neuron. In the case of myelinated fibers, whose sheath acts as an insulator and covers most of the membrane, impulses travel along gaps in the membrane's sheath (Fig. 3–4). Approximately once every millimeter, the myelin sheath does not completely cover the axon. These

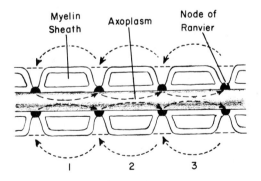

Fig. 3–4.   Saltatory conduction along a myelinated axon. (From Guyton, A.C.: Basic Human Physiology: Normal Function and Mechanisms of Disease. Philadelphia, W.B. Saunders Co., 1971.)

gaps in the sheath are called nodes of Ranvier. Even though ions cannot flow to a large extent through the thick myelin sheaths, they can flow readily from node to node during depolarization. In fact, at the node of Ranvier, the axon membrane is 500 times more permeable than the membranes of most unmyelinated fibers.

This increased permeability allows a more rapid passage and flow of ions along the fiber. The conduction of ions in this manner from node to node is called saltatory conduction. The advantages of saltatory conduction are that higher velocities of nerve transmissions are possible and that less energy is needed because only the nodes depolarize, not the entire axon. The velocity of conduction in nerve fibers varies with the fiber's diameter. In small fibers of 0.3 μ in diameter (1 μ = .001 mm.), the conduction is about 0.5 m./sec., but in larger fibers of 17 μ in diameter, the conduction may be as high as 130 m./sec.

THE SYNAPSE

A synapse is the junction where one neuron electrically excites another neuron. This excitation is either temporarily increased or temporarily decreased. In most neurons, the membrane potential (or polarity) is not changed by one excitatory event at the synapse. For a signal to pass from one neuron to the next, the sum of all synaptic activity to that neuron must be a threshold value or more. Figure 3–5 shows a motor neuron with many fibers from other neurons. None of these fibers is from the same neuron. Excitation occurs when the sum of all the activity at the synapses reaches the threshold level of the neuron.

Figure 3–6 shows the anatomy of a synaptic junction. The neuron conducting a signal toward a synapse via its axon is called the presynaptic neuron. At the fibril end of the axon there is a slight enlargement called the synaptic knob. The neuron conducting impulses away from the synapse is called the postsynaptic neuron. The space separating the two neurons is the synaptic cleft, which prevents the direct propagation of signals from one neuron to the next.

Almost all synapses function in one direction, which is determined by a chemical substance stored only in small vesicles in the synaptic knob. The signals traveling to the synaptic knob depolarize it, thereby releasing the chemical transmitter into the synaptic cleft. The chemical diffuses across and affects the permeability of the postsynaptic cell, which lies directly under the synaptic knob. If the strength of the impulse reaches a

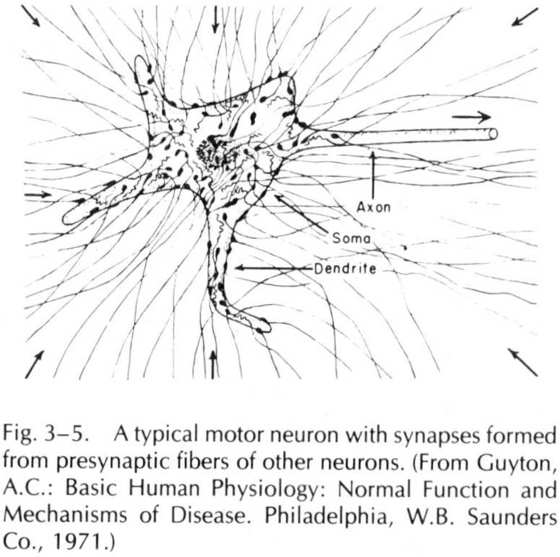

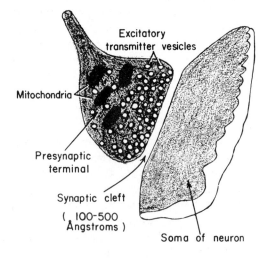

Fig. 3–5. A typical motor neuron with synapses formed from presynaptic fibers of other neurons. (From Guyton, A.C.: Basic Human Physiology: Normal Function and Mechanisms of Disease. Philadelphia, W.B. Saunders Co., 1971.)

Fig. 3–6. A synaptic junction. (From Guyton, A.C.: Basic Human Physiology: Normal Function and Mechanisms of Disease. Philadelphia, W.B. Saunders Co., 1971.)

threshold level, the membrane potential changes in the postsynaptic cell, causing depolarization and transmission of impulses. Signals do not pass between neurons when the chemical transmitter is transformed or leaves the area of the synaptic cleft.

Excitatory Synapse

There are two different types of synapses, and they are classified according to their effects on the postsynaptic cells. These types are either excitatory synapses or inhibitory synapses. When an excitatory synapse is activated, the membrane potential of the postsynaptic cell either reaches or comes close to a threshold value. Even when the stimuli are not great enough to reach threshold, they may nevertheless slightly depolarize the postsynaptic cell and, thus, bring its membrane closer to threshold.

The excitation of a single presynaptic terminal is seldom sufficient to cause excitation of the neuron. Before a postsynaptic cell can be excited, either many presynaptic terminals must be activated simultaneously or one presynaptic terminal must be repeatedly activated. The phenomenon whereby many presynaptic terminals are stimulated to excite another neuron is called spatial summation. When only one presynaptic terminal is continually activated so that an action potential is at threshold value, the phenomenon is called temporal summation. Action potentials are usually a result of both spatial and temporal summation.

Convergence and Divergence

The relationships between the thousands of synapses in the body take different forms. When many different presynaptic cells end on a single postsynaptic cell, the relationship is called convergence (Fig. 3–7A). When the axon of a nerve cell branches out so that all its fibers synapse and excite many other cells, the relationship is called divergence (Fig. 3–7B). All the terminal branches of a single presynaptic cell do not synapse with the same postsynaptic cell; they end on many different cells. In most cases, a single active synapse cannot cause an action potential in the postsynaptic cell by itself. The anatomic arrangement of cells in patterns of convergence and divergence is necessary for integrated neural activity of complex movement. Of course, for signals to pass from neuron to neuron, a single neuron must be postsynaptic to one group of cells and presynaptic to another.

Facilitation

As a consequence of convergence of neural pathways, a postsynaptic neuron either can be excited to the extent that threshold is reached and an action potential is spread throughout the cell or cannot be sufficiently excited to reach threshold. In the latter situation, the membrane of the postsynaptic neuron is slightly depolarized and can reach threshold with a small additional amount of excitation. When the excitatory postsynaptic potential brings the membrane closer to threshold, neural activity has undergone "facilitation." Postsynaptic neurons that have been facilitated can reach threshold with less excitatory input than would have been needed before facilitation. Both temporal summation, during which individual presynaptic fibers fire faster, and spatial summation, during which many of the presynaptic fibers to the same neuron fire together, produce facilitation.

Inhibitory Synapse

For neural integration to occur so that desired movements are achieved, some neurons must be excited and others must be inhibited. Signals are inhibited from moving from one cell to another in two ways: (1) direct postsynaptic effects on the permeability of the cell membrane and (2) presynaptic inhibition, which eventually affects the permeability of the cell membrane at a postsynaptic site. Inhibition that occurs at the postsynapse is brought about by a reduction of membrane permeability. This reduction lessens the likelihood that the cell will be depolarized to cause an action potential.

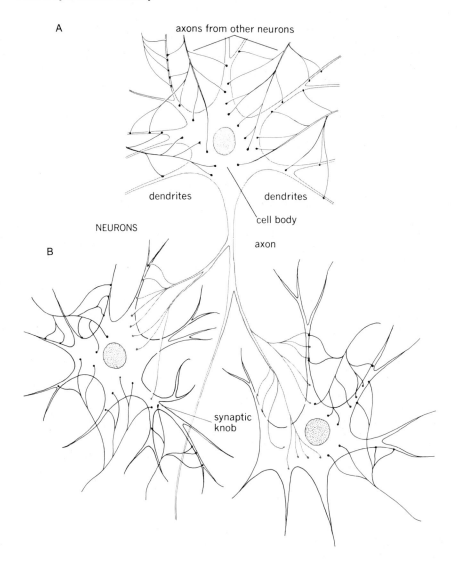

Fig. 3–7. Convergence *(A)* and divergence *(B)* relationships among neurons. (From Vander, A.J., Sherman, J.H.,and Luciano, D.S.: Human Physiology—The Mechanisms of Body Function. New York, McGraw-Hill, Inc., 1975. Used with permission of McGraw-Hill Book Co.)

Changes in cell permeability are brought about by a chemical transmitter that acts on the membrane of the postsynaptic cell. Whereas excitation in a postsynaptic neuron occurs when relatively greater amounts of positively charged sodium ions pass into the cell through the membrane than positive potassium ions pass out of the cell to cause depolarization, the inhibition of a postsynaptic neuron occurs when its membrane becomes permeable only to potassium ions. Consequently, the greater amount of potassium ions passing out of the neuron cell both increases the negativity inside the cell and increases the positivity outside the cell. When this happens, the neuron is less likely to achieve an action potential because its membrane electrical potential is moved farther from the threshold level. As a result, a stronger stimulus is needed to achieve an action potential.

In the other kind of synaptic inhibition,

the site of inhibition is the presynapse. When inhibition occurs at the presynapse, it is called presynaptic inhibition. Although direct activation of an inhibitory synapse is characteristic of postsynaptic inhibition, it is not characteristic of presynaptic inhibition. The site of inhibition is the synaptic knob of an excitatory synapse where the amount of released chemical transmitter is reduced. Consequently, the changes in permeability of the postsynaptic cell are smaller and the threshold level is less likely to be reached. The reduction of chemical transmitter at an excitatory synapse is illustrated in Figure 3–8. In presynaptic inhibition, when the synaptic junction between the presynaptic terminal of one neuron (neuron A) and the synaptic knob of the second neuron (neuron B) is activated, the membrane of the synaptic knob is slightly depolarized. The depolarization is not sufficient to cause an action potential in neuron B, but it does raise membrane permeability so that a smaller action potential will be needed to reach threshold in the synaptic knob. Before proceeding, one must understand the positive relationship between the amount of chemical transmitter secreted at the synapse and the amplitude of action potentials at the synaptic knob. The greater the amplitude of an action potential necessary to reach threshold in the synaptic knob (B), the larger the amount of chemical transmitter released from the knob to the neuron (C). Consequently, when neuron A is activated and produces a slight depolarization in neuron B, the action potential necessary to reach threshold and excite neuron B is less than it would be otherwise. As a result of a smaller action potential in neuron B, less chemical transmitter is released from the synaptic knob (B), and the permeability changes in the postsynaptic cell (neuron C) are smaller. Consequently, the postsynaptic cell (C) is less likely to reach threshold.

Presynaptic inhibition is important because it permits only desired movements by discarding inputs that do not contribute to performance. If the many terminal fibers to a nerve cell were all excited without selective inhibition, movements would be quite chaotic. But, by permitting some to excite and others to inhibit, coordinated and necessary movements are possible. Whereas presynaptic inhibition depresses only certain inputs to the postsynaptic cell and allows other inputs to excite, postsynaptic inhibition depresses all information to the cell. During presynaptic inhibition, activity of the cell is not necessarily depressed, but is excited only by a select group of inputs. The undesirable inputs are inhibited.

Synaptic Fatigue at the Neuromuscular Junction

Under normal exercise conditions, fatigue probably does not occur at the junction between the motor neuron and the muscle fiber. This was demonstrated when a muscle, voluntarily contracted to exhaustion, was stimulated electrically via its motor neuron. The action potentials in the muscle were not diminished from their original state when the muscle was not fatigued.[1] If the neuromuscular junction had been fatigued, the action potentials in the muscle would not have been maximal. This phenomenon occurs even when the force capacity of a voluntary effort is zero.

CENTRAL NERVOUS SYSTEM

The human nervous system consists of the brain, the spinal cord, and all the nerves,

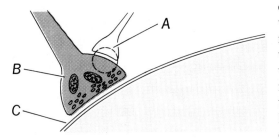

Fig. 3–8. Presynaptic inhibition on neuron A acting on neuron B to decrease chemical transmitter released on neuron C. (From Vander, A.J., Sherman, J.H., and Luciano, D.S.: Human Physiology—The Mechanisms of Body Function. New York, McGraw-Hill, Inc., 1975. Used with permission of McGraw-Hill Book Co.)

both sensory and motor, that regulate the function of muscle and internal organs (Fig. 3–9). The brain and spinal cord, which form the central nervous system (C.N.S.), are protected by a bony skull and vertebral column. The nerve cells or parts of nerve cells that are located outside the skull or vertebral column are known collectively as the peripheral nervous system.

The bony cavities enclosing the brain and the spinal cord are called the cranium and the vertebral column. Surrounding the brain and spinal cord is the cerebrospinal fluid. Probably the most important function of this fluid is to support the brain and spinal cord within the skull and vertebral column by providing a buoying effect. This buoyancy prevents the nerves and blood vessels entering and leaving the nervous system from stretching too much during rapid move-

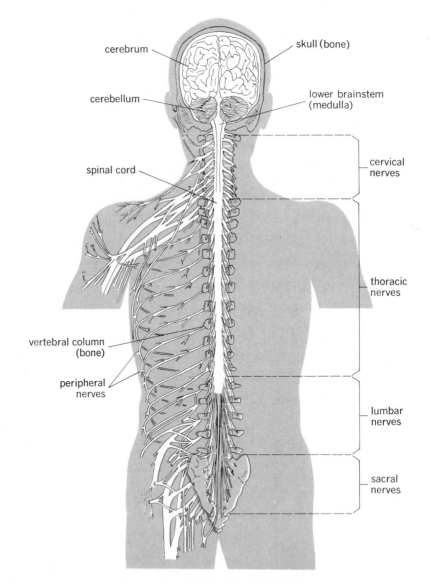

Fig. 3–9.   The central and peripheral nervous systems. (From Vander, A.J., Sherman, J.H., and Luciano, D.S.: Human Physiology—The Mechanisms of Body Function. New York, McGraw-Hill, Inc., 1975. Used with permission of McGraw-Hill Book Co.)

Table 3-1.

The Main Divisions and Subdivisions of the Central Nervous System

---

I. Brain
   A. Cerebrum
      1. Cortex
      2. Basal ganglia
      3. Thalamus
      4. Hypothalamus
   B. Cerebellum
   C. Brain stem
      1. Medulla
      2. Pons
      3. Midbrain
II. Spinal Cord

---

ments of the head. The control of substances passing into the brain, such as food nutrients and other necessary substances, is provided by blood passing through capillaries. The C.N.S. is covered by three membranes (from inside out: pia mater, arachnoid, and dura mater), which act as connective tissue helping to support the structures. The term used to describe all these membranes is meninges.

The brain consists of three main parts: the cerebrum, the cerebellum, and the brain stem. The main divisions and subdivisions of the C.N.S. are presented in Table 3-1. The brain and the spinal cord have unique functions even though both detect and process information from within and without the body and control movements by stimulation and/or inhibition of muscle contractions.

BRAIN

The three primary divisions of the brain are shown in Figure 3-10. These divisions

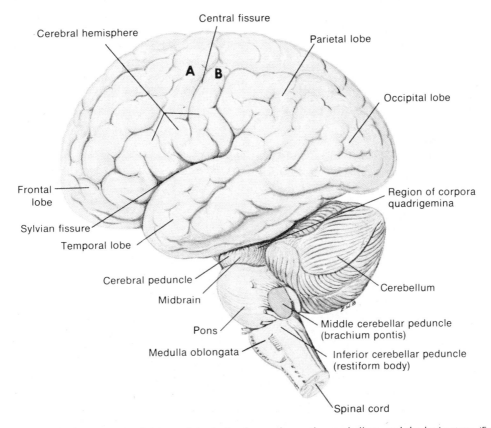

Fig. 3-10. The three primary divisions of the brain: the cerebrum, the cerebellum, and the brain stem. (From Schottelius, B.A., and Schottelius, D.D.: Textbook of Physiology. 18th Edition. St. Louis, The C.V. Mosby Co., 1978.)

are intimately related to carry out the nervous functions that sustain life. All the nerve fibers relaying signals from afferent receptors and sending signals in the other direction by efferent output pass through the brain stem, where the spinal cord and higher brain centers are joined. Coordinated functions among the three divisions are essential for appropriate bodily movement.

Cerebrum

The cerebrum is a large mass of nervous tissue located in the cranium. It consists of the cerebral cortex and subcortical centers called the basal ganglia, the thalamus, and the hypothalamus. The outer gray layer of the cerebrum, the cerebral cortex, primarily contains bodies of nerve cells. Below this layer is the white matter, which consists mostly of processes or fibers emanating from bodies of nerve cells. The white appearance comes from the myelin (fatty material) coating around the fibers.

Cerebral Cortex

The cerebral cortex is about .25 in. thick and contains about 14 billion neurons. It stores a large volume of information concerning past experiences and patterns of motor responses. Certain areas of the cortex control specific functions by receiving stimuli from sensory nerves and acting on them by motor nerves. Distinct areas of the cortex are involved with eliciting movement of the skeletal muscles. The motor regions of the cortex are in the posterior part of the frontal lobe (Fig. 3–11). Each has a particular function, depending on its position in the cortex. Moving from the top of the brain down the side, the cortical neurons are located so that neurons affecting movements of the toes and feet are at the top of the brain, followed by neurons controlling muscles of the leg, trunk, arm, hand, fingers, neck, and face. The amount of cortex devoted to the control of these muscles is proportional to the size of each of the body parts shown in Figure 3–12. The cortical areas representing the hand and face are the largest, which is why humans have a fine degree of motor control over these parts. Some of the axons of these cortical neurons pass directly (without synapsing) to motor neurons whereas others link up with many other neurons before following pathways to motor neurons. Fibers that pass directly to the vi-

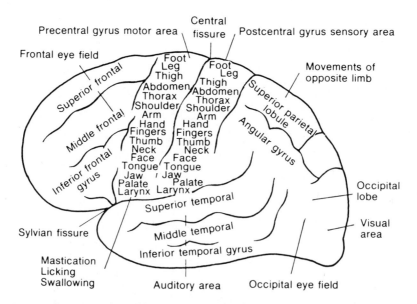

Fig. 3–11. Motor and sensory regions of the cerebral cortex. (Schottelius, B.A., and Schottelius, D.D.: Textbook of Physiology. 18th Edition. St. Louis, The C.V. Mosby Co., 1978.)

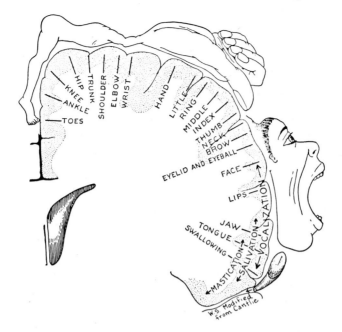

HIP
KNEE
TRUNK
ANKLE
SHOULDER
ELBOW
WRIST
TOES
HAND
LITTLE
RING
MIDDLE
INDEX
THUMB
NECK
BROW
EYELID AND EYEBALL
FACE
LIPS
JAW
TONGUE
SWALLOWING
MASTICATION
SALIVATION
VOCALIZATION
W.S. Modified from Cantlie

Fig. 3–12.   Motor regions of the cortex and the muscles they control. The representation of the body parts in the cortex is indicated. (From Gray's Anatomy of the Human Body. 29th Edition. Revised and edited by Charles M. Goss. Philadelphia, Lea & Febiger, 1973.)

cinity of the motor nerves in the spinal cord form the corticospinal pathway or the pyramidal system. Their nerve cells in the cortex are shaped like pyramids (Fig. 3–13). Other descending fibers from the pyramid system branch away in the brain stem to contact motor neurons whose axons innervate, via the cranial nerves, the muscles of the eye, face, tongue, and throat. The pathways originating from the right and left sides of the cerebral cortex cross the spinal cord at the junction of the cord and brain stem to descend on the opposite side of the spinal cord. Thus, the skeletal muscles on the right side of the body are controlled by the neurons in the left side of the brain and vice versa.

Cortical neurons that form multineuronal pathways before they reach the motor neurons provide the second type of motor control by the cortex. These neurons, combined with the subcortical centers and the fibers descending from them, make up the multineural system or extrapyramidal system (Fig. 3–14). This system sets into mo-

tion patterns of neural interaction that are developed in lower control centers of the C.N.S. The cortex initiates the signals and guides the movement, but the actual neural mechanisms involved operate at subcortical levels. Information conveyed by the extrapyramidal system is continually modified at each synaptic junction between the neurons in the pathway. These neurons may or may not fire, depending on the synaptic input they receive. All movements, especially voluntary, require the continual and coordinated interaction of both the pyramidal and extrapyramidal systems. Cortical motor neurons are stimulated to send signals in these descending pathways by input information from a variety of sensory receptors throughout the body. Input comes from vision, joint movement, smooth and skeletal muscles, and the brain stem of the C.N.S. and goes to different areas of the cortex. The sensory cortex then sends signals to the motor cortex to initiate motor responses via the two descending pathways.

The area of the cerebral cortex that re-

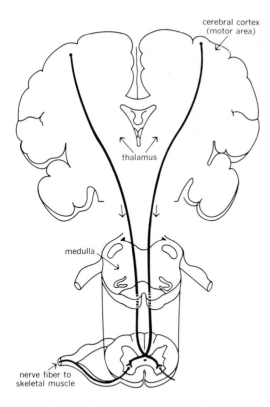

Fig. 3–13.   Pyramidal system or corticospinal pathway. (From Vander, A.J., Sherman, J.H., and Luciano, D.S.: Human Physiology—The Mechanisms of Body Function. New York, McGraw-Hill, Inc., 1975. Used with permission of McGraw-Hill Book Co.)

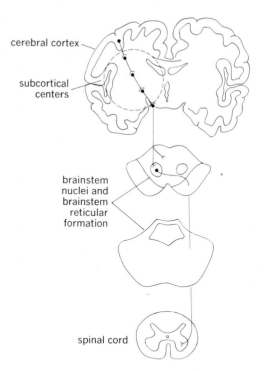

Fig. 3–14.   Extrapyramidal system or multineuronal pathway. (From Vander, A.J., Sherman, J.H., and Luciano, D.S.: Human Physiology—The Mechanisms of Body Function. New York, McGraw-Hill, Inc., 1975. Used with permission of McGraw-Hill Book Co.)

ceives pathways carrying information about mechanical changes in the skin and underlying tissues, movement in the joints, and temperature changes, is called the somatic (refers to body walls) sensory or somatosensory cortex (see Fig. 3–11). Distinct areas of the somatosensory cortex correspond to specific body parts. They identify the particular point at which a stimulus is applied in the body. But, as is the case with motor pathways, the sensory pathways in the right side of the body pass to the left brain at the spinal cord or brain stem and vice versa. The body parts and the extent to which they are sensitive are represented in Figure 3–15 according to the area covered in the somatosensory cortex.

Subcortical Centers

The area of the brain below the cortex and within the center of the brain contains subcortical nuclei that contribute to the coordination of muscle movements. The basal ganglia, thalamus, and hypothalamus are located in this area. These portions of the cerebrum receive input and convey output from a variety of sources. One such source is the reticular formation, which is a core of tissue running through the entire brain stem. This interconnecting network of reticular cells includes integrating centers for respiration, cardiovascular function, afferent and efferent systems, and states of consciousness in sleeping and waking.

The basal ganglia receive sensory input from the reticular formation. With input

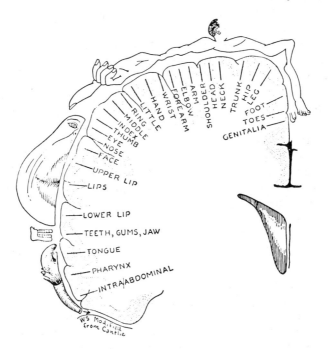

Fig. 3–15.   Sensory regions of the cortex and the representative body parts from which stimuli are detected. (From Gray's Anatomy of the Human Body. 29th Edition. Revised and edited by Charles M. Goss. Philadelphia, Lea & Febiger, 1973.)

from the extrapyramidal pathway and some input from the pyramidal pathway, the basal ganglia process and integrate this information to control mechanisms in the brain stem for complex movements. They do this by influencing motor control mechanisms at the spinal cord level to either facilitate or suppress motor activity. In addition, the basal ganglia influence the pyramidal system via the thalamus. Output goes to the cortex from the thalamus to affect the motor neurons of the pyramidal system.

The thalamus conveys to the cortex information other than that provided by the basal ganglia. It receives sensory input from all sources, except smell, and integrates this information before passing it to the cortex. Because a portion of the thalamus is made up of the reticular system, it is also involved in sleeping and waking. The hypothalamus, which lies directly below the thalamus, initiates and coordinates motor movement of the internal organs by way of the autonomic nervous system.

Cerebellum

The cerebellum is located on top of the brain stem (see Fig. 3–10). It is involved in the unconscious control of skeletal muscles because it influences other regions of the brain responsible for motor activity. Movement is not initiated in the cerebellum, but is greatly affected by its interpretive function. Sensory input is received from a variety of sources, such as the afferents of the skin, muscles, joints, equilibrium apparatus in the inner ear (vestibular system), and visual and auditory mechanisms. In addition, the cerebellum receives information about what the muscles should be doing from the multineuronal pathway and from the branches of fibers in the direct corticospinal pathways. After completing a movement, information about what actually happened is picked up via the spinal cord from the muscle, stretch receptors, tendon organs, and cutaneous receptors. Any discrepancies in what was done and what should have been done are noted by the cerebellum. Adjustments to be made to eliminate the error begin with the cerebellum, which sends the information to the motor-coordinating centers. Influence is exerted over the motor neurons to the muscles by modifying the activity of cells in the cerebral cortex and subcortical centers, from which the descending motor pathways to the spinal cord rise.

Brain Stem

The brain stem is composed of the medulla oblongata, pons, and midbrain (see Fig. 3–10). All the nerve fibers conveying signals from afferent input and efferent output pass through the brain stem and form the connection between the higher brain centers and the spinal cord. Cell bodies of motor neurons that control the skeletal muscles of the head are contained in the brain stem. The parasympathetic nerve fibers that affect the function of internal organs either pass through the brain stem to the smooth muscle and glands of the head and thoracic and abdominal organs or locate in the brain stem their cell bodies that have fibers going to the heart. Many afferent fibers from the head and visceral cavities pass into the brain stem.

The reticular formation of the brain stem is involved in the control of spinal reflexes and in the coordination of muscular activity during movement. It contains short fibers that diffuse throughout much of the midbrain. The reticular formation also includes neurons with long fibers extending downward to the spinal cord. Input comes from a variety of sources via small nerve fibers of afferent pathways. Output is conveyed by descending fibers at the spinal cord level, where spinal motor mechanisms are controlled.

Stimulation of the reticular formation strongly affects motor activity in terms of facilitating or inhibiting movement. Much of this influence comes from its regulation of gamma motor nerves, which control the discharge of muscle spindle afferents. These spindles are sensory receptors located in skeletal muscle. Gamma motor nerves directly stimulate the spindles. The reflex response is a contraction of the muscle in which the spindles are located. Muscle spindles will be covered in more detail later in this chapter.

SPINAL CORD

The spinal cord is a small cylinder, about .5 in. in diameter, that extends from the base of the skull to the upper lumbar spine (see Fig. 3–9). It is divided into a central gray area and a white peripheral area. The gray area consists primarily of interneurons, motor neurons, cell bodies, dendrites, and the entering fibers of afferent neurons. Cell bodies of neurons in the gray matter that have similar functions band together to form groups called nuclei. The peripheral region of the spinal cord, or white region, is comprised of nerve axons, which send signals between different levels of the spinal cord or between the spinal cord and brain. The white appearance of the region is caused by the fatty myelin coating covering the nerve fibers. Fibers are divided into bundles in the white matter. These bundles are called pathways or tracts. They are organized according to their function and are comprised of fibers that convey the same kinds of information. The spinal white matter has many tracts that descend to carry signals from the brain to the spinal cord. Other tracts transmit signals in the opposite direction.

The spinal cord gives off 31 pairs of spinal nerves, which supply the trunk and limbs. These spinal nerves are made up of both the dorsal (back) root and the ventral (front) root, which unite directly outside the spinal cord (Fig. 3–16). The major portion of the peripheral nervous system is formed by spinal nerves. Afferent fibers enter the spinal

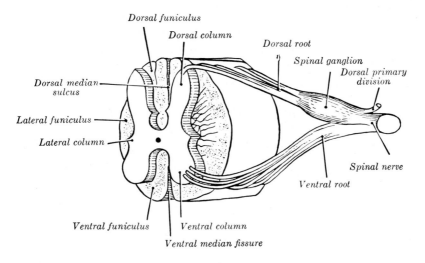

Fig. 3–16.   Cross section of the spinal cord with one pair of spinal nerves. (From Gray's Anatomy of the Human Body. 29th Edition. Revised and edited by Charles M. Goss. Philadelphia, Lea & Febiger, 1973.)

cord by the dorsal roots and efferent fibers by the ventral roots.

PERIPHERAL NERVOUS SYSTEM

The nerves outside the C.N.S., including those whose cell bodies arise from the C.N.S., comprise the peripheral nervous system (Table 3–2). These nerves travel from the C.N.S. to various parts of the body. Some of the nerve fibers (afferent fibers) conduct information from sensory receptors to the C.N.S. whereas others (efferent fibers) send signals from the C.N.S. to effector organs, such as the skeletal muscles. Nerve cell bodies are found in the peripheral nervous system as well as in the C.N.S. Outside the C.N.S., the nerve cell bodies collectively form ganglia where synapses are made with other fibers to transmit signals to various parts of the body.

Table 3–2.
The Peripheral Nervous System

   I. Afferent division
  II. Efferent division
    A. Somatic nervous system
    B. Autonomic nervous system
      1. Sympathetic nervous system
      2. Parasympathetic nervous system

There are two divisions of the peripheral nervous system: the afferent division and the efferent division. These divisions involve input and output information, respectively, to regulate and control internal and external bodily tissues and organs.

Afferent Division

Information is conveyed from the sensory receptors, located throughout the body, to the C.N.S. But, before signals from the receptors can be carried along sensory fibers, they must be translated into the language of action potentials. Each receptor is best stimulated by a specific form of energy. When excited, the receptor membrane depolarizes by becoming less negative inside the cell and less positive outside. As the stimulus intensity increases, depolarization increases. When the membrane is depolarized to the threshold level, an action potential is propagated along the afferent axon to the C.N.S. In this way, the body is constantly informed about which motor responses are made.

Sensory Receptors

The anatomic structures of receptors may take the form of nerve endings of afferent neurons or may be separate cells connected at the end of afferents, such as the sensory organs of vision or sound. In any event, these receptor endings may be activated by several different forms of energy if the stimuli are intense enough, even though they respond best to a specific stimulus. For example, eye receptors are usually stimulated by light but can be excited by a mechanical stimulus, such as a poke in the eye. The actual process involved in exciting a receptor ending varies somewhat for different receptors. Nevertheless, a generalization may be made about these processes. From the application of a stimulus to a sensory receptor to the discharge of nerve impulses in its fibers, there are intervening events, outlined as follows:

Stimulus→ Local change (in permeability)→ Generator current (charge transfer)→ Local depolarization (generator potential)→ Action potential along sensory axon

The stimulus to a receptor results in a transfer of charge across the nerve membrane that produces a depolarization. This transfer of charge is called the generator potential. When depolarization reaches threshold value, action potentials are conducted along the nerve fiber. Generator current initiated by the stimulus may be produced by spatial summation when two or more weak stimuli, which are delivered to separate sites on the receptor, are sufficiently intense to depolarize the membrane to a firing level. Or, the receptor may

Table 3–3.
Sensory Receptors and Their Stimuli

Stimulus	Location of Receptor	Input Information
Mechanical force	Skin and underlying tissues, skeletal joints	Touch pressure. Position of limbs and trunk.
	Skeletal muscle and tendon	Unconscious sensation for controlling muscle length and tension.
	Cochlea	Hearing.
	Vestibular apparatus	Equilibrium.
	Carotid (artery) sinuses	Blood pressure.
	Cervical vertebra	Equilibrium.
Heat (or lack of)	Skin (thermoreceptors for warmth and cold)	Temperature.
	Hypothalamus	
Light	Eye	Vision.
Chemical		
Water-soluble or lipid-soluble chemicals	Taste buds in tongue	Taste.
Odorous substance	Olfactory mucosa	Smell.
O_2 lack	Arterioles	Unconscious sensation for controlling blood flow.
CO_2 excess		
Acidity of blood	Carotid bodies	
Extremes of mechanical force, heat or cold, and certain chemicals	Nociceptors	Pain.

be depolarized by temporal summation when repeated stimuli are delivered to the same site on the receptor. Stimuli take the various forms shown in Table 3–3. Examples are given of various kinds of receptors and the stimuli by which they are most easily activated. Note that a particular stimulus, such as mechanical force, has an effect on receptors located at a variety of sites both deep within the body and on the body's surface. The same holds true for chemoreceptors, which stimulate receptors in the mouth and nose and also within arteries at the neck (carotid artery). The energy form of light, however, only stimulates the photoreceptors of vision in the eye.

Knowledge of the world external to the nervous system is gained only through these receptors. Forms of energy for which no human receptors exist, such as radioactivity, television waves or microwaves, or infrared light, are not detected by the body.

However, when stimuli evoke a receptor, the response may take a variety of forms either at a conscious level or at an unconscious level. Responses to sensory input that are unconscious, although consciousness of the response may or may not occur after the response, involve nervous reflexes in the C.N.S. at levels below the cerebral cortex. In fact, simple reflexes never go beyond the spinal cord. As more complex reflexes are elicited, higher levels of the C.N.S. become involved.

Reflexes Evoked by Sensory Receptors

Serving a tennis ball or performing a somersault is a complex act involving many muscle groups and movements. These complex movements are made up of simple movements that are coordinated to accomplish a task. The coordination and combination of simple movements to achieve complex motor acts are accomplished, re-

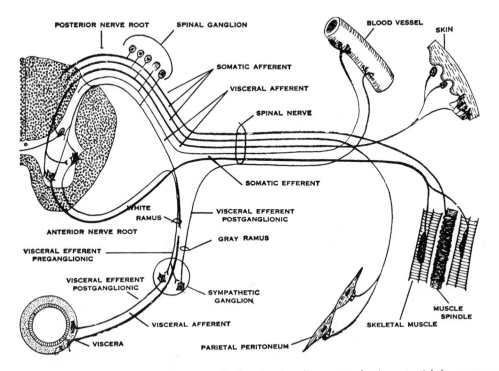

Fig. 3–17. Structure of a typical spinal nerve. A reflex loop involves the passage of action potentials from a sensory receptor to an afferent fiber, then to the central nervous system, over an efferent fiber, to the muscle. (From Gray's Anatomy of the Human Body. 29th Edition. Revised and edited by Charles M. Goss. Philadelphia, Lea & Febiger, 1973.)

spectively, at the lower levels of the C.N.S. in the spinal cord and at the higher levels of the C.N.S. by means of reflex activity.

During movements of large muscles, reflex activity is initiated by a variety of sensory receptors that usually function simultaneously and continuously. They constantly provide feedback information to the C.N.S. where it is deciphered and acted on reflexly by the motor nerves. Nerve impulses in a reflex response follow a loop pattern. Impulses are initiated at a sensory receptor, consequently pass to the C.N.S., and finally return to the muscle or effector via a motor neuron (Fig. 3–17). Reflexes are fixed reactions evoked consistently and rapidly by certain stimuli. Prior experience or learning is not required for reflexes to occur because they are innate.

Although each reflex involves a unique pattern of movement, all reflexes have basic common aspects: (1) each reflex adjusts the body to its external and internal environment. For example, if the hand touches a hot stove, the elbow flexes rapidly to remove the hand. The same movement happens when the foot steps on a sharp object. The knee flexes reflexly to pull the foot away. But, the elbow and knee must flex without losing body balance; thus, other muscles come into play. In the case of the knee, when the foot is withdrawn from the ground, body weight is shifted to the other leg. The muscles in the opposite leg reflexly contract with more force to adjust to their increased load. This example leads to the second aspect of reflexes: (2) Reflex reactions consist of not a single reflex but rather of movement patterns that involve the coordinated activity of several muscle groups and reflexes. Some of these are evident when the muscle antagonistic to the agonist or contracting muscle is reflexly relaxed to minimize resistance to movement. At the same time, there is reflex contraction of synergists, which are muscles whose action enhances or facilitates movements produced by a particular muscle. When the arm is contracted with

great force while lifting a load, muscles in the legs also contract and act as synergists to help to lift the weight. And, lastly: (3) Each reflex is ordinarily evoked by a particular stimulus and usually by no other. In the body, in particular, some sensory receptors in the arteries are only stimulated by stretch. Others are only excited by excess carbon dioxide or insufficient oxygen. The reflex activity initiated by these stimuli affect heart action or respiration.

Although reflex activity occurs in the entire C.N.S., more simple reflexes function at the level of the spinal cord and more complex reflexes function at the upper levels. Generally the interneurons in the C.N.S. are less involved when reflexes are confined to the spinal cord, but, in more complex reflexes, the interneurons carry messages up and down through all levels when connecting afferent input to efferent output.

Proprioceptors

Sensory receptors that receive information from the stimulation of the body surface and deep-lying tissues and structures within the body are called somatic senses. They may be classified according to the sites in the body from which the stimuli arise. In this classification, receptors in the skin are referred to as exteroceptors; those in the deep tissues and organs are interoceptors; and those in skeletal muscle, tendons, joints, and vestibular apparatus are proprioceptors. Proprioceptors are of most concern because they are activated by movements of skeletal joints and muscles during work and exercise.

The proprioceptors are end-organs stimulated by actions of the body itself. They lie within skeletal muscles, tendons, joints, skin, the labyrinth of the inner ear, and the upper cervical vertebrae of the neck. These receptors are stimulated by mechanical force. The effect of stimulation is a reflex response that is made possible in the gray area of the spinal cord. In fact, all reflexes function at the spinal cord level and/or at the brain stem regardless of where in the body the sensation originates.

Muscle Proprioceptors

There are two kinds of muscle proprioceptors: the muscle spindles, which lie within muscle tissue and are stimulated by stretch; and the Golgi tendon organs, which are located in tendons and respond to tension. Both function by reflex action. Impulses generated by the stimulation of these sensory receptors are conveyed by axons to the spinal cord. Interneurons within the C.N.S. carry the impulses to motor neurons, which then elicit responses in the appropriate muscles. Coordinated movements largely result

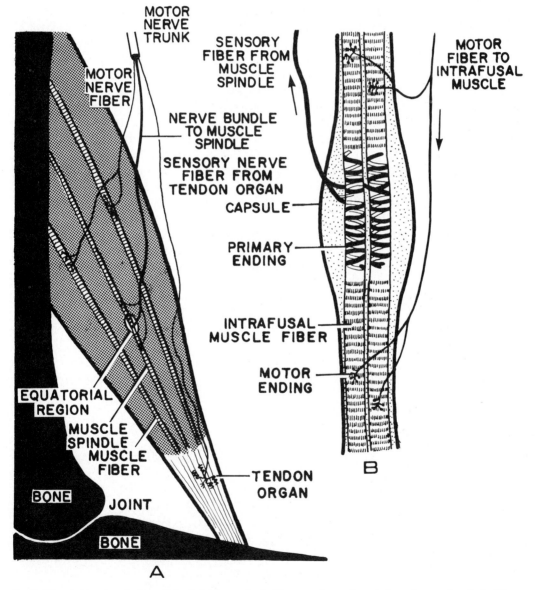

Fig. 3–18. *A,* Muscle spindles within skeletal muscle. *B,* Diagram of an enlarged view of a muscle spindle. (From Merton, P.A.: How we control the contractions of our muscles. Sci. Am., *226*:30. Copyright 1972 by Scientific American, Inc. All rights reserved.)

from the interacting functions of these muscle proprioceptors.

Muscle Spindles. Proprioceptors located within skeletal muscle and stimulated by muscle stretch are called muscle spindles (Fig. 3–18). They are fluid-filled capsules enclosing several small and modified muscle fibers. Their diameters are smaller than those of skeletal muscle fibers and vary from 10 to 24% of their size.

The nuclei of muscle spindles are located more in the center of the fibers; they are not distributed throughout the fiber as are the nuclei of skeletal muscle. The contractile portions of these fibers are restricted to their polar ends. The muscle fibers of spindles are called intrafusal fibers whereas fibers in skeletal muscle are called extrafusal. There are two kinds of intrafusal fibers, and they are distinguished from each other by their length and diameter, by the makeup of their central nuclei, and by their innervation. The larger fibers are usually called nuclear bags; the smaller fibers are nuclear chain intrafusal fibers (Fig. 3–19). Most spindles are supplied with two kinds of sensory nerve fibers: one primary afferent neuron of large diameter, which spirals around the central portion of both types of spindles, and one to five small secondary afferent neurons, which are found only on chain intrafusals and are located more distally on the nuclear region. The primary afferents of all spindles

are stimulated by the rate and degree of stretch. Secondary afferent nerves on chain intrafusals are only stimulated by degree of stretch.

Each spindle is innervated by 7 to 15 small motor neurons, called gamma neurons, whose end-plates lie on the distal portions of the fiber, where the contractile properties of the spindle are located. The cell bodies of gamma neurons are located in the brain stem. However, these gamma neurons are not the same as the motor neurons that directly activate skeletal muscle. Motor neurons to skeletal muscles are larger than gamma neurons and are called alpha motor neurons.

Stretching and consequently exciting a muscle spindle occur reflexly in two ways: (1) by simply lengthening the skeletal muscle and the spindle within, or (2) by stimulating the gamma motor neurons, which causes the muscle tissue at the distal ends of the spindle to contract, thus stretching the middle portion of the spindle as shown in Figure 3–18.

Stimulation of the spindles may occur from an external force, such as a weight that stretches the extrafusal muscle. This stretch is referred to as external stretch. When the spindles are stimulated by the gamma efferents, the stretch is called an internal stretch. Whether stimulation occurs by external or internal stretch, impulses are conveyed by the primary afferent neurons and

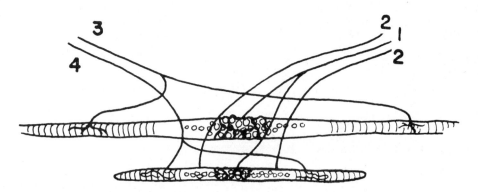

Fig. 3–19.   A nuclear bag intrafusal fiber and a nuclear chain fiber with their afferent and gamma efferent innervations. (From Gardner, E.B.: Proprioceptive reflexes and their participation in motor skills. Quest, *12*:1, 1969. Permission granted by Human Kinetics Publishers, the copyright holder.)

secondary afferent neurons to the C.N.S., where synaptic connections are made with the alpha motor neurons of the extrafusal fibers. The muscle then contracts to relieve the spindle stretch. At the same time, interneurons in the spinal cord carry signals from the spindle afferents to alpha motor neurons of other skeletal muscles that assist in the performance.

Contractions occur in skeletal muscle by direct stimulation of alpha motor neurons via the spindle afferents. But, the greatest stimulation of spindles is evident when the extrafusal fibers are stretched. As the muscle shortens, excitation of the spindles, caused by lengthening, is diminished. However, there is always some stimulation because of the continuous action of the gamma efferents. Even at rest, there is always some muscle tone caused by gamma activation of spindles.

When stimulated by external stretch of the muscle or by contraction of intrafusal fibers owing to gamma activation, the primary afferent neuron sends signals into the C.N.S. and, by monosynaptic connections with alpha motor neurons of its own muscle, produces a contraction of just enough force to relieve spindle stretch. In addition, the primary afferent neuron sends branches from its axon to two or more interneurons, which excite synergistic muscles and inhibit antagonistic muscles. The effects of primary afferent stimulation are shown in Figure 3–20.

The two distinct responses of primary afferents to their stimuli (velocity of spindle stretch and intrafusal length at a given time) are shown in Figure 3–21. By measuring the electrical activity of extrafusal muscle and recording the response with electromyograms after applying loads to an outstretched arm, one can distinguish the involvement of the two stimuli. Without a load added to the arm, the elbow flexors show a steady discharge of electrical activity (A).

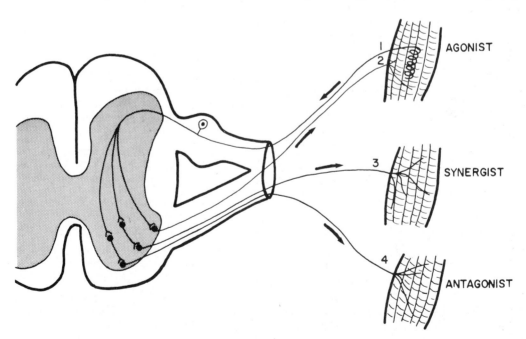

Fig. 3–20. Stimulation of the primary afferents (1) in the agonist muscle sends excitatory signals to an alpha motor neuron of the same muscle (2). Simultaneously, an excitatory disynaptic connection is made with an alpha neuron of the synergistic muscle (3), and an inhibitory disynaptic connection is made with the alpha neuron of the antagonistic muscle (4). The inhibitory effect on the antagonistic muscle as the agonist contracts is an example of reciprocal innervation. (From Gardner, E.B. Proprioceptive reflexes and their participation in motor skills. *Quest 12:*1, 1969. Permission granted by Human Kinetics Publishers, the copyright holder.)

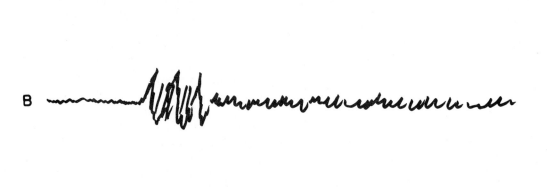

Fig. 3–21.   Electromyograms showing the electrical activity of muscle under three loaded conditions. *A,* the arm is held flexed at 90°. *B,* load is added abruptly to the hand. *C,* the same load is added, but more slowly. In both B and C, the increase of stretch in the muscle from the load is the same. The heightened activity after the addition of the load is caused by the greater stretch in the extrafusal fibers. (Adapted from Gardner, E.B.: Proprioceptive reflexes and their participation in motor skills. Quest, *12*:1, 1969. Permission granted by Human Kinetics Publisher, the copyright holder.)

After a load is added, electrical activity immediately increases. The extent of the increase depends on how abruptly the load is added (B and C). The load applied to the arm and the amount of stretch are the same in both B and C. The different levels of electrical activity are related to the time taken to add the loads. A fast loading (B) stimulates the spindles more than does a gradual and slower loading (C); consequently, more muscle fibers initially contract in the former. Soon afterward, however, the electrical activity is the same for both loading conditions (B and C) because the load on the arm further stretches the muscle and intrafusal length to stimulate primary afferents.

As more load is added to the muscle and, in turn, a greater stretch occurs, increased muscle force meets the added stress as a result of stimulating primary afferents. This spindle response allows muscles to adjust to a variety of loads. Therefore, the right amount of force is applied to accomplish a task efficiently and to protect the ligaments and other tissues around the joints from injury. If muscle force did not increase rapidly

with additional loads, the stress on the skeletal joints could be excessive, causing injury. The continued activation of spindles, even after an abrupt addition of load to the muscles, ensures the maintenance of muscle force at a functionally safe level.

Secondary spindle afferent neurons are activated simultaneously with primary afferents, but have different effects on the muscles. They have smaller neurons and less sensitivity to stretch than do the primary afferents. After impulses enter the C.N.S. over their axons, the secondary afferent neurons enhance muscle activity in the flexor muscles and inhibit muscle activity in the extensors. These actions occur regardless of the type of muscle in which the spindles lie. That is, secondary afferents of flexor muscle spindles, when stimulated by degree of stretch (not velocity of stretch), enhance contraction of the flexors. When secondaries of extensor muscle spindles are stimulated, they inhibit contraction in their own muscles but produce cocontraction in antagonistic flexors. Secondaries in flexor muscles enhance the contractile effects of primary afferents. The many secondary afferents in antigravity extensor muscles suggest that they provide an important mechanism for stabilizing the weight-bearing joints in movement. Their cocontraction effect results in both the flexors and extensors of the same joint contracting together in a balancing fashion to maintain a desired posture. Such balancing is a constant concern of the antigravity muscles.

When initiating and controlling movement under conscious direction, much of the coordination among muscles is unconscious. Precision of control at the unconscious level is largely owing to gamma efferent innervation of spindles. Gamma activity continuously stimulates intrafusal muscle fibers. Consequently, muscle contraction is maintained at varying levels of force. This variable state of contraction is known as gamma bias. The sensitivity of the spindle afferents to external stretch is increased when gamma bias is high. The gamma efferent system is excited mainly by certain regions in the brain stem that receive input from the cerebellum and the cerebral cortex. The importance of this system is indicated by the large number of gamma neurons, which comprise about one third of all motor neurons to the skeletal muscle.

The gamma system controls extrafusal contraction to achieve a desired muscle length. When the preferred length is reached, the spindles fire minimally. Apparently, the muscle automatically seeks out the degree of contraction that will reduce to a minimum the firing frequency of its stretch receptors. Apparently, involuntary movement of the spindle mechanism can regulate the amount and rate of muscle shortening. In a tennis serve, the individual decides on the desired position of the joints and muscles to perform the task well. He thereby sets the spindle length corresponding to the desired muscle length and proceeds to match the two. When the spindles are minimally stimulated during the serve, the muscles are at their desired length and contraction force. If the effect is not what was expected, i.e., a poor serve, the spindles are "reset" for the next serve. The subsequent serve then results in different muscle lengths and forces to accommodate the new spindle setting. Although this phenomenon occurs in voluntary movement and involves setting by the gamma system, the actual adjustments in muscle force and length to produce the right effect in the serve are reflex in nature. They occur in the spindles of both agonists and antagonists, each of which have different settings for muscle length.

Coordination of muscles through the entire course of a movement is assured by spindles. As movement occurs, continuous feedback is provided by the changing lengths of the muscles that contain the spindles.

Golgi Tendon Organs. Golgi tendon organs are the second type of muscle proprioceptors. They are located at the junction of muscle fibers and their tendons and respond to forces provided by the contracting muscle (Figs. 3–18 and 3–22). When activated by a strongly contracting muscle, sensory signals are sent from the tendon organs to the spinal cord where, by disynaptic or polysynaptic interneurons, the agonist muscles are inhibited from contracting and cause a reduction in force while the antagonistic muscles are facilitated to contract.[2] The effects are opposite to those from the spindle primary afferents because the Golgi tendon organs inhibit their own muscles and synergists and facilitate their antagonists. Tendon organs generally function as safety mechanisms to protect the muscles from overextension and to prevent consequent damage. The threshold for stimulation of tendon organs is considerably higher than that for muscle spindles when the tendon is stretched passively. But, some research evidence has shown that, during rapid voluntary movement in human beings, the interneurons in the spinal cord connecting the Golgi afferents to the alpha and gamma neurons are inhibited.[3] This discovery means that the tendon organs are not functional in fast movement. It has been suggested that the tendon organ not

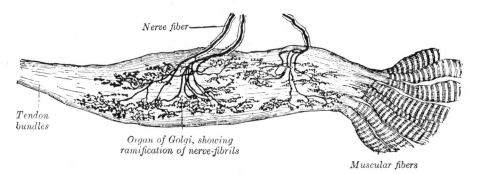

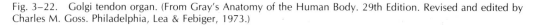

Fig. 3–22.   Golgi tendon organ. (From Gray's Anatomy of the Human Body. 29th Edition. Revised and edited by Charles M. Goss. Philadelphia, Lea & Febiger, 1973.)

only protects muscle from overloading, but also acts as a transducer (a device that is activated by power from one system and supplies power to another system) in a continuous feedback system that regulates muscle tension, just as the muscle spindle is the transducer in the system that regulates muscle length.[4]

The advantage to having a control system to regulate muscle tension is that it permits the exact amount of muscle force necessary to accomplish a particular task. The Golgi tendon organ regulates muscle tension by responding to any tension that is greater or less than the desired value. Tension on the organ varies as a function of muscle length, velocity of shortening, and fatigue level. When tension falls below the "set" control value, the inhibiting effect on the motor neurons by the organ lessens. Likewise, if the tension goes beyond the "set" control value, the tendon organ inhibits the motor neurons to the muscle.

Muscle Proprioceptive Reflexes as a Positional Control System. The Golgi tendon organs work with the muscle spindles to provide a positional control system involving coordinated movement of muscles antagonistic to each other. The control system involves a change-of-length detector (muscle spindles) in each muscle. This detector, when activated, facilitates the muscle in which it is located and inhibits the antagonistic muscle. In addition, the system has a tension detector (Golgi tendon organ) in each muscle tendon which, when activated, leads to inhibition of the agonist muscle and facilitation of the antagonistic muscle.

During the operation of the control system, when an extensor muscle contracts, the flexor muscle passively stretches and relaxes as the joint extends. The relaxation comes about by the inhibition of motor nerves to the flexor muscles as the extensors contract. This phenomenon is called reciprocal innervation and is initiated by a contracting muscle. The primary afferents of spindles within the contracting muscle are activated by the gamma system. Signals are sent from the spindles to the spinal cord, where the alpha neurons to the agonist muscle are excited and, thereby, match the contraction force to the load lifted. At the same time, the alpha neurons to the antagonist muscle are inhibited and, consequently, cause the muscle to relax. The effect is a smooth and controlled contraction with minimum resistance from the antagonistic muscles. In all muscle contractions, whether in sports or work, reciprocal innervation is always operating.

To prevent overextension of a joint, the tension detector of the positional control system is activated. The Golgi tendon organs of the extensor muscle and the muscle spindles of the flexor muscle are excited by stretch. Near the end of extension, the activity of these two receptors leads to inhibition of the extensor motor neurons and facilitation of the flexor motor neurons. That is, the extensor muscles relax from stimulation of their tendon organs and the flexor muscles contract from their spindle excitation. This happens, for example, when throwing a baseball fast. Just before releasing the ball by extending the arm, the previously relaxed elbow flexors and muscle spindles are excited by stretch to contract the flexors. At the same time, the Golgi tendon organs of the extensors are excited and cause relaxation of the extensors. A smooth transition takes place in the involved muscles to allow the execution of an explosive movement without joint damage.

Vestibular Apparatus

Sensory receptors are located in a membranous sac, called the vestibular apparatus, which is within the bony labyrinth of the skull (Fig. 3–23). The apparatus forms three semicircular canals, a utricle, and a saccule on each side of the skull. A specialized fluid, called endolymph, fills all these structures. The actual receptors of the vestibular apparatus are hair cells that are located at the ends of the afferent neuron.

When the head moves, the endolymph fluid presses against and, thus, stimulates the hair cells. The extent and velocity of the movement determine how much the hairs

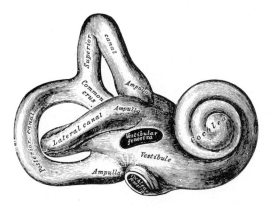

Fig. 3–23. The vestibular apparatus. (From Gray's Anatomy of the Human Body. 29th Edition. Revised and edited by Charles M. Goss. Philadelphia, Lea & Febiger, 1973.)

bend and their level of excitation. The semicircular canals are stimulated by movements different from those that stimulate the utricles and saccules. Angular acceleration stimulates the semicircular canals whereas linear acceleration and head position relative to gravity stimulate the utricles and possibly the saccules. The afferent nerve fibers from the semicircular canals and the utricles enter the brain stem. Some of the fibers also end there, but others go to the cerebellum. From these locations, secondary fibers go to the spinal cord interneurons, subcortical centers, and cerebral cortex, the areas involved in controlling the motor systems.

Vestibular Reflexes. The vestibular apparatus provides information for two purposes. The first purpose is to control eye movement so that, regardless of head position, the eyes can remain fixed on the same point. When the head is turned to the right, the balance of afferent input from the vestibular apparatus is altered so that the ocular muscles controlling eye movement are affected differently. The muscles turning the eyes to the left are activated while their antagonists are inhibited. The second purpose of vestibular input is to maintain upright position. However, even before an individual can assume an upright position (e.g., a young infant), the vestibular reflexes are evident in a primitive and highly predictable form known as the tonic labyrinthine reflex (TLR). Positioning of an infant's head in reference to the body produces specific reflex responses.[5] In the supine position, the TLR is extension in all limbs and inhibition in flexion, whereas, in the prone position, the opposite responses occur, i.e., flexion of limbs and inhibition of extensors. Lying on the side induces reflex activity of extension for the under limbs and flexion of the upper limbs with inhibition of antagonists (Fig. 3–24). As the child develops, the TLRs are supplanted by more complex reflexes that primarily orient the head with gravity by action of the neck muscles so that an upright position is possible. The vestibular ap-

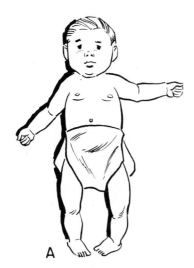

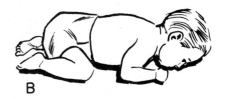

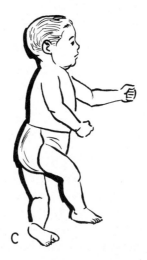

Fig. 3–24.   Tonic labyrinthine reflex (TLR) in an infant. In a supine position, all limbs are extended *(A)*; when prone, limbs are flexed *(B)*. When lying on a side, the under limbs are extended and the upper limbs flexed *(C)*. (From Gardner, E.B.: Proprioceptive reflexes and their participation in motor skills. Quest, *12*:1, 1969. Permission granted by Human Kinetics Publishers, the copyright holder.)

paratus plays a role with other proprioceptive reflexes in the postural fixation of the head, orientation of the body in space, and reflexes associated with locomotion. Generally, it facilitates extensor motor neurons to prevent the limbs from collapsing. Other reflexes cooperating with the vestibular reflexes to maintain posture arise from stimulation of visual, skin, and neck receptors. As development proceeds in the child, reflexes that evoke muscular responses to maintain body balance gradually dominate the simple postural reflexes. The muscular responses maintaining equilibrium involve moving the body segments to keep the center of gravity above the base of support or shifting the base of support under the center of gravity.

Neck Receptors

Sensory receptors located in the first three cervical vertebrae are stimulated by movement of the head. These receptors are called neck receptors. When activated, they cause reflex responses that are designed to maintain body posture and balance. Reflexes initiated by neck receptors are called tonic neck reflexes (TNR). Coordination of limb movements to accomplish desired movement patterns of the entire body is a result of both the TLR and TNR; the former acts more on the lower limbs, and the latter acts more on the upper limbs.[5a]

The TNR, like the TLR, is also present in a primitive form at birth. This presence is shown when an infant moves the neck by ventriflexing the head (flexion of neck), dorsiflexing the neck (extension of neck), or rotating the head. In a supine position, when the head is ventriflexed, the reflex response is flexion of the arms and extension of the legs. When the head is dorsiflexed, the arms extend and the knees flex. Rotating the head to the left extends the left arm and leg and flexes the right arm and leg. Rotating the head to the right causes the opposite movements to occur (Fig. 3–25). In later life, these primitive reflexes are gradually modified by changes in synaptic facilitation and by inhibition of motor neurons to the muscles involved in the reflex pattern of responses. Although these reflexes modify or subdue with age, they can be recalled in certain situations.[6,7,7a,7b] For example, if an individual stands in a doorway, presses the backs of the hands forcefully against the door frame for about a minute, and then steps forward out of the doorway, the arms raise, even when the individual tries to relax the muscle (neural motor transmission continues after relaxing, thus, converting from an isometric contraction to a concentric contraction). A TNR pattern is shown in a responsive individual when the head is rotated to one side. Turning to the right side facilitates the muscles of that shoulder and inhibits the left shoulder. Therefore, the right arm raises higher than the left arm.

Joint Receptors

Sensory receptors located in ligaments, joint capsules, and adjacent connective tissues of skeletal joints, when stimulated, initiate reflexes to modify muscle activity by way of the alpha and gamma systems. Most joint receptors are pacinian corpuscles that are surrounded by layers of cells which, when deformed by mechanical pressure, activate nerve terminals. Other sensors have either free nerve endings with no particular receptor structure or more complex nerve endings called flower-spray endings or organs of Ruffini. Some receptors seem to respond only to acceleration, such as the pacinian corpuscles in ligaments and Ruffini end-organs in joint capsules. Both of these receptors are highly sensitive to movement. Pacinian corpuscles around tendons and joints also are stimulated by pressure per se.

Some receptors are only stimulated by joint angle. These receptors are located throughout joint capsules and discharge continuously, although all are not stimulated simultaneously. At any joint angle, some sensors are intensely stimulated, others are only mildly stimulated, and others are not at all stimulated. These receptors make known the exact position of all body parts. Afferent neurons of joint receptors send impulses to

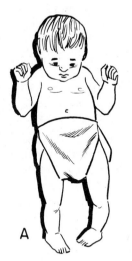

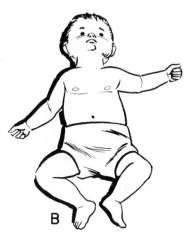

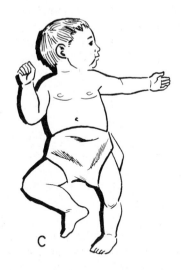

Fig. 3–25.   Tonic neck reflexes (TNR) in an infant. When head is ventriflexed, arms are flexed and knees are extended *(A)*; when dorsiflexed, arms are extended and knees are flexed *(B)*. In head rotation to the side, arm and leg are abducted and extended to that side, whereas the opposite limbs are adducted and flexed *(C)*. (From Gardner, E.B.: Proprioceptive reflexes and their participation in motor skills, Quest, *12*:1, 1969. Permission granted by Human Kinetics Publisher, the copyright holder.)

the spinal cord where they interconnect with many interneurons. In fact, these afferent neurons contact more interneurons than do the muscle proprioceptors. Consequently, their influence is more diffuse. When stimulated, they not only modify acitivity in the same limb, but also affect the activity of other limbs. For example, clenching the fists before jumping has a facilitative effect on the legs to enhance muscle force. There is even a facilitative effect of joint movement on the vestibular apparatus so that, when walking and standing, the limbs are more stable and strong. Activation of the vestibular system sends signals to the spinal cord, where motor neurons to the lower limbs are stimulated to contract with more force.

Because the impulses from joint receptors find their way to the sensory cortex, which is not the case with muscle spindles and Golgi tendon organs, they provide body awareness of the position and movement of all the joints. Consequently, kinesthesis or body awareness primarily results from the information supplied by the joint receptors. In athletics and dancing, desired movements are accomplished by assessing kinesthetic awareness and making adjustments to future movements.

Cutaneous Receptors

Sensory receptors in the skin and subcutaneous tissues affect both alpha and gamma neurons. Stimulation is provided by touch, pressure, heat, cold, and tissue damage. These receptors function both as somesthetic exteroceptors and as proprioceptors. As exteroceptors, they provide information to the sensory cortex for conscious awareness. As proprioceptors, they contribute to the reflexes involved in righting the body by providing information about surface contacts.

There is a variety of different types of afferent receptors in the skin. Most of the receptors are free nerve endings whose distal parts have no myelin covering. Their endings are located both on the skin surface (epidermis) and just below the skin surface (dermis). Other receptors are encapsulated structures, such as pacinian corpuscles and Meissner's corpuscles, and still others have naked terminals that are covered by connective tissue capsules shaped like bulbs or discs.

The traditional theory of sensitivity holds that each particular kind of nerve ending responds to a specific stimulus that is either mechanical or chemical. However, if stimulus intensity is high, both kinds of stimuli may elicit an action potential in a receptor. Free nerve endings are thought to be primarily responsible for pain and have a large dispersion in the skin for such a purpose. Pacinian and Meissner's corpuscles respond to touch, especially on hairless areas of the skin. In areas with hair, the sense of touch is mediated by free nerve endings that are wrapped around hair follicles and are excited by movement. There are many unanswerable questions about the physiology of sensory receptors in cutaneous tissue in terms of their response to specific stimuli and of the relationship of their physical structure to these stimuli. In particular, the physiology of pain is poorly understood. Nevertheless, the organism's response to pain is well known.

The body's response to pain is unique. Such stimuli as touch-pressure, temperature, light, and sound, give rise to sensation, but a pain stimulus results in a sensation and a reaction. The response to pain is reflex in nature and does not require any prior deliberation at the level of the cerebral cortex. Similarly, when the afferent receptors in the skin and subcutaneous tissues function as proprioceptors, responses involve reflex pathways in the nervous system that occur below the conscious level.

Skin receptors have a broad effect on the alpha neurons to the skeletal muscles and the gamma neurons to the spindles. The reflex response from stimulation of the skin receptors is rarely limited to the muscles that are close to the stimulus or to the muscles directly involved. For example, pulling the hand away from a hot stove involves reciprocal inhibition where the antagonist muscles are inhibited so that a faster response is possible by the agonist muscles. In addition, impulses are sent to the opposite limb and assist in moving the body away from the painful stimulus. Some reflexes are especially associated with the subcutaneous receptors in the soles of the feet and involve extension of both knees or extension of one knee and flexion of the other.

Extensor Thrust Reflex. When the soles of the feet strike the ground, the sensory receptors in the cutaneous tissue are stimulated by pressure and send signals by their afferents to the spinal cord. Action potentials travel to the alpha motor neurons supplying the knee extensors. The extensors contract to prevent the knee from overflexing. This kind of reflex, involving the receptors in the feet and the knee extensors, is called an extensor thrust reflex (Fig. 3–26). The reflex contraction of the extensors may be primarily concentric, as happens in walking, or, if an individual jumps off a high place, the response is first a strong eccentric contraction to absorb the weight of the body followed by a concentric contraction. In the latter reflex response, the contraction is more forceful because of the greater stimulation of the receptors.

Crossed Extensor Reflex. Another reflex initiated by the receptors in the feet is more complex and involves an extensor thrust reflex with one foot and a flexor reflex with the opposite limb. This reflex is initiated by stepping on a stimulating object, such as a tack. The immediate response is knee flexion to withdraw the affected foot from the tack. At the same time, the opposite limb extends at the knee to move the entire body away from the stimulus. The total reflex is called a crossed extensor reflex (see Fig. 3–26). The reflex circuit goes from the receptors in the foot to the spinal cord. The motor neurons going from the spinal cord to the knee flexors are excited whereas the neurons going to the knee extensors are inhibited (reciprocal inhibition). Simultaneously, impulses are sent by interneurons

to the opposite limb where the motor neurons to the knee extensors are excited and the neurons to the flexors are inhibited.

Other reflexes arising from pressure receptors in the skin evoke responses that orient the body when in space or when in contact with the ground. Such responses maintain the proper relationship among the head, body, and limbs so that equilibrium is maintained.

Proprioceptive Reflexes in Skilled Movement

The primary goal in learning a skilled movement is to perform the details of the movement with minimal conscious awareness. If every move used to swing a tennis racquet required conscious and detailed concern over all the body parts and what they were doing, strategy in play would greatly suffer. The desire is to free the cerebral cortex from thinking about movement details so that more attention can be given to strategy. In athletic competition that requires great concentration before the unleashing of one quick movement, such as in golf or the shotput, the cortex should be free to concentrate on the total movement. When skill is acquired in a motor act, smooth and coordinated movements of body segments are evident and are assured by the self-regulating control of proprioceptive feedback. These proprioceptive responses are conditioned so that each movement provides the stimulus for the next movement.

Learning a motor skill requires putting a group of simple movements into complex combinations. Neuromuscular pathways between receptors and effectors must be developed before learning can happen. New neuromuscular patterns must be formed and synchronized in an appropriate sequential order. During the early phases of learning a difficult task, the learner must be consciously aware of the individual parts of the total pattern. Early errors are often the result of interference between conscious direction of movement by the cerebral cortex and smooth functioning of activity at subcortical levels. As a result, many wasteful

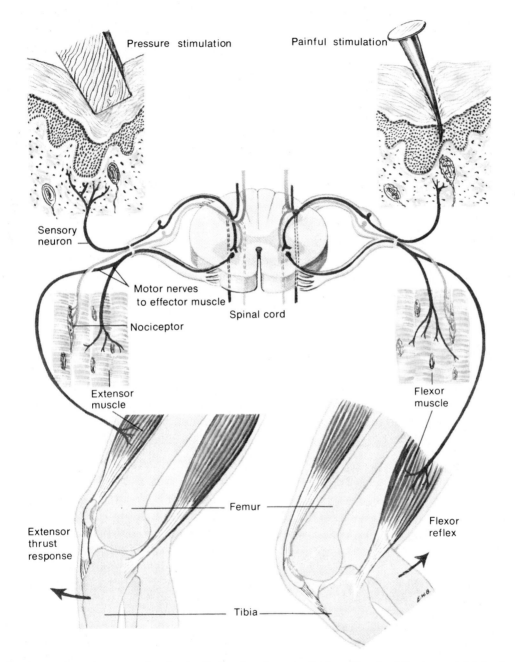

Fig. 3–26.   Crossed extensor reflex showing flexion of one leg and extension of the other following a painful stimulus. (From Schottelius, B.A., and Schottelius, D.D.: Textbook of Physiology. 18th Edition. St. Louis, The C.V. Mosby Co., 1978.)

movements occur. Later, as learning progresses, the cortical control of the movement patterns involved gradually reduces. When the skill is learned and established within the receptor-effector pathways, only one single conscious stimulus or thought at the cortex level is needed to set off the chain of events leading to its performance. The learning process changes movement control from primarily the cerebral cortex to physiologic mechanisms operating in the peripheral nervous system and at subcortical levels. The main feedback for regulating activity is provided by the proprioceptors.

Reflexes of Muscle Spindles and Golgi Tendon Organs in Motor Performance

In all movements, spindles and tendon organs either facilitate, reinforce, or inhibit muscle contraction. These effects, of course, occur simultaneously so that some muscles are reinforced to contract with more force, others are prepared to contract with a little more encouragement by nerve impulses (facilitation), and still others relax by inhibition of their motor nerves. Reinforcement of contraction occurs by stretching before contracting a muscle. In this way, the spindles are activated by external stretch so that the motor neurons to the extrafusal fibers are excited. This effect is added to the length-tension phenomenon (see Fig. 1–17), which results in still more muscle force. The external stretch of a muscle directly activates the spindles, whose afferents carry impulses to the alpha neurons and to the gamma neurons. The gamma neurons, in turn, further excite the spindles and, thereby, enhance muscle force. The amount of muscle force augmented by spindle activity is related to spindle activation. As previously mentioned, stimulation of spindles is provided by the degree of stretch and by the velocity of stretch. Maximum stretch with high velocity increases involuntary discharge to the muscle so that when the voluntary command is given, muscle force is greatest.

The advantage to stretching a muscle before movement is shown by the various backswings assumed in tennis and handball and by the crouches taken just before high jumping. For any movement that requires a high force, stretching as much as possible at high velocity, without jeopardizing skill, is necessary. To further enhance muscle force, a minimum hesitation between the stretch and the concentric contraction should be taken; otherwise, the spindle effect from velocity of stretch is lost.

When the primary concern of the forward movement is accuracy rather than force, the effect of spindle stimulation should be minimized. In this case, the backswing is slower and shorter, and a pause is taken before moving forward. Throwing darts at a target is a good example of a movement that emphasizes accuracy rather than force. After spindle activity is minimized by a slow stretch and by hesitation in the backswing, a slower forward movement allows more last-second adjustments in direction and distance.

Some movements require both a high degree of force and accuracy, such as batting and pitching. Practicing to improve performance should emphasize both force and accuracy; force should be stressed more as skill improves. This is especially true for baseball pitchers who must throw hard most of the time. Participants in racquet sports should achieve a happy balance between force and accuracy. For some strokes, such as a smash, more emphasis should be given to force. However, when playing the net, as in tennis, the emphasis is greatest on meeting the ball and placing it accurately on the opponent's court.

Before any movement occurs, gamma neurons are activated by impulses initiated in the consciousness of the cerebral cortex. Consequently, the spindles are held in a variable state of contraction known as gamma bias. The greater the gamma bias, the greater the sensitivity of the spindle afferents to external stretch. Once the movement is initiated, the response occurs more rapidly than it would occur otherwise. In preparing to perform an explosive movement, such as during a racing start, the "get set" position should be used to obtain optimal gamma bias. The runner in this position responds more quickly and forcefully to the gun.

Applying force too early when swinging a baseball bat or racquet can reduce the force with which a ball is struck. The inhibiting effect on the contraction force of the agonist muscles by stimulation of the tendon organs in the early phases of the swing diminishes force. To maximize the impact of the striking implement on the ball, the initial swing should be more gradual so that muscle force does not reduce and can be optimal on contact. In addition to the inhibiting effect on muscle force by the tendon organs, a greater contraction in the antagonistic muscles occurs because of reciprocal innervation. This effect further contributes to the reduced impact of the racquet on the ball.

The activity of spindles may be controlled to eliminate muscle spasms or cramps. Evidence shows that an overly worked muscle tends to remain in a contracted state of spasm.[8,9,9a] These spasms may be caused by increased contractions, which prevent adequate blood flow for a complete recovery from fatigue. A symptom, pain, is usually felt 24 to 48 hr. after exercise. This pain is different from that experienced during or immediately after training, which subsides in several hours. and from pain that is caused by a muscle or connective tissue tear, which is immediate and prolonged. The spasm is diminished by stretching the muscle slowly and maintaining the position for several minutes. The slow stretch minimizes activation of the spindles and lessens firing of the alpha motor neurons to the muscle.[10] Consequently, blood flow increases, the muscle relaxes[10,11] and the soreness diminishes.[12,13] Further relaxation of the affected muscle occurs by eliciting the reflex of reciprocal inhibition. Contracting the antagonistic muscle inhibits the activity of motor neurons to the agonist and decreases fiber activity.

Reflexes of the Neck and Vestibular Apparatus in Motor Performance

The position of the head provides stimulation to the neck receptors, which exert a great influence on the trunk and limbs. Certain movements and head positions reinforce contractions of arm muscles. When the head is flexed forward (ventriflexion), the arm flexors can contract with more force. If the head is extended (dorsiflexion), force in arm extension increases. The influence of head position on force was shown in a study that found that young adult males were able to apply more force in a benchpress exercise when their heads were dorsiflexed than when their heads were level with the trunk. The same individuals were able to apply more force in elbow flexion when their heads were ventriflexed.[14] During the last phase of the shot put, when the arm extends to propel the ball, the head is dorsiflexed to maximize extension force. Performing a handstand is easier with the head dorsiflexed because of the added strength to arm extension.

Head position may either enhance or inhibit some performances, especially during the early stages of learning. The position of the head that facilitates trunk and limb flexion in the forward somersault is ventriflexion; in the layout backward somersault, dorsiflexion facilitates extension. But, in some stunts and dives, the natural tendency for a beginner is ventriflexion when dorsiflexion is required or vice versa. This tendency occurs because the tonic neck reflexes are not completely eliminated in the child or adult. Beginning divers often tend to raise their head because they lose their balance in the air as a result of the headrighting reflex. The result is either a "belly flop" or a feet-first entrance. Young children, when learning the forward somersault tend to dorsiflex the head as the hands touch the mat. Pressure on the hands elicits the extension reflex and the corresponding dorsiflexion of the head. Teaching emphasis is placed on instructions to "tuck" or ventriflex the head to avoid possible injury to the neck.

The vestibular apparatus functions with the neck receptors and integrates information from cutaneous receptors, vision, and other proprioceptors to provide an awareness of body position in space. In human beings, the vestibular apparatus provides input for the motor control of the eye muscles and for posture when the body is not completely steady, as occurs often in land sports and when under water. However, during resting conditions, upright posture is maintained primarily by other proprioceptors, cutaneous sensation, and vision. In fact, individuals whose vestibular apparatus has been destroyed have little difficulty in maintaining balance during everyday activities provided that their visual system and their joint and cutaneous receptors are normal. Nevertheless, complex movements (where the body is continually moving and assuming a variety of balanced postures) require a normal functioning vestibular system.

Vision assists in balance when the eyes first focus on a point by fixating the head and stabilizing the gravitational effects on the vestibular apparatus. The steady inflow of information from these and other receptors helps to maintain the desired position. The neck reflexes continually operate to align the body with the correct posture of the head. Coordinated reflex activity between the vestibular system and the neck receptors is essential for achieving high levels of balance in relatively static body postures, such as balancing on the toes in dancing, or in dynamic postures, such as those encountered during most sport activities that require the body to continually change its posture. Both kinds of balance, static and dynamic, are achieved when the line of gravity (an imaginary vertical line passing through the weight center of the body) is above the base of support. Activities of a dynamic nature, such as basketball or football, provide situations to which athletes must adjust to maintain balance. Bodily contact with opponents teaches athletes how to maintain the line of gravity over the base of support. In football, the offensive lineman learns to lean forward to block his opponent. Sometimes, the athlete actually moves the line of gravity beyond the base of support in the direction of an oncoming force. When contact is made, the line of gravity is pushed back above the base so that balance is maintained. When the line is pushed beyond the base, the athlete loses balance and falls.

As with the neck receptors, some skilled movements require the inhibition of vestibular reflexes for optimal performance. These skills involve movements in opposition to righting and equilibrium reflexes and are controlled by the vestibular apparatus, e.g., somersaults, cartwheels, and most dives. In the early stages of learning, instructions emphasize the inhibition of reflexes that detract from correct performance. As learning progresses, the conscious inhibition of the undesired reflexes lessens because unconscious synaptic inhibition begins to play a more dominant role in controlling undesirable moves. The effectiveness of teaching motor skills depends largely on recognizing the reflexes that both enhance and inhibit learning and applying this information to firmly establish new motor patterns.

Reflexes of Joint and Cutaneous Receptors in Motor Performance

Proprioceptors of joint and cutaneous tissue operate reflexly and simultaneously with all other proprioceptors. The specific effects of either joint or cutaneous receptors in controlling movement are difficult to isolate but, certainly, feedback from these receptors contributes to overall regulation. Input information from joint receptors is important in the coordination of arms and legs. By means of irradiation from joints during movement, impulses are sent to primary muscles and to other skeletal muscles to augment force. Apparently, impulse outflow proceeds over subconscious pathways to the motor synapses of prime mover muscles in the central nervous system. In fact, the phenomenon of irradiation, during which impulses diffuse out to other motor neurons from activated proprioceptors, is believed to be a normal concomitant in the development of motor skills.[6,7] This has been shown by the increase of force in one muscle after a strong contraction in another muscle. Clenching the fists or gritting the teeth when leaping in the long jump increases impulse flow to primary muscles used in jumping.

Joint receptors provide input information in movements involving pattern sequences. In this way, feedback controls not only unconscious but conscious reflex activity by kinesthetic awareness. Once the proper joint angulations and their movement velocities are kinesthetically known, the "feel" of body position on the ground or in the air provides the feedback for making necessary adjustments in sequential moves. A gymnast or diver times a movement by the "feel" of the body in the air and coordinates muscle contractions to achieve the desired move. A dancer uses a mirror for visual feedback and coordinates this information with limb and trunk joint receptors to perform as desired. Later, as learning occurs, the movements can be repeated without visual feedback.

Cutaneous receptors are stimulated in movement by contact with a variety of objects. Stimuli are provided by contact with the external environment, e.g., the floor, diving board, water, or trampoline; by contact with sport implements, such as a ball, golf club, racquet, or bat; and by contact between body parts. The intensity and nature of the contact determines the response. Movements in such sports as tumbling, diving, football, golf, and baseball provide the nervous system with information at the instant of impact. Many of the responses involve the extensor thrust reflex, which is initiated by pressure on the sole of the feet. As movement continues, the changing contact with the surface or sport implement and the contact between body parts provide feedback that is acted on at both the conscious and unconscious levels, depending on how much learning has been acquired. The more skilled the individual, the less need for conscious response to feedback.

Efferent Division

The efferent division of the peripheral nervous system puts into effect information from sensory input. Movement is either increased or decreased in the end-organs, depending on the degree of stimulation they receive from their effector nerves. When effector signals are frequent and involve a large number of motor units, the effector organ is highly active. In some situations, effector nerves may be inhibited to slow down or to prohibit responses in organs or muscles. The efferent division controls activity by either stimulating or inhibiting end-organs. There are two subdivisions of the efferent division: the system affecting the internal viscera, called the autonomic nervous system; and the system affecting the skeletal muscles, called the somatic system. The motor neurons of the somatic system connect the central nervous system with skeletal muscle fibers and have their cell bodies in the brain stem and spinal cord. Their axons go directly from the cell bodies to innervate the skeletal muscles.

Autonomic Nervous System

Innervation of the internal viscera by the autonomic nervous system is arranged differently. The axons that directly connect to the end-organs, such as smooth muscle, cardiac muscle, and adrenal gland, have cell bodies entirely outside the central nervous system. The cell bodies of these outlying neurons are grouped together in peripheral ganglia. The synaptic connections with axons, whose cell bodies are located in the central nervous system are made in the ganglia. Innervation of the viscera always occurs by the interruption of the pathway from the central nervous system to the effector organ by peripheral ganglia.

The autonomic nervous system has two

separate divisions: the sympathetic and the parasympathetic. Each division's motor neurons originate in different sites of the central nervous system. The location of their peripheral ganglia also differs, and, when one division increases its activity, the other division decreases its activity at most end-organs.

Sympathetic and Parasympathetic Divisions. The two divisions of the autonomic nervous system have motor axons that leave the central nervous system at different levels. The sympathetic division fibers leave from the middle portions of the spinal cord whereas the parasympathetic fibers leave from the brain and lower part of the spinal cord (Fig. 3–27). Most glands, smooth muscle, and the heart are innervated by fibers from both divisions. Generally, the sympathetic fibers stimulate end-organs and the parasympathetic fibers slow them down. However, there are exceptions, e.g., the sympathetic fibers in the smooth muscle of the intestinal wall reduce contraction and the parasympathetic fibers cause contraction. In any event, dual innervation of most visceral organs provides a fine degree of control.

Figure 3–27 shows fibers leaving the central nervous system and passing to the synapses in the ganglia and fibers leaving the ganglia and going to the effector organs. Fibers moving from the central nervous system to the ganglia are called preganglionic fibers; fibers moving from the ganglia to the effectors are called postganglionic fibers. The chemical transmitter at the synapses of the ganglia, which is secreted by the terminal endings of the preganglionic fibers of both divisions, is acetylcholine. But, the chemical transmitter secreted by the postganglionic fibers at the effectors differs according to the division in which the fibers belong. Most parasympathetic fibers release acetylcholine whereas practically all sympathetic fibers release norepinephrine in the postganglionic fibers. One exception to this rule is the acetylcholine secreted by some sympathetic fibers to the smooth muscle of arterioles in skeletal muscle. The effect is to relax the smooth muscle and thereby to cause the blood vessels to dilate. However, most sympathetic nerves to smooth muscle around arterioles release norepinephrine, which contracts muscle and constricts blood flow. The role played by the acetylcholine sympathetic fibers is described in more detail in Chapter 5. There are no parasympathetic fibers to arterioles; consequently, there is no dual control by the autonomic nervous system.

The sympathetic system is greatly stimulated by work and/or emotional stress whereas the parasympathetic system is most active during rest. The effects in the body of sympathetic stimulation are more widespread than the effects of parasympathetic stimulation for several reasons. Each preganglionic sympathetic fiber synapses in the ganglion with many more postganglionic fibers than does each preganglionic parasympathetic fiber. In fact, a parasympathetic fiber may only innervate four or five postganglionic fibers. The sympathetic division also stimulates many organs and tissues by way of its activation of the adrenal gland. When the sympathetic fibers stimulate the adrenal gland, epinephrine is released from the adrenal medulla and enters the circulating blood. Epinephrine is similar to norepinephrine in chemical makeup and effects. As a result, the epinephrine transported throughout the body by the blood produces an effect that resembles the simultaneous discharge of all sympathetic fibers. Organs directly activated by the norepinephrine released from their sympathetic nerves are stimulated additionally by the epinephrine circulating in the blood. For example, norepinephrine released at the heart increases contraction force and heart rate, but, when epinephrine also reaches the heart, the effects are further increased.

Somatic Nervous System

The nervous system of the efferent division of the C.N.S. consists of central and peripheral parts that innervate skeletal muscles and is known as the somatic nervous

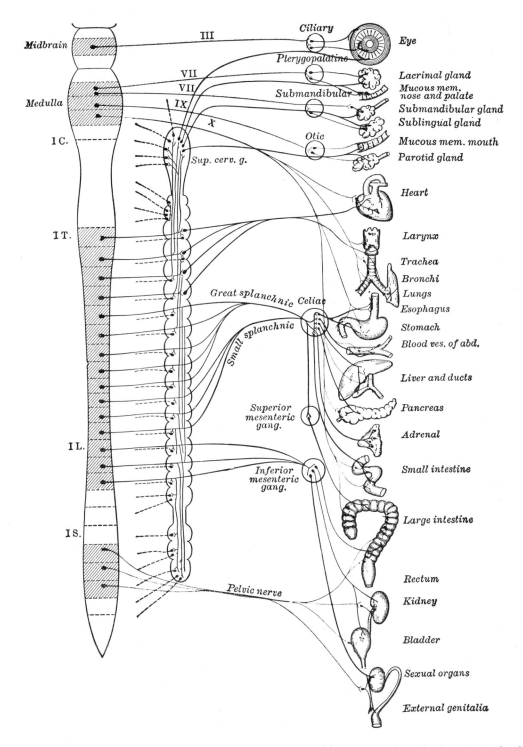

Fig. 3–27. The autonomic nervous system. (From Gray's Anatomy of the Human Body. 29th Edition. Revised and edited by Charles M. Goss. Philadelphia, Lea & Febiger, 1973.)

system. Cell bodies of these motor neurons are located in the brain stem and spinal cord. Their fibers directly connect the C.N.S. to the skeletal muscle fibers. Thus, this system differs from the autonomic nervous system whose connector neurons, which go directly to end-organs, lie outside the C.N.S. Motor neurons of the somatic nervous system can be excited by proprioceptors, as in a simple reflex, or by pathways descending from higher brain centers.

Cell bodies of motor neurons are located specifically in the ventral horn of the spinal cord. Their axons leave the cord by ventral roots and pass directly to skeletal muscle. There are more than 5,000 fibers at each level of the spine. Each fiber receives signals from a variety of such sources as the skin, muscles, joints, cerebellum, vestibular apparatus, brain stem, basal ganglia, and cerebral cortex. Motor neurons innervating a particular muscle are usually called a motor neuron pool. Neurons representing a pool possess different characteristics in terms of their size and related functions. The number of cells in a pool varies, depending on the size and function of the muscles that their neurons innervate. The cell bodies of a pool lie in a column that may extend over one level of the spinal cord, in the case of small muscles, or may be represented at two or three levels of the cord, in the case of large muscles. The axons passing out of the cord to the muscles leave by one, two, or three ventral roots. There are two types of motor fibers in a ventral root: alpha fibers and gamma fibers. Each of the thousands of alpha cell bodies can have as many as 10,000 synaptic connections; thus, motor function in performing voluntary or involuntary movements is quite complex.

Several functional characteristics are common to all motor neurons: they transmit signals, they are excitable, and they may be inhibited. However, the extent to which they carry out these functions depends on their size. Axons vary in diameter and, consequently, in the effect they have on their muscles. Axons of large diameter innervate motor units that develop large muscle force, whereas axons of small diameter innervate motor units that produce smaller muscle force. This effect occurs because axons of larger diameter transmit impulses of greater amplitude. Motor neurons respond to stimuli in various ways, depending on their size. Generally, the smaller neurons in a pool are excited by a lower intensity of stimulation. The size of a motor neuron determines its threshold level. In fact, the relative excitability of a cell is inversely related to its size. The susceptibility of motor neurons to inhibition is also related to cell size. Generally, the larger neurons are most likely to be inhibited.

Each motor neuron integrates all its input before making a response. The net effect of cell size, excitatory input, and inhibition in a motor neuron pool produces a response that is appropriate to the situation.

MOTOR PERFORMANCE IN EXERCISE AND SPORTS

In athletic performance and exercise, the initiation of movement is voluntary and begins at the cerebral cortex. But, as soon as movement begins, speed, force, range, direction, and termination of activity must be regulated. Even though movements are initiated voluntarily, the fine details of the performance are largely controlled at the unconscious level. Unconscious regulation occurs in the central nervous system at the lower brain stem and the spinal cord. All movement is a combination of conscious and unconscious aspects that function in coordination to achieve desired responses.

Cerebral Cortex and Motor Control

When learning a skilled activity, such as tennis, an individual begins to recognize correct and incorrect moves. This recognition occurs when the repeated practice of tennis skills has imprinted the correct movement patterns in the "memory bank" of the brain (the sensory cortex). With each tennis stroke voluntarily initiated by the cerebral cortex, the feedback information from the sensory receptors, primarily the proprioceptors, match the motor response to the sensory memory. Any discrepancies between the two are considered errors. Modifications in motor responses are made in subsequent moves to avoid repeating the error.

The kinds of motor responses made depend on which specific area of the motor cortex transmits the impulses. In the early stages of learning, when every move is contemplated, the specific area of the motor cortex primarily involved is the pyramidal system (see Fig. 3–13). A beginning learner is consciously aware of the hand grip on the racquet and of the position of the limbs and trunk in preparation for the stroke. When a stroke is taken, movement occurs largely by the activation of motor neurons of the pyramidal system. These neurons usually go to the spinal cord and then directly to the skeletal muscles of the hand, limbs, and trunk, in this case. As learning progresses, involvement shifts toward the extrapyramidal system in controlling motor activity (see Fig. 3–14). Whereas the stimulated pyramidal system produces specific muscular movements, the extrapyramidal system produces more general movement patterns that are associated with the more advanced stages of learning. When the neuromuscular pathways of the extrapyramidal system have been developed by practice, the tennis player is not consciously aware of detailed movements. Consequently, more attention is given to game strategy because the conscious and voluntary aspects of movement are confined mostly to initiating moves.

Cerebellum and Motor Control

When a tennis player voluntarily activates the motor cortex during a tennis serve, a complex chain of nervous events occurs. Impulses descending from the pyramidal and extrapyramidal pathways go to the muscles used in the serve and also pass to the cerebellum on the way down. During movement, the proprioceptors in the muscles, joints, tendons, cutaneous tissue, and

vestibular apparatus are stimulated. Their afferent nerves carry impulses to both the cerebellum and the sensory area of the cerebral cortex, reporting what the muscles are doing. Other input regarding the correctness of the serve is provided by auditory and visual sensory receptors. Because of the close connection between the cerebral cortex and the reticular formation in the brain stem, the basal ganglia, and the thalamus, both the cortex and cerebellum receive input regarding the serve. The cerebellum integrates all this input to determine how closely the actual serve came to the desired serve. The results of this integration are sent to the motor cortex so that the next serve can be modified, if necessary.

The cerebellum prevents a limb from going beyond a reasonable follow-through, e.g., a forehand tennis stroke. As the stroke commences, input to the cerebellum predicts the location of the limb as it continues on its course. To achieve the desired movement, the cerebellum initiates signals that eventually result in the inhibition of the agonist muscles and the excitation of the antagonist muscles. Movements involving equilibrium and balance must cooperate closely with the sensory receptors of the vestibular apparatus and the cerebellum. Movements of the head from running send signals from the vestibular apparatus to the cerebellum. After integrating this information with other input, the cerebellum initiates the stimulation of motor neurons going to the posture muscles.

Interrelationships Between the Autonomic Nervous System and the Somatic Nervous System in Motor Control

The initiation of muscular contractions comes from the cerebral cortex and/or from other subcortical areas, but the somatic efferent system directly activates skeletal muscle. The motor neurons, whose cells lie in the brain stem and ventral horn of the spinal cord, and the axons that lead from the motor neurons to muscles make up the somatic system and provide the connecting link between the C.N.S. and the "outside world," where muscles act on the external environment. But, proper muscle function requires a "support system." Muscles need an adequate blood flow and the life-giving substances it carries, such as oxygen and cell nutrients. In addition, waste products from the cells must be taken away. The organs that keep the blood flowing and enrich it with oxygen are the heart, blood vessels, and lungs. To coordinate the functions of these organs with the metabolic needs of muscle tissue requires a model that receives and interprets sensory input and subsequently acts on it through all the effector outputs. The effector systems that interact with each other to coordinate function so that movement is possible are the autonomic nervous system and the somatic nervous system. Because both systems are motor outflows from a common central nervous system, the afferents from all body parts activate the same centers that integrate responses of the effector outflows. The concern here is with the neural interactions between the somatic-autonomic systems in work and exercise.

The nerves that connect afferent input to efferent outflow, via the C.N.S., are responsible for the coordination between these systems. Information is continually fed back to the C.N.S., where it is integrated and interpreted. Impulses are then initiated along motor nerves to produce specific muscular responses. The nature of the motor response further stimulates the sensory receptors. In this way, movement is constantly monitored and adjusted to accomplish the work at hand. The operating relationship between afferent and efferent neurons in coordinating the functions of the somatic and autonomic systems in exercise is illustrated in Figure 3–28.

Muscle contractions in exercise are effected by activation of the somatic system and have a stimulating effect on the pro-

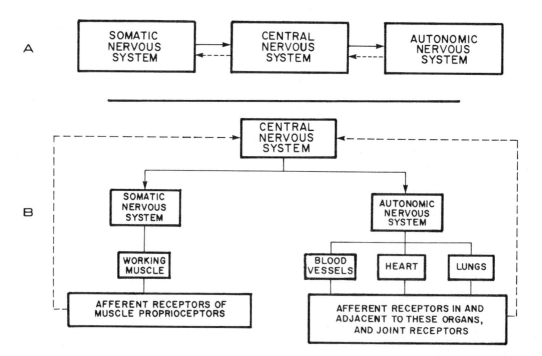

Fig. 3–28.   *A,* Interrelationships between the somatic and autonomic nervous systems during exercise. *B,* the specific systems involved with the afferent receptors that control them.

prioceptors lying within the muscles and surrounding the joints. Stimulation of the joint receptors affects the autonomic nervous system by activating ventilation, heart rate, and blood pressure. Muscle proprioceptors control the force of contractions through the afferent-central nervous system-efferent loop and have little effect, if any, on the autonomic system. The relationship through the joint receptors between the somatic system and the autonomic system is depicted in Figure 3–28A. This relationship is overly simplified in the figure, but points out the association. The autonomic system is often activated by the cerebral cortex before exercise begins. Merely thinking about the anticipated effort signals the ventilation and circulatory systems and the skeletal muscles to get ready. Nevertheless, the autonomic system usually receives its greatest stimulation from the working muscles.

The nervous pathways connecting the somatic-autonomic systems are presented in greater detail in Figure 3–28B. The sequence of events is initiated at the higher levels of the C.N.S., such as happens when an individual first begins to exercise. The skeletal muscles contract by stimulation of their somatic efferents. Movement of the skeletal joints activates their proprioceptors. Afferent signals are conveyed to the C.N.S. where they activate the autonomic system. Efferent signals are sent to the muscles of the heart, blood vessels, and ventilation to increase their activity. The amount of stimulation to these organs via the autonomic nerves depends on how hard the skeletal muscles are working, which is logical because the primary purpose of the somatic-autonomic systems is to supply the muscles with the necessary nutrients and to take away the waste products. As these organs function in exercise, their performance is continually monitored by afferent receptors located within or adjacent to them. The feedback provided leads to modifications in subsequent function so that a balance with the metabolic demands of working muscle is achieved. The roles of the heart, blood vessels, and lungs in exercise are presented in detail in subsequent chapters.

Reaction Time and Movement Time in Performance

The time that elapses from the application of a stimulus to a sensory receptor until the first muscular contraction is detected in response to the stimulus is reaction time (RT). The shortest pathway from the sensory receptor along the afferent neuron to the central nervous system and then, usually by way of interneurons, to the motor neurons of the muscle results in the smallest RT. If interneurons do not join the afferent and efferent neurons in the spinal cord, such as occurs in a simple reflex, RT should be even shorter. During athletic performance, which requires quick and coordinated movements for success, there is no awareness of reflex activity in the body. Proprioceptors in muscles and joints and reflex mechanisms regulating the heart, the circulatory system and other organs function reflexly below the level of consciousness. But, some responses in sports are initiated at a conscious level, either by a sound stimulus, such as in the start of a running race, or by vision, such as when an athlete responds to the movements of an opponent. Often the athlete with the fastest RT is most successful in sports that require quickness.

RT is just one part of a total response. The second part is movement time (MT), which is the time span between the first move (the end of RT) until the completion of the move. Response time, therefore, equals the sum of RT and MT. The importance of RT and MT in a physical task or sport depends on MT relative to RT. Obviously, the ratio of MT to RT is smaller in a 10-yard run than in a 50-yard run. In short races, RT is highly important, but, as the distance increases, the relative importance of RT decreases. Consequently, sprint runners spend much more time practicing starts than do long-distance runners.

The importance of RT and MT varies within one sport, depending on whether an athlete is playing defense or offense. Defensive linemen in football are more likely to make a tackle if they can react quickly to the snap of the ball. A fast movement once the reaction is made is also essential. However, an offensive lineman does not need to react initially as quickly as a defensive lineman because he can anticipate the starting signals. This gives him a "jump" on his opponent. But, as the play develops, both offensive and defensive players must rely equally on RT and MT in response to their opponent's moves.

Relationship Between Reaction Time and Movement Time. Few research studies have proved that the ability to react quickly (RT) is related to the ability to move quickly (MT). However, in most of these studies, the subjects knew where to move before a stimulus was presented. Responses made under this testing condition are referred to as simple RT and simple MT. Often, however, an athlete does not know in which direction to move and must chose one of several directions. Responses under this testing condition are called choice RT and choice MT. In one study that examined the relationship between choice RT and MT, 15 subjects moved the entire body 5 ft. either left, right, forward, or backward in response to a visual stimulus. When choice RT and MT were compared, a significant relationship was found. However, when the study was repeated using test conditions to obtain simple RT and MT, no relationship was found. Apparently, there are mental processes common to both RT and MT that operate under choice stimulus conditions.

Reaction Time and Movement Time Among Different Body Parts and Movement Directions. Reacting or moving quickly with the arms does not guarantee that the legs can also move with the same relative quickness.[16-18] A fast response in limb extension is not necessarily an indication of a relatively fast response in limb flexion.[19,20]

A handball player's hands may respond quickly to a ball, but his legs may not move quickly enough to reach the ball, or vice versa. The same reasoning holds true for a boxer who can punch with great speed but cannot move his feet rapidly enough to advance toward or retreat from his opponent. These relationships were brought out clearly by Loockerman and Berger,[15] who measured hand RT and MT and compared them to total body RT and MT. Hand movement was 11 in. and movement of the total body was 5 ft. A comparison between hand RT and total body RT showed that the ability to predict one from the other is possible. However, accuracy is low. When MT of the hand and MT of the total body were compared, neither could predict the other with any accuracy. These results held true whether RT and MT were initiated under simple stimulus conditions or under choice stimulus conditions.

Because RT and MT are specific to a body part, athletic performance can be predicted accurately only when the movements and limbs measured are identical to those involved in the game. If running speed is essential for success both in moving straight ahead and in dodging between players, the best predictor of those abilities is RT and MT in performing those specific moves. The specificity of RT and MT also has implications for training. To more directly improve RT and MT for a particular sport, the specific moves involved in a game should be practiced. Thus, training on the practice field has the best carry-over to the game situation.

Reaction Time and Movement Time with Age and Sex. The ability to react quickly and to move rapidly can be learned to some degree. By training for athletic sports, an individual learns how to respond faster to stimuli. With practice, the linebacker in football can interpret and respond faster to the movements of opponents. When preparing to run a sprint race, the track athlete learns from training how to get off the blocks faster.

Factors other than learning determine response time. These factors largely set the limits in speed performances for most athletes. Two of the most important factors that relate both to RT and MT and to performances involving quick movements are age and sex. Even though an individual may achieve a high level of speed from training, the young athlete may not reach the optimal level until complete physical maturity is attained. An older athlete, who has passed his "prime," may notice a decline in response time. Both RT and MT become slower with age[20a,21,22] and are often reflected in poorer athletic performance. From the ages of approximately 10 to 20 yr., response time increases. Beyond approximately the age of 30, response time gradually slows down. An example of this increase and decrease is shown in Figure 3–29, where the response was based on a circular movement of 36 in. using the hand and arm. Even when move-

ments are relatively simple and involve an 11-in. forward movement of the hand, similar results are shown.[19]

Changes in RT and MT with age follow a similar pattern for both males and females. However, the male generally has a faster MT, but only a slightly faster RT. This conclusion was based on hand movements of various complexities during one study that used an auditory stimulus[21] and another study that used a visual stimulus.[23] Males often exceed females in MT partly because of their greater force capacity. Because significant relationships between strength and MT[19] have been found, one might expect that the strongest males, on the average, move fastest. However, the reason for the differences between the sexes in RT is not as easily explained because no evidence exists indicating that nerve impulses travel faster in one sex than in the other. Perhaps the

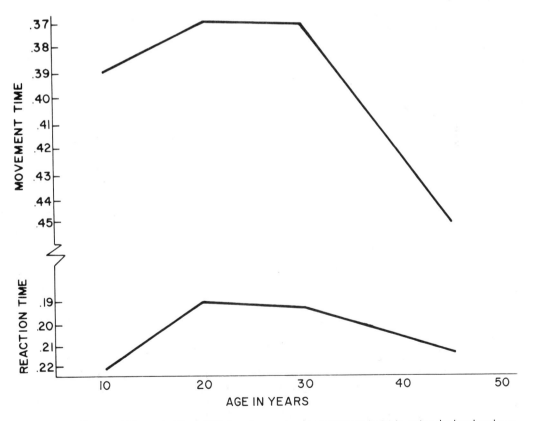

Fig. 3–29.   Changes with age in RT and MT based on a circular movement in 36 in. using the hand and arm.

differences are a consequence of sport participation. The more frequent involvement of males than of females in sports in the United States may have a conditioning effect favoring quicker RT among males.

Cross Transfer Effects from Nervous Activity

Exercising a limb by overload training with heavy loads, such as in weight lifting, improves strength of the opposite or contralateral limb.[24-26] Apparently, the contracting and working muscle sends afferent signals to the spinal cord and then to the motor neurons of the opposite limb to facilitate firing. The continuous and repeated stimulation of these motor neurons, in time, produces a greater force capacity in the muscle of the opposite limb. This phenomenon is primarily a neural effect that is initiated by the exercised limb. Because the muscle of the opposite limb is not contracting with a force approaching a threshold level, any increases in strength are not a direct effect of overloading. A study by Berger and Davies showed that not only does the opposite limb increase in strength, but the cross-transfer effects follow a pattern similar to the increases found in the exercised limb (Fig. 3–30).[24] Note that, where the largest strength increases occurred in the exercised leg as a result of training on an isokinetic device, there was a

parallel but smaller increase in the strength of the opposite limb. In this study, training continued for a nine-week period, three times weekly.

The phenomenon of cross transfer has also been observed during the recovery period following work. When one limb is exercised to exhaustion, strength recovery of the exhausted limb is enhanced by working the opposite limb.[26a] Young adult males performed a dumbbell press with a 25-lb. weight for a maximum number of times using the dominant arm. Immediately after, maximum repetitions were performed with the opposite limb. After 2 min., the dominant arm again lifted the same dumbbell for maximum repetitions. On another occasion, the same procedure was followed except the nondominant arm rested between the two trials involving the dominant arm. When the nondominant arm was worked rather than rested, the dominant arm exhibited more strength and endurance recovery. Apparently, the nondominant limb had a cross transfer effect on the dominant limb. This effect probably involved greater innervation or facilitation of the motor nerves to the muscles of the dominant arm. Similar results were found in another study that exercised the opposite arm with a relatively light load while the dominant arm was worked to exhaustion.[27] After the muscles of the oppo-

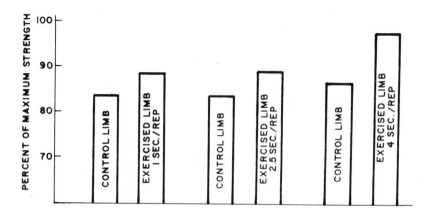

Fig. 3–30.   Knee extension strength of unexercised limbs after nine weeks of overload training the other limbs at various movement velocities (see Fig. 1–31). Note that the largest cross transfer effect of strength occurred in the control limb whose opposite pair had the greatest training effect.

site limb had worked, the force of contraction of the dominant arm was significantly raised.

PRINCIPLES FOR TRAINING

1. When success in an athletic event depends on high muscle force, performance is improved when (a) the backswing is fast, (b) the hesitation between the backswing and forward swing is minimal, and (c) the backswing is long. A fast backswing stimulates the muscle spindles in the stretched muscle. Additional stimulation is provided when the backswing is long, thereby increasing the length of the stretch. With a short hesitation between muscle stretch and concentric contraction, force is increased because more motor units are fired. Any prolonged hesitation between the stretch and the contraction results in reduced force of contraction.[28] The hesitation causes the firing frequency of spindle afferents to subside and, consequently, their subsequent effect on alpha neurons diminishes.

2. If the primary objective of a forward movement is accuracy, the backswing should be slower and shorter. The slower and shorter backswing provides less stimulation to the spindles and, in turn, to the alpha neurons supplying the muscle. The effect is less force and, as a result, better control of coordinated movements because more contraction time permits discriminative adjustments to be made to maximize accuracy.

3. Force can be increased in a specific muscle by contracting other muscles. A high jumper may increase the force with which he pushes off the ground by contracting muscles other than those of the hips and legs. Competitive weight lifters contract the muscles of the face and even the little toes when lifting with the arms and shoulders. The afferent nerves from these supportive muscles send impulses via the interneurons in the spinal cord to the primary muscles performing the work and facilitate their firing.

4. Anticipating a quick and explosive movement by "getting set " maximizes the movement effect. As the athlete assumes the starting position in a race, the stretching and contraction of muscles increases the activity of the gamma motor neurons to the muscle spindles. When this increase occurs, the spindles become more sensitive to stimulation. Therefore, when the starting gun is fired, a maximum number of spindle afferents are activated. This results in the stimulation of more motor neurons to the running muscles and in greater force capacity.

5. Applying force too early in a striking movement may diminish the striking force. When swinging a bat forward to hit a baseball, too much force applied too soon may stimulate the Golgi tendon organs to inhibit muscle force. As a result, when contact is made with the ball, the bat is not swinging with optimum velocity. The bat should be swung with less initial acceleration and gradually increased until it strikes the ball. By avoiding a sudden initial movement, one can minimize the activation of the tendon organs and their inhibiting effect on the contracting muscles.

6. Skillful movement develops when feedback information from the proprioceptors is matched to the correct technique. During a physical performance involving skill, the athlete is consciously aware of the "correct" movements. He matches his perceptions to the feedback received from the joint receptors and modifies subsequent movement to correct for errors. Learning occurs when what is perceived as correct agrees with what is said by the proprioceptors. The neuromuscular patterns of the skill become more permanently ingrained in the nervous system because of the facilitation and inhibition of the right muscles. When the perception of the movement is incorrect in the athlete's mind and the feedback is conformed to this perception, poor performance results. This can be avoided by proper and correct instruction of the athlete so that perception is correct.

7. Frequent practice and repetitive movements are necessary to learn a skilled activity so that innate reflexes may be inhib-

ited. Some skills take longer than others to learn because of the inhibiting effect provided by some reflexes. The righting and equilibrium reflexes controlled by the vestibular apparatus must be inhibited before certain skills can be learned effectively. To learn skills involving somersaults and other rotational moves, such as those encountered in gymnastics and diving, the individual must consciously impose inhibition on these reflex responses. The student must apply muscular contractions that are antagonistic to the reflex response. As learning progresses and synaptic inhibition of the reflex circuits occurs, conscious contraction of the antagonistic muscles is unnecessary. Regular practice and repetitive movement are essential for overcoming reflexes that hinder the learning of a physical skill.

8. Muscle force can be enhanced by the position of the head in reference to the rest of the body. Certain moves in athletic sports can be improved when muscle force is augmented by the position of the head. In diving and tumbling, ventriflexion of the head facilitates trunk and limb flexion for the foward somersault, and dorsiflexion facilitates extension for the layout backward somersault. More muscle force is possible in these moves when facilitation is provided by neck position. When lifting barbells, more weight can often be raised in the supine bench press when the head is dorsiflexed; ventriflexion of the head increases the force of the elbow flexors. To achieve optimal performance in skills that require high muscle force, one must position the head to augment force provided, of course, that movement form is not adversely affected. When skill can be maintained while the head is positioned to achieve maximum force, a better performance results.

9. Stretching a muscle relieves muscle cramps, minimizes soreness after exercise, and increases joint flexibility. Stretching a muscle with a steady pull may initially stimulate the muscle spindles, but muscle activity reduces shortly after the stretch is main-

tained. Further relaxation of the stretched muscle is possible when the antagonist is contracted. Then, the reflex pattern of reciprocal inhibition becomes involved, causing still more relaxation (by inhibition) in the stretched muscle. A general rule to follow for the alleviation of muscle cramps, the reduction of muscle soreness, and the increase in joint flexibility, is to forcefully contract the muscle that is antagonistic to the muscle of concern. As indicated, such a contraction relaxes the muscle optimally and further reduces its resistance to stretch.

10. Balance is maintained when the line of gravity is over the base of support. To improve balance, the base of support is enlarged and the weight center of the body is lowered. The vestibular apparatus maintains the desired balance of the body by initiating the right contractions in the effector muscles. The response to the movement of the proprioceptors in the joints and skin provides feedback to correct for later moves if necessary. If the main concern is balance, the body assumes all the positions to maximize this quality. But, if the primary concern is graceful movement, such as in dancing, the individual may have to sacrifice balance for aesthetic movement. In any event, sensory input is always matched with the desired motor output.

11. To improve RT and MT, one should practice and train for the specific moves required by an activity. Specificity of training, as it applies to RT and MT, means that training effects are highly specific to and are a consequence of the movements made in practice. Logically, then, the best way to enhance RT and MT in a particular sport is to practice the exact movements that must be improved. In this way, the most appropriate neuromuscular patterns are developed so that, when stimuli present themselves, less time is needed to respond and to move the body for the completion of a task. With the right kind of practice, the responses to stimuli become less conscious as they are initiated in the higher brain centers.

Quick movements, in particular, are a result of a reduction in decision time at the level of the cerebral cortex. But, to achieve largely subcortical control of RT and MT, one must train with specificity.

12. A limb prevented from moving because of a cast or other restriction can be given an exercise effect by training the opposite limb. The synergistic effects on unexercised muscles, brought about by working muscle, are associated with an increase in force and endurance. Within the central nervous system, interneurons carry action potentials from spindles of exercised muscle to motor neurons leading to the opposite limb. As a result, some of the motor neurons are activated to contract in the inactive limb while other motor neurons to the limb are facilitated. Thus, their threshold level lowers. Consequently, atrophy of muscle around inactive joints can be minimized. Periodic and regular overload training of healthy muscles, where the loads are heavy for about 10 repetitions, seems the best way to guarantee a training effect in the impaired muscles of the opposite limb.

REFERENCES

1. Merton, R.A.: Voluntary strength and fatigue. J. Physiol., *123*:553, 1954.
2. Jansen, J.K.S., and Rudjord, T.: On the silent period and Golgi tendon organs of the cat. Acta Physiol. Scand., *62*:364, 1964.
3. Hufschmidt, H.J.: Demonstration of autogenic inhibition and its significance in human voluntary movement. *In* Muscle Afferents and Motor Control. Edited by R. Grant. New York, John Wiley & Sons, 1966.
4. Houk, J., and Henneman, E.: Responses of Golgi tendon organs to active contractions of the soleus muscle of the cat. J. Neurophysiol., *30*:466, 1967.
5. Brunnstrom, S.: Historical approach. *In* Approaches to Treatment of Patients with Neuromuscular Dysfunction. Edited by C. Sattely. Dubuque, William C. Brown Book Co., 1974.
5a. Latimer, R.: Utilization of tonic neck and labyrinthine reflexes for facilitation of work output. Phy. Ther. Rev., *33*:39, 1953.
6. Hellebrandt, F.: Physiological effects of simultaneous static and dynamic exercise. Am. J. Phys. Med., *35*:106, 1956.
7. Hellebrandt, F., and Waterland, J.: Motor patterning in stress. Am. J. Phys. Med., *41*:56, 1962.
7a. Hellebrandt, F., Schode, M., and Carns, M.: Methods of evoking TNR in normal individuals. Am. J. Phys. Med., *41*:90, 1962.
7b. Kinesiology and Biomechanics Research Laboratory, Sargent College of Allied Health Professions, Boston University, 1968. Unpublished study.
8. Norris, F.H., Jr., Gasteiger, E.L., and Chatfield, P.O.: An electromyographic study of induced and spontaneous muscle cramps. Electroencephalogr. Clin. Neurophysiol., *9*:139, 1957.
9. Petajan, J.H., and Eagan, C.J.: Effect of temperature and physical fitness on the triceps surae reflex. J. Appl. Physiol., *25*:16, 1968.
9a. Talaq, T.S.: Residual muscular soreness as influenced by concentric, eccentric, and static contractions. Res. Q., *44*:458, 1973.
10. Hunt, C.C.: The effects of stretch receptors from muscles on the discharge of motor neurons. J. Physiol., *117*:359, 1952.
11. Inman, V.T., et al.: Relation of human electromyogram to muscular tension. Electroencephalogr. Clin. Neurophysiol., *4*:187, 1952.
12. de Vries, H.A.: Prevention of muscular distress after exercise. Res. Q., *32*:117, 1961.
13. de Vries, H.A.: Electromyographic observations of the effects of static stretching upon muscular distress. Res. Q., *32*:468, 1961.
14. Berger, R.A.: Tonic neck reflexes in muscular strength. Unpublished study. Biokinetics Research Laboratory, Temple University, 1973.
15. Loockerman, W.D., and Berger, R.A.: Accuracy of predicting reaction and movement times of a gross motor performance from the dominant hand under simple and choice stimulus conditions. Percept. Mot. Skills, *33*:1326, 1971.
16. Lotter, W.S.: Interrelationships among reaction times and speeds of movement in different limbs. Res. Q., *31*:147, 1960
17. Lotter, W.S.: Specificity or generality of speed of systematically related movements. Res. Q., *32*:55, 1961.
18. Seashore, L.H., and Seashore, R.H.: Individual differences in simple auditory reaction times of hands, feet, and jaws. J. Exp. Psychol., 29:342, 1941.
19. Henry F.M., Totter, W.S., and Smith, L.E.: Factorial structure of individual differences in limb speed, reaction, and strength. Res. Q., *33*:70, 1962.
20. Smith, K.E.: Reaction time and movement time in four large muscle movements. Res. Q., *32*:88, 1961.
20a. Fleishman, E.A.: The structure and measurement of physical fitness. Englewood Cliffs, N.J., Prentice-Hall, Inc., 1964.
21. Henry, F.M.: Stimulus complexity, movement complexity, age, and sex in relation to reaction latency and speed in limb movements. Res. Q., *32*:353, 1961.
22. Mendryke, S.: Reaction time, movement time, and task specificity relationships at ages 12, 22, and 48 years. Res. Q., *31*:156, 1960.
23. Bartell Associates, Inc.: The study of police women competency in the performance of sector police work in the City of Philadelphia. State College, Pa., 1978.

24. Berger, R.A., and Davies, A.: Cross transfer effects as a function of force changes in the opposite limb. Unpublished study. Biokinetics Research Laboratory, Temple University, 1976.
25. Carlson, B.R.: Cross transfer during flexor serial isometric trials. Am. Correct. Ther. J., *27*:36, 1973.
26. Darcus, H.D., and Salter, N.: The effect of repeated muscular exertion on muscle strength. J. Physiol., *129*:325, 1955.

26a. Berger, R.A.: Comparison between two methods of recovery from muscular fatigue. Am. Correct. Ther. J., *24*:73, 1970.
27. Karpovich, C.V.: Physiological and psychological dynamogenic factors in exercise. Arbeitsphysiol., *9*:626, 1937.
28. Gardner, E.B.: Proprioceptive reflexes and their participation in motor skills. Quest, *12*:1, 1969.

4

The Heart in Work and Exercise

The heart is a four-chambered pump that moves blood throughout the body. The pumping action occurs by the alternating contraction and relaxation of the heart muscle. During rest, the heart beats slowly because the metabolic needs of the body are minimal. But, when the skeletal muscles are doing heavy work and need a large supply of oxygen, the heart may beat almost three times faster to increase blood flow. The coordination between energy needs of the skeletal muscle and cardiac activity permits man to function continuously over relatively long periods of time. With increased metabolism of muscle and the corresponding accumulation of chemical by-products that must be discarded, the need for more blood flow is greatly increased. To maintain an adequate source of ATP energy over an extended time period, adequate quantities of oxygen must also be conveyed by the blood to the working muscles. Moving blood to achieve a balance between energy input and output is the function of cardiac tissue.

Because of the close relationship between muscle metabolism and heart function, heart rate is used to estimate the stress placed on the vascular system during work or exercise. The cardiovascular fitness of individuals can be compared by the response of heart rate to a given amount of work. In addition, heart rate can be used in exercise to achieve a desired stress level.

STRUCTURE AND FUNCTION OF THE HEART

The heart muscle is similar to skeletal muscle in some aspects. Both contract con-

centrically to perform work; both need oxygen for prolonged activity; both of their muscle fibers are under nervous control; and both use the same nutrients to maintain life. However, these muscles differ largely in function. Although both need oxygen for long and continued activity, skeletal muscle can work without oxygen for a short period of time. The heart cannot sustain an oxygen debt. Although the heart and skeletal muscle are under nervous control, only the heart can contract without nervous stimulation. Although heart tissue never rests for more than a second, skeletal muscle can rest for hours. Some of these differences in function are reflected in structural variations between skeletal and heart muscle.

Cardiac Tissue

The heart is a muscle located in the chest (Figs. 4–1, 4–2). Its walls are mostly composed of a muscle whose structure is different from either skeletal or smooth muscle. But, in some respects, heart and skeletal muscle have the same characteristics. They both have myofibrils consisting of actin and myosin filaments that interdigitate and slide among each other during contraction. Heart muscle is referred to as myocardium. The lining of the inner surface of the myocardium, in contact with the blood in the heart chambers, is composed of a thin layer of cells called the endocardium. The outer layer is lined with a thin membrane referred to as the epicardium. The heart is covered by a fibrous sac called the pericardium.

The walls of the heart vary in thickness because of the differences in blood pres-

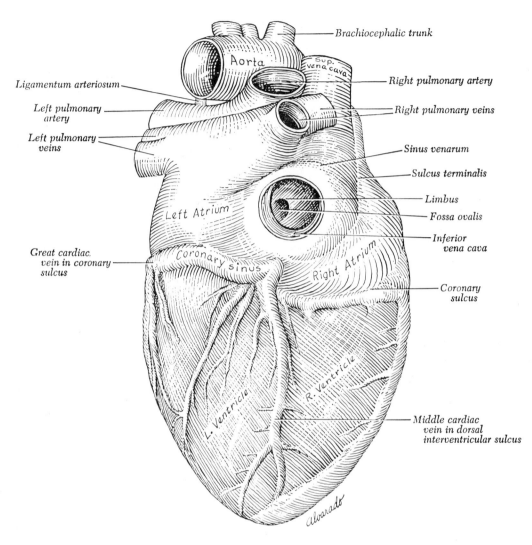

Fig. 4–1.   The heart viewed from the front (ventral). (From Gray's Anatomy of the Human Body. 29th Edition. Revised and edited by Charles M. Goss. Philadelphia, Lea & Febiger, 1973.)

sures and resistance to blood flow among the chambers. Blood passing out of the left ventricle must overcome the large pressure and resistance in the aortic artery. To accomplish this, the left ventricle contracts with more force than do the muscles of the other chambers. As a result, the left ventricular wall hypertrophies more. The relative differences in blood pressures among the chambers indicate the muscle forces required to move blood through the heart. The blood pressures between the two lower

chambers (the ventricles) can differ by as much as fivefold. The blood pressures in the two upper chambers (the atria) can be up to 50 times less than pressures in the left ventricles.

The four-chambered heart has four one-way valves that form the openings between the atria and the ventricles and between the great arteries and the ventricles (Fig. 4–3). The two valves between the atria and ventricles are called atrioventricular valves (AV valves) and permit blood to flow from atrium

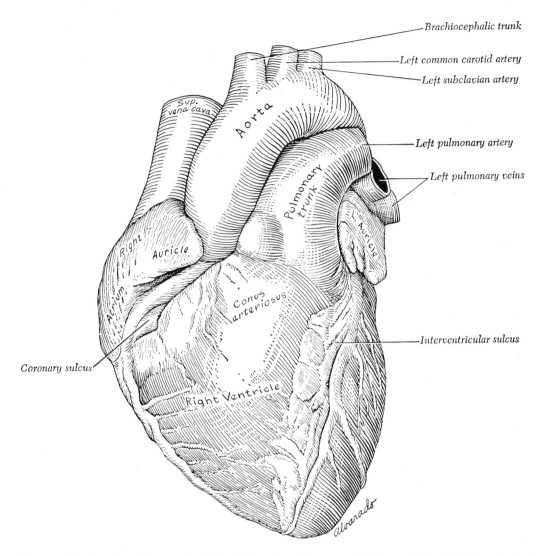

Fig. 4–2.   The heart viewed from the back (dorsal). (From Gray's Anatomy of the Human Body. 29th Edition. Revised and edited by Charles M. Goss. Philadelphia, Lea & Febiger, 1973.)

to ventricle, but not back again. The valves between the right ventricle and pulmonary artery and between the left ventricle and aorta artery are called semilunar valves. There are no true valves through which the blood flows from the large vein into the right atrium, nor through which the pulmonary veins direct blood into the left atrium. To prevent blood flow in the wrong direction, the valves are fastened by fibrous strands to muscular projections of the ventricular walls. Valves are not opened or closed by

these muscular projections; they are just prevented from eversion.

The individual muscle cell of cardiac tissue is striated and contains both thick myosin and thin actin filaments, as does skeletal muscle (Fig. 4–4). Cardiac cells are shorter than skeletal fibers and have several branching processus. The processus of the cells lying next to each other are joined end to end at structures known as intercalated disks. The membranes of adjacent cells are fused within these disks so that action poten-

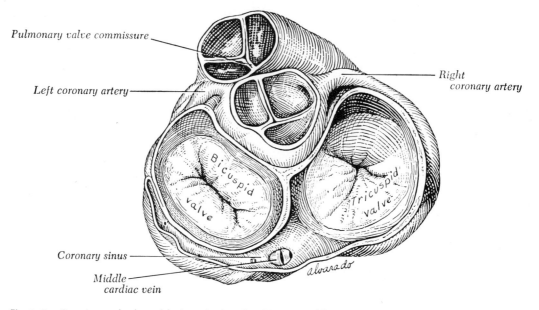

Pulmonary valve commissure

Left coronary artery

Right coronary artery

Bicuspid valve

Tricuspid valve

Coronary sinus

Middle cardiac vein

alvarado

Fig. 4–3.   Openings and valves of the heart in closed position viewed from above after removal of atria and arteries. (From Gray's Anatomy of the Human Body. 29th Edition. Revised and edited by Charles M. Goss. Philadelphia, Lea & Febiger, 1973.)

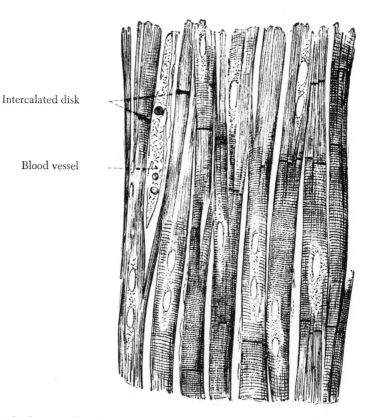

Intercalated disk

Blood vessel

Fig. 4–4.   Longitudinal section of cardiac muscle fibers. (From Gray's Anatomy of the Human Body. 29th Edition. Revised and edited by Charles M. Goss. Philadelphia, Lea & Febiger, 1973.)

tials can be transmitted from one cell to another. The points at which membrane fusion occurs are called nexuses. In addition to the usual type of cardiac muscle, certain areas of the heart contain specialized muscle fibers that have a different appearance. These fibers are essential for normal excitation of the heart and make up a network known as the conducting system. They contact other cardiac fibers to form nexuses, which transmit action potentials from cell to cell.

Cardiac Hypertrophy

The increased pressure within the left ventricle, as a result of forcing the blood into the high pressure of the artery, eventually produces more hypertrophy there than in any other chamber wall. When the heart is subjected to the vigors of exercise over prolonged periods, additional hypertrophy occurs. This effect is shown when thickness of the left ventricular wall and heart volume are compared in athletes and nonathletes. The average athlete generally has a ventricular wall that is thicker than that of a nonathlete. Athletes may exceed nonathletes in thickness by 1%, on the average, to 30% or more.[1] The extent of the thickness may be related to the nature of the training overload. In endurance athletes, who train by long sustained activity during which cardiac output is maintained at maximum or near-maximum levels, the ventricular thickness does not appear to increase as much as does the ventricular thickness in athletes who participate in activities that require brief but high muscular efforts, such as wrestling.[1] Apparently, the large elevation in blood pressure during an explosive effort requires a greater force of cardiac contraction to overcome the increased arterial pressure. This effect places more overload on the left ventricle and results in greater hypertrophy.

Cardiac Volume

Physical training also influences volume of the ventricular cavity. Individuals who constantly train by stressing the heart and circulatory system develop larger heart volumes.[1] These changes are more pronounced in endurance athletes than in power athletes, such as football players and weight lifters. Because ventricular volume partly determines how much blood is pumped out of the heart, training that enhances heart volume also increases stroke volume (the amount of blood pumped each beat). This relationship was shown after subjects trained for seven weeks, two to three days per week, on a bicycle ergometer.[2] Heart volume increased about 13% and stroke volume during exercise rose about 25%. The proportionally greater increase in stroke volume than in heart volume was probably owing to another factor that enhances stroke volume during training. This factor is ventricular force, which results in a greater emptying of blood in the left ventricle.

Heart volume, on the average, is larger in males than in females by about 40% among untrained individuals.[2] This difference in volume is partly the result of the difference in body size between the sexes. Generally, larger individuals have greater heart sizes. However, after strenuous training when heart volumes of males may rise 18% and of females 29%, the difference between the sexes drops from 40% to about 18%.[2] This 18% reflects more closely the body weight differences between males and females.

Blood Flow in the Heart

Blood is moved from one chamber of the heart to the other chamber by pressure changes caused by the contracting heart. When the atria contract, the pressure on the blood within the atria exceeds the pressure within the ventricles and causes blood flow. After the ventricles fill with blood and the atria relax, the ventricles contract, and the blood pressure within them increases. When ventricular pressure exceeds arteriolar pressure, the blood is forced into the vessels of the circulatory system.

The sequence of blood flow in the heart begins in the right atrium, where venous return comes from two large veins: the superior vena cava which brings blood from the upper body, and the inferior vena cava which carries blood from the lower body (Fig. 4–5). The blood moves from the right atrium into the right ventricle through the AV valve (or bicuspid) by the contracting atrium. From here, the blood is pushed out by the contracting right ventricle through the semilunar valve into the pulmonary artery. The blood picks up oxygen and releases carbon dioxide in the lungs and returns to the left atrium by way of the pulmonary vein. The contracting atrium moves the blood through the other AV valve (or tricuspid) to the left ventricle, where it is then forced out by contraction through the other semilunar valve into the aorta artery. The right and left atria contract simultaneously as do the right and left ventricles. The contraction of the atria begins slightly before that of the ventricles (0.08 to 0.12 sec.). The effect is a continuous and equal flow of blood from both the atria and ventricles. The output into all the arteries is the same.

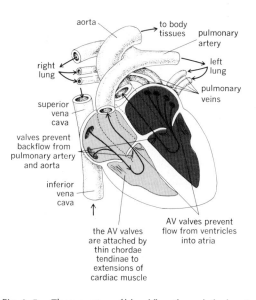

Fig. 4–5.   The sequence of blood flow through the heart. (From Vander, A.J., Sherman, J.H., and Luciano, D.S.: Human Physiology —The Mechanisms of Body Function. New York, McGraw-Hill, Inc., 1975. Used with permission of McGraw-Hill Book Co.)

Blood Vessels of the Heart

The heart must be continuously supplied with oxygen and metabolic fuels to replace the energy used in work. A balance between energy used and energy restored is achieved when the working heart slows down to match work output to energy input. Energy is restored in the heart by the substances in the blood that flow through the heart in the coronary blood vessels. The by-products of metabolism are likewise carried away by blood flow. The exchange of substances between the blood and the cardiac cells occurs in the capillaries just as it does in skeletal muscle. The sequence of flow moves from the coronary arteries to the arterioles, capillaries, venules, and then to the veins. Venous blood from the coronary vessels flows into the heart directly above the AV valve in the right atrium.

The coronary arteries encircle the heart like a crown (hence, the term coronary) set upon the brow of the ventricles (see Figs. 4–1 and 4–2). The two coronary arteries

arise from the left and right sides of the aortic sinus and branch off into the heart muscle. These branches provide a profuse network of vessels to all the cells. As a result, the distance between the blood and the active contractile fibers is small. This probably accounts for the large amount of oxygen extracted from the blood in the capillaries. In fact, at rest, approximately 75% of the oxygen is extracted from this blood. This amount is significantly larger than the 5% of oxygen extracted from the blood in skeletal muscle at rest.

The coronary vessels fill with blood during ventricular diastole and empty during systole. From 3 to 10% of the entire systolic output of blood passes through the heart. In heavy work or exercise, coronary blood flow may increase fivefold. The consequence of strenuous exercise over a long training period is an increase in mitochondrial mass, which plays a significant role in enhancing oxidative capacity of the heart.[3] Whether or not biochemical adaptations in respiratory enzyme levels occur in cardiac tissue from physical training is not clear. The indication is that training does not significantly increase the enzymes (expressed per gram weight of cardiac tissue) of the mitochondrial respiratory chain,[4] perhaps because enzyme levels are normally about five times higher in the heart than in the skeletal muscle. Therefore, heart muscle may be functioning within its respiratory limits even during strenuous work.

Physical work may open more blood vessels in the heart.[5-9] Collateralization occurs in the arterial tree as a probable consequence of increased blood flow from vasodilatation during exercise. Myocardial collateralization is more pronounced in hearts that are so occluded by atherosclerosis that hypoxia (diminished oxygen supply) occurs in the surrounding tissue. This situation was shown in animal studies when coronary circulation was impeded.[5] As a result of hypoxia, the ratio of capillary vessels to ventricular muscle fibers increased after training. The effect was reduced hypoxia because of enhanced blood flow and oxygen absorption by the heart muscle.

TRANSMISSION OF HEART IMPULSE

When motor nerves to skeletal muscles are severed, muscles cannot contract. This situation does not occur with cardiac muscle. When the nerves connecting the central nervous system to the heart are cut, the heart can still contract. The stimulation for a heart contraction, when innervation is absent, is provided by the volume and velocity with which blood enters the cardiac chambers. Regulation of cardiac pumping by a mechanism other than nervous activity is referred to as intrinsic autoregulation. When at rest, control of the heart is provided by both intrinsic autoregulation and neural stimulation. During heavy work or exercise, however, intrinsic autoregulation begins to play a larger role. Under normal conditions, the initiation of an impulse in the heart oc-

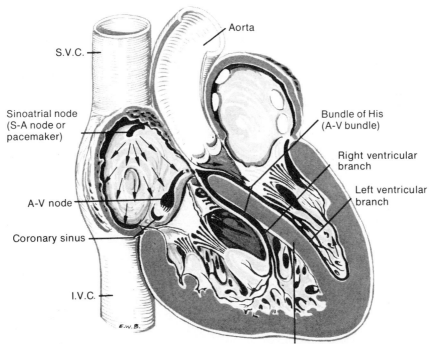

Fig. 4–6.   The sinoatrial node (SA node) and impulses that emanate to all parts of the heart. (From Schottelius, B.A., and Schottelius, D.D.: Textbook of Physiology. 18th Edition. St. Louis, The C.V. Mosby Co., 1978.)

curs at the sinoatrial (SA) node, which is located in the posterior wall of the right atrium near the opening of the superior vena cava (Fig. 4–6). The node is only 3 mm. wide and 1 cm. long. Impulses spread from the SA node to the muscle fibers of the atria, causing them to contract. At the same time, impulses are transmitted to the atrioventricular (AV) node and to the bundle of fibers called the atrioventricular bundle (bundle of His). From here, the impulses are conveyed to the ventricles, causing them to contract. A delay of approximately 0.10 sec. permits the propagation of an impulse through the AV node to the bundle of His, thereby allowing the atria sufficient time to complete a contraction before ventricular contraction begins (Fig. 4–7). Impulses travel rapidly along the AV bundles (1 m/sec.) so that all the muscle fibers of the ventricles receive the impulses at approximately the same time. The SA node is called the pacemaker of the heart because it controls the beat of the heart. Although the AV node and AV bundle may initiate impulses under abnormal conditions, the impulses are usually controlled by the SA node. The rate of impulse discharge is greater at the SA node than at both the AV node and AV bundle. When two joined cells contract autonomously at different rates, the faster cell sets the pace for the slower cell. This phenomenon is responsible for the SA node's role as pacemaker of the heart.

All-or-None Principle of Heart Muscle

The all-or-none principle for heart muscle is the same as that for skeletal muscle but with one exception. In skeletal muscle, only individual fibers receiving impulses at their threshold values contract. But, in cardiac muscle, where the muscle fibers are not insulated from each other by sarcolemma, an impulse can travel from an excited fiber to all the other fibers. As a result, the all-or-none principle applies to the whole heart rather than to a single fiber, as in skeletal muscle.

Electrical Activity and Mechanical Events of the Heart

The electrical activity of the heart varies during contraction and relaxation. A recording of this activity is called an electrocardiogram (ECG). Electrical signals are picked up by electrodes attached to the surface of the skin. The ECG is the electrical sum of all cardiac fibers during depolarization and repolarization. Each beat of the heart results in an electrical wave form that is similar from beat to beat. The parts of the wave correspond to different stages of depolarization and repolarization of the atria and ventricles. The upper portion of Figure 4–8 is an electrocardiogram that shows the wave form of a single heart beat.

The P wave represents depolarization of the atria; the QRS interval reflects depolari-

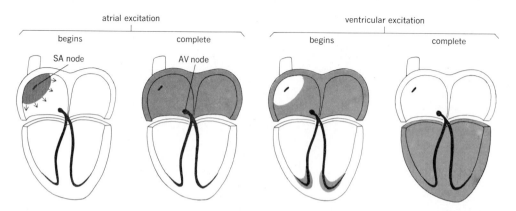

Fig. 4–7.   Cardiac excitation begins and ends in the atria before excitation begins in the ventricles. (From Vander, A.J., Sherman, J.H., and Luciano, D.S.: Human Physiology—The Mechanisms of Body Function. New York, McGraw-Hill, Inc., 1975. Used with permission of McGraw-Hill Book Co.)

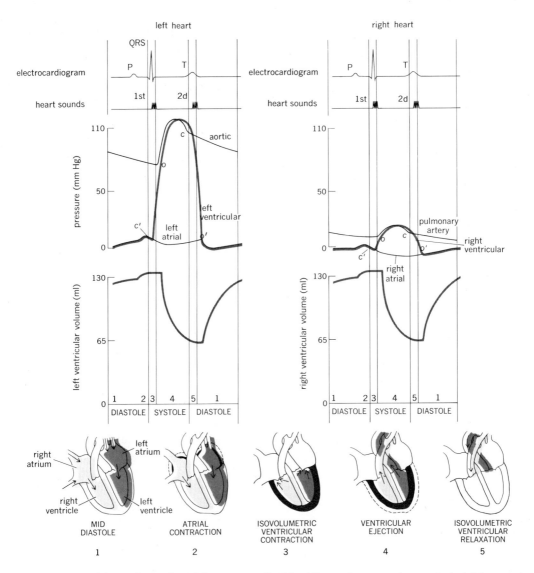

Fig. 4–8. Stages of the cardiac cycle and the corresponding blood flow and pressure changes. In the left heart and aorta, the AV valve closes at C' and opens at O'. At O, the aortic valve opens and, at C, it closes. The parts of the heart contracting are in black. In the right heart and pulmonary arteries, the AV valve closes at C' and opens at O'. At O, the pulmonary valve opens and, at C, it closes. (From Vander, A.J., Sherman, J.H., and Luciano, D.S.: Human Physiology—The Mechanisms of Body Function. New York, McGraw-Hill, Inc., 1975. Used with permission of McGraw-Hill Book Co.)

zation of the ventricles and repolarization of the atria; and the T wave represents the repolarization of the ventricles. The ECG is related to the mechanical events of the cardiac cycle that occur as a consequence of the pressure changes of blood brought about by cardiac contractions. The ECG and the corresponding changes in blood flow and pres-

sure in the heart are summarized in Figure 4–8. This figure looks formidable but, when studied in stages, can help the reader to understand the exact relationship between the ECG and the mechanical events of the heart. The cardiac cycle is presented first for the left heart and then for the right heart. Recall that diastole is the name of the period of ventricular relaxation. The various stages of the cardiac cycle are presented, beginning with late diastole when the left atrium and ventricle are both relaxed; moving to systole when the ventricular muscle contracts; and ending with early diastole after which the ventricular muscle relaxes.

Mid-Diastole. Although both the left atrium and ventricle are relaxed, left atrial pressure begins to exceed slightly left ventricular pressure because of the blood entering the atrium from the pulmonary veins. As a result, blood passes from the atrium to the ventricle before atrial contraction. In fact, about 80% of the blood filling the ventricle occurs before atrial contraction, and most of this amount occurs during early ventricular diastole. The aortic valve between the aorta and left ventricle is closed because ventricular pressure is greater than aortic pressure as blood flows from the atrium into the ventricle.

Atrial Contraction. At the end of atrial diastole, the SA node discharges and depolarizes the atrium, as shown by the P wave, to cause contraction. The quantity of blood in the ventricle just before ventricular systole is called the end-diastolic volume.

Isovolumetric Ventricular Contraction. The wave of depolarization passes from the atrium through the ventricle, as indicated by the QRS wave of atrial repolarization and ventricular depolarization, and sets off ventricular contraction. As the ventricle contracts, it pushes against the blood and causes pressure to rise steeply. The increased pressure closes the AV valve to prevent backflow into the atrium. For a brief period, blood does not flow out of the ventricle because aortic pressure still exceeds ventricular pressure. This early phase of ventricular systole is called isovolumetric ventricular contraction because ventricular volume remains constant during this period. In this phase, the length of cardiac muscle fibers remains constant, as in an isometric skeletal muscle contraction.

Ventricular Ejection. When ventricular pressure exceeds aortic pressure, the aortic valve opens and blood ejects into the aorta. The ventricle does not empty completely. The amount remaining after ejection is called the end-systolic volume. Aortic pressure continues to rise with ventricular pressure as blood is squeezed out by systole. At the same time, atrial pressure rises as blood flow continues from the pulmonary veins.

Isovolumetric Ventricular Relaxation. After ventricular systole, the ventricle relaxes rapidly and pressure falls below aortic pressure. Consequently, the aortic valve closes. This phase is represented by the T wave of repolarization. However, ventricular pressure remains larger than atrial pressure and the AV valve remains closed. This early phase of ventricular diastole is called isovolumetric relaxation. This condition ends when ventricular pressure falls below atrial pressure and the AV valves open to allow blood to fill the ventricle. As previously indicated, ventricular filling is almost complete during early diastole, thereby ensuring that filling is not seriously diminished during times of rapid heart rate even though the duration of diastole is greatly reduced.

Electrocardiogram and Pulmonary Circulation Pressures. The relationships between the electrical activity and the pressures in the right side of the heart are summarized in Figure 4–8. The events in the right heart occur simultaneously with those in the left heart, and the patterns of response are similar. The big difference between the right and left hearts is ventricular and arterial pressures, which are considerably lower in the former. The left side of the heart must apply more pressure by contraction than the right side to force out the blood into a relatively higher pressure system. This additional pressure accounts for the thicker muscular walls of the left ventricle. But the pulmonary circulation of the right heart is a low-pressure system because the pulmonary artery provides relatively little pressure resistance to blood flow. Even though pressure differs between the right and left ventricles, both ventricles eject the same quantity of blood at each heart beat.

HEART ACTIVITY IN REST AND WORK

The function of cardiac tissue is unique in several ways. It repeatedly contracts with relatively little rest; contractions occur without any conscious effort; the pattern of movement is basically identical from one contraction to the next; its main purpose is to push blood through vessels; it hardly ever fatigues; and it meets all kinds of work demands. Skeletal muscle cannot work continuously without becoming exhausted and contractions are not always initiated at an unconscious level. Also, the sequence of pattern of contraction in skeletal muscle varies, depending on the load to be moved and the direction of the move. A major distinction between heart muscle and skeletal muscle lies in their primary functions: skeletal muscle moves the bones at the joints and supports the joints; heart muscle moves blood throughout the circulatory system. The activity of the heart can be understood by studying the functional characteristics unique to the heart and how these characteristics vary according to training, sex, and age.

Cardiac Cycle

The time from the end of one heart contraction to the end of the next contraction is called the cardiac cycle. Each cycle is initiated by an impulse at the SA node in the right atrium. During a cycle, the heart contracts and relaxes. The relaxation phase of atrial contraction (diastole) at rest lasts more than seven times longer than the contraction phase (systole). In the ventricles, the diastolic phase is about 25% longer than the systolic phase at rest.

Heart Rate

The number of ventricular beats per minute is heart rate (HR). Heart rate is usually determined from pulse rate, which is the number of pressure waves per minute along the carotid artery at the neck or the radial artery at the wrist. In normal individuals, HR equals pulse rate. The time period from one heart beat to the next is the interval between cardiac cycles. Control of HR at rest and during work is maintained by the blood entering the heart and by the autonomic nervous system. Stimulation of the vagus nerves to the heart slows down (bradycardia) HR whereas stimulation of the sympathetic nerves speeds up HR (tachycardia).

At rest, HR is about 75 for nonathletes and 53 for athletes who train primarily aerobically. The decreased HR at rest for athletes is a consequence of physical training that is carried out continuously and over a long time span. The cause of resting bradycardia is related to the effects of training on the autonomic nervous system that are particularly reflected in the vagus nerves (parasympathetic division) to the heart. Training may either increase parasympathetic inhibition of HR (result of greater stimulation), decrease sympathetic stimulation, or affect both. The present research findings indicate that resting bradycardia is primarily the result of inhibition of HR by increased stimulation of the parasympathetic fibers.[10,11]

Although HR is about the same for males and females during rest, HR does not remain the same during work. Among young adults, working at 50% of maximum oxygen consumption ($\dot{V}O_2$ max), males have lower HR values than do females.[12] These values are about 130 for males and 140 for females. At maximum work, differences between the sexes in HR are not apparent. However, maximum HR decreases for both sexes with age. At age 10, HR is about 210 and drops steadily to 165 at age 65.[13,14] The relationship between HR and age is shown in Figure 4–9.

Stroke Volume

The amount of blood that a ventricle ejects in one heart beat is called stroke volume (SV). Aerobic training increases SV when training is strenuous and is carried out for a prolonged period. As expected, SV differs among trained and untrained individuals at rest and during work. Untrained

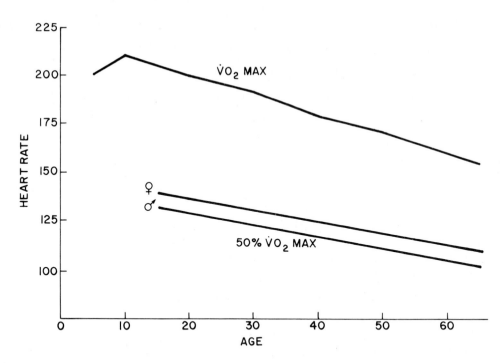

Fig. 4–9. Changes in heart rate with age and sex.

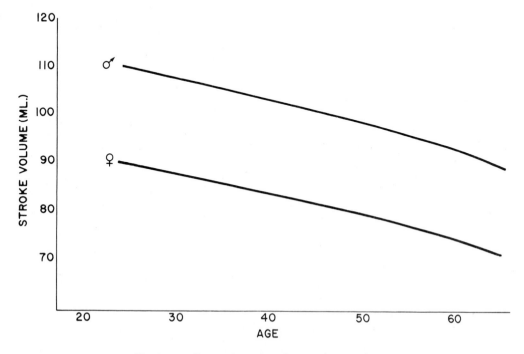

Fig. 4–10. Changes in stroke volume with age and sex.

young adults at rest pump about 80 ml. of blood per beat; the trained pump 110 ml. During maximum work, the SV for the untrained group rises to 110 ml; the SV for the trained group reaches 160 ml. Some athletes with high aerobic capacity have SVs of 220 ml. or more.

SV differs with age and between sexes (Fig. 4–10). The SV in work of the average young adult male (110 ml.) declines to 88 ml. in a 65-year-old male. Similar declines with old age are observed with females. Such declines can be attributed partly to inactivity in old age. On the average, females have lower SVs than do males at all ages. In the young adult at rest, the average female has an SV of 60 ml., and the male has an SV of 80 ml. During exercise, the values rise to about 90 ml. in females and 110 ml. in males. Most of the differences between males and females are owing to body size.

Cardiac Output

The amount of blood that the heart pumps into the circulatory system in one minute is cardiac output ($\dot{Q}$). $\dot{Q}$ can vary depending on how much blood is pumped each beat (SV) and on the number of times the heart beats in a minute (HR). The formula for $\dot{Q}$ is

$$\dot{Q} = SV \times HR$$

Based on the average values previously presented for SV (80 ml. and 110 ml. for untrained and trained males, respectively) and on the maximum HR for males (195), $\dot{Q}$ is

(untrained) $\dot{Q} = 110$ ml. $\times\ 195 =$
$$21.50\ \text{l/min.}$$
(trained) $\dot{Q} = 160$ ml. $\times\ 195 = 31.20$ l/min.

Because both SV and HR decrease with age, $\dot{Q}$ also diminishes with age for both sexes. The relationships between $\dot{Q}$ and age for males and females are shown in Figure 4–11. The $\dot{Q}$ values for females were based on the HR and SV values previously presented. Males were expected to have higher $\dot{Q}$s than females because of their larger body

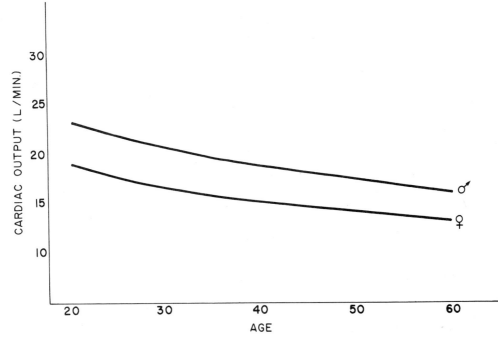

Fig. 4–11. Changes in cardiac output with age and sex.

size. However, when $\dot{Q}$ is expressed in terms of body weight, the difference between sexes is negligible. Although $\dot{Q}$ does not differ significantly between males and females when expressed per pound of body weight, differences do exist between sexes in oxygen consumption per unit body weight (see Fig. 4–11).Because body weight is usually the largest work load in most exercises and sports, females are at a disadvantage in terms of the utilization of oxygen in maximum work.

REGULATION OF CARDIAC OUTPUT

A heart at rest may pump 4 to 6 l. of blood each minute but, during heavy exercise, it may pump 5 times this amount. The heart can increase output by this amount during exercise because of the stimulating effects of increased metabolic activity on SV and HR. Even before exercise begins, stimulation of the sympathetic nerves to the blood vessels and heart increases the availability of blood in the systemic circulation and simultaneously increases HR. When exercise begins, these effects on the cardiovascular system are further enhanced and occur quite rapidly. The increase in $\dot{Q}$ upon the initiation of exercise is pronounced and happens so quickly that it cannot be solely explained by the metabolic activity of working muscles. $\dot{Q}$ increases rapidly and then levels off, usually in less than one minute, but the plateau reached depends on the work load or on the metabolic needs of the contracting muscles. The early and rapid increase in $\dot{Q}$ is primarily caused by the shifting of blood from the viscera and nonworking muscles to the peripheral circulation. Because $\dot{Q}$ is a product of SV and HR, the interacting relationships between these factors ultimately control $\dot{Q}$. A knowledge of the mechanisms that control SV and HR leads to an understanding of $\dot{Q}$ regulation.

Control of Stroke Volume

Two mechanisms are primarily responsible for controlling SV: (1) the volume of blood entering the heart and (2) the extent of neural stimulation by the autonomic nervous system. Control by blood flow is referred to as intrinsic control because of the internal effect produced. As blood rushes into the heart, the increased pressure stretches the myocardium. The extent of the stretch determines the contraction force of systole. The larger the quantity of blood, the more forceful the contraction. The combination of more blood and greater contractile force of cardiac muscle produces an increase in SV. When the sympathetic nerves to the heart are also stimulated, which commonly occurs in exercise, SV is further enhanced. The involvement of the autonomic nervous system in this way is referred to as extrinsic control of SV.

Intrinsic Control of Stroke Volume

Control of SV by intrinsic factors involves the effect of blood volume on cardiac function. But, before discussing these factors, one must know how greater quantities of blood are shifted from other parts of the body to the heart during exercise. When one exercises, large quantities of blood are shunted from the viscera and nonworking muscles into the peripheral circulation. This action increases the amount of blood flowing through the circulatory system to the working muscles. Blood is shifted by vasoconstriction, which is effected by the activation of sympathetic nerves to the smooth muscle of blood vessels. In this way, blood is pushed out from the viscera in the abdomen and thorax. The amount of blood moved from these regions depends on the severity of exercise. During heavy work, up to 80% of the blood supply in the viscera is removed,[15] whereas in moderate work the reduction is about 40%.[16] The effects of strenuous exercise on the distribution of blood in the body are shown in Figure 4–12. Redistribution of blood occurs in all tissues except the brain. Note how most of the increases in blood flow occur in the tissues that are directly involved in exercise, such as the heart and skeletal muscle tissues, and in the skin where excessive heat is removed from the

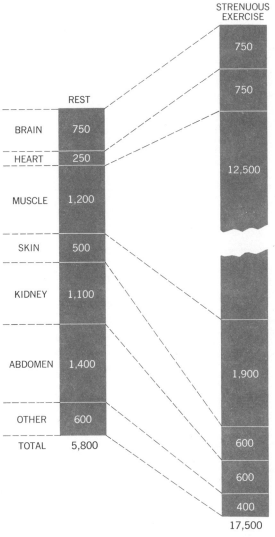

STRENUOUS EXERCISE

750
750
12,500
1,900
600
600
400
17,500

REST

BRAIN	750
HEART	250
MUSCLE	1,200
SKIN	500
KIDNEY	1,100
ABDOMEN	1,400
OTHER	600
TOTAL	5,800

Fig. 4–12. Distribution of blood flow to various tissues and organs during rest and strenuous exercise. The numbers refer to blood flow in ml. per min. (From Vander, A.J., Sherman, J.H., and Luciano, D.S.: Human Physiology— The Mechanisms of Body Function. New York, McGraw-Hill, Inc., 1975. Used with permission of McGraw-Hill Book Co.)

the muscles provides more oxygen and removes excessive metabolites. In exercise, blood flow in the muscle increases about threefold.

Movement of blood during exercise is expedited by respiratory activity, which increases venous pressure and, thereby, assists in pushing the blood through the veins and into the heart. Venous pressure is also increased by the "pumping" action of skeletal muscle on the veins. One-way valves in the veins allow the blood to move toward the heart in only one direction when the muscle contracts and squeezes on a vein. Pressure within the heart chambers, provided by the blood pushing on the walls, distends the myocardium. The response, in terms of a contraction force in systole, depends on the extent of the stretch. The greater the stretch, the greater the force of contraction. A similar phenomenon occurs in skeletal muscle, where force of a contraction is enhanced by stretch. The relationship between the length of cardiac muscle fibers and contraction force was expounded by Frank and Starling and associates in 1914.[17] As a result, during the first half of this century, most explanations for variations in SV during different levels of work were based on several rules: (1) $\dot{Q}$ is determined by the amount of venous return; (2) SV is determined by venous return when HR is constant; (3) SV depends directly on end-diastolic filling; (4) tension of resting fibers depends on their length; (5) diastolic filling and volume of the ventricles depends on the filling pressure; and (6) the mechanical energy released when heart muscle contracts depends on the length of the myocardial fibers.[18] Later research with new techniques concluded that SV and $\dot{Q}$ were not solely the result of changes in ventricular blood volume, as had been assumed by those accepting the Starling concept. Investigators demonstrated that the end-diastolic volume of the heart was relatively constant during rest and exercise.[19] If so, increased SV in exercise is caused by the greater force of systolic contraction, which empties the ventricles

body. Although the quantities of blood in different organs and tissues of the body are controlled by vasoconstriction produced by the sympathetic nerves, control of blood flow in the working muscles is provided by the end-products of metabolism, which cause vasodilatation. The increased blood flow to

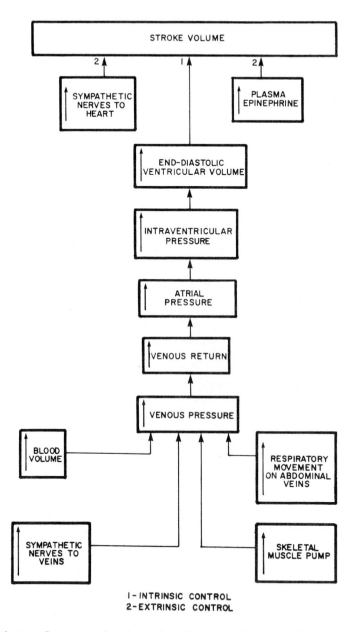

Fig. 4–13.   Major factors influencing stroke volume. (From Vander, A.J., Sherman, J.H., and Luciano, D.S.: Human Physiology—The Mechanisms of Body Function. New York, McGraw-Hill, Inc., 1975. Used with permission of McGraw-Hill Book Co.)

more completely. Other factors also have regulating effects on SV and $\dot{Q}$, such as tachycardia (increased HR) and sympathetic stimulation of the myocardium. These factors of HR and neural effects are presented later in this chapter. Nevertheless, Starling's law is one of several factors regulating SV.

The amount of blood pumped by the heart, or SV, depends specifically on the contraction force of the left ventricle during systole and the end-diastolic ventricular volume. The intrinsic factors that determine end-diastolic ventricular volume are illustrated in Figure 4–13. Because SV and venous return must be equal, an increase in one also increases the other. By the same token, end-diastolic ventricular volume is determined by the amount of venous return. For venous return to increase during exercise, the force driving the blood, or venous pressure (the pressure difference between the veins and right atrium), must be increased. The factors that increase blood volume to the heart, such as activity of the sympathetic nerves and movements of skeletal muscle, enhance venous pressure. As a consequence, more blood is forced into the right atrium to increase atrial pressure. Thus, intraventricular pressure increases and, consequently, end-diastolic ventricular volume is maintained. The greater tension on the ventricular walls, although volume may not increase significantly, stretches the myocardial fibers and, as a result, enhances systolic force. The final outcome is increased SV.

Extrinsic Control of Stroke Volume

Control of SV by extrinsic means refers to the neural participation of the autonomic nervous system in heart activity (Fig. 4–13). The sympathetic system is responsible for activating cardiac function, but the exact nature of the activation at the beginning of exercise is unclear.[20]

Nevertheless, neural involvement in exercise is essential for high levels of performance. Studies have shown that, when sympathetic stimulation is absent, physical performance is greatly impaired.[20a,21] The accelerator nerves of the sympathetic system, when stimulated, effect an increase in atrial and ventricular force through their action at the SA node and in the myocardial cells. The increased force results in more complete emptying of the left ventricle and in a greater SV. A similar effect on SV is also brought about by the action of the sympathetic nerves on the adrenal medulla gland. Stimulation of this gland by the sympathetics causes a secretion of epinephrine (80%) and norepinephrine (20%), which pass into the blood and then to the heart. The effect at the heart is the same as the effect when the accelerator nerves are stimulated: force of systolic contraction and HR are enhanced.

The role of the sympathetic nervous system in controlling SV is not limited to the heart. Stimulation of the sympathetics by exercise affects both the heart and blood vessels. As HR increases, the blood vessels in nonworking muscles and in the viscera constrict. More blood volume is pushed into the systemic circulation thus increasing venous return and SV. Even before exercise begins, venous return is increased by the overall decline in the resistance of blood vessels to flow in practically all skeletal muscle. This effect continues several seconds into exercise. Most of the resistance to blood flow is reduced because of vasodilatation in working muscles, which is primarily a local effect caused by the increase of certain metabolites from work. The effect is related to the metabolic needs of the muscle. As the severity of work increases, the resistance to blood flow in the muscle decreases.[22] The reverse occurs as work diminishes. Local vasodilatation in working muscles is as important as sympathetic stimulation for increasing venous return. When only sympathetic stimulation of the heart and blood vessels is involved, $\dot{Q}$ is doubled. But, when local vasodilatation is added to the effects of sympathetic stimulation, as happens in exercise, Q̇ increases to four times its resting level.

Control of Heart Rate

HR is controlled intrinsically by the quantity and velocity of blood flow and extrinsically by the autonomic nervous system. Although rhythmic stimulation of the SA node is affected intrinsically by blood flow, HR is largely controlled by neural activity (Fig. 4–14). The parasympathetic and sympathetic fibers of the autonomic nervous system end on the SA node and on various parts of the myocardium. The two parasympathetic nerves, called vagi, slow down HR (bradycardia) by releasing acetylcholine at their endings. The accelerator nerves of the sympathetic system release norepinephrine to speed up HR (tachycardia) and to increase the force of cardiac contraction. At any given time, HR depends on whether the sympathetic or the parasympathetic nerve fibers dominate control.

A variety of afferent receptors in the body affect HR by their actions on the autonomic nervous system (Fig. 4–15). Their influence also affects circulatory and ventilatory mechanisms via the autonomic nervous system (see Fig. 3–28). These receptors are stimulated to a greater or lesser degree, depending on the metabolic needs of skeletal muscle either at rest or work. In exercise, the needs of muscle fibers for more oxygen and for the removal of metabolic waste products are made known to specific recep-

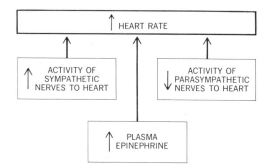

Fig. 4–14.   Neural control of heart rate by the autonomic nervous system. Stimulation of the sympathetic nerves to the adrenal medulla increases plasma epinephrine. (From Vander, A.J., Sherman, J.H., and Luciano, D.S.: Human Physiology—The Mechanisms of Body Function. New York, McGraw-Hill, Inc., 1975. Used with permission of McGraw-Hill Book Co.)

tors in the body. For example, the oxygen and carbon dioxide content of blood during exercise is detected by arterial receptors located near the heart (chemoreceptors). If either oxygen is in low supply or carbon dioxide is too plentiful, these receptors convey the information to the control regions of the brain stem. The response is greater activation of the sympathetic fibers to increase HR. Other receptors responding to exercise that modify HR are located in the arteries to the lungs and in the branches of arteries directly above the heart (baroreceptors). These receptors are stimulated by high blood pressure and have an inhibiting effect on HR at rest, but not during exercise.[23] Atrial receptors, located at the junctions

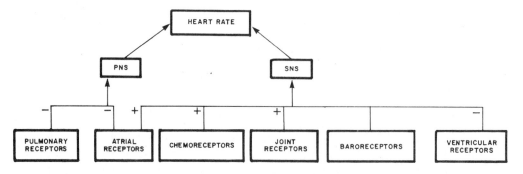

Fig. 4–15.   Afferent receptors influencing heart rate during exercise.

where the veins enter the right and left atria, are excited by increased amounts of blood in exercise. Consequently, the parasympathetic fibers are inhibited and the sympathetic fibers to the heart are excited.[23a] At the same time, there is probably a "vagal brake" on the heart that prevents too much HR (excessive tachycardia) by the activation of the afferents in the left ventricular wall.[24-26] This activation is brought about by the large quantities of blood entering the heart. If HR is too high, ventricular filling and SV drop. As a result, oxygenated blood is reduced and the amount reaching the working muscles is less. The reduction of oxygen to the working muscles impairs performance.

The lungs have receptors that respond to stretch. These receptors accelerate HR by primarily inhibiting the vagus nerves to the heart.[20] At the same time, the vasomotor sympathetic fibers to the exercised muscles are inhibited.[10] Even movement of the skeletal joints plays a part in regulating HR. Joint proprioceptors are stimulated in exercise and, as a result, activate the autonomic nervous system to excite the sympathetic accelerator nerves of the heart.[27,28] While these receptors are being excited during exercise and, consequently, are accelerating HR, stimulation of the adrenal medulla gland by sympathetic fibers and by secretion of the hormone, epinephrine, into the blood adds further to increased HR. Other factors affecting HR are temperature, plasma electrolyte concentrations, and some hormones, but these factors are less important than the effects related to, and initiated by, the working muscles.

HR responds rapidly to work and may double after only 15 sec. of severe exertion. The great increase in HR at the beginning of exercise is probably caused by a reduction in stimulation of the vagi nerves to the heart and an increase in sympathetic activity.[29] These neural responses are reflex in nature, as shown by their rapidity and overshoot effect. At the beginning of moderate exercise, HR peaks rapidly. It then drops several beats and levels off. As work continues, the increased heat produced adds to the rise in HR.

Relationship Between Stroke Volume and Heart Rate in Cardiac Output

The effects of both SV and HR on $\dot{Q}$ are shown in Figure 4–16. Note that sympathetic stimulation increases HR and SV by enhancing myocardial force. Although the acute effects of exercise on HR are well known, the effects on SV are not known. HR is fairly independent of such factors as venous return and myocardial force, whereas SV is not. The interacting effects of venous return, cardic force in systole, and HR influence SV. If venous return at the initiation of exercise is increased more rapidly than HR, SV increases above the resting level. However, if HR increases more rapidly than SV, SV may actually decrease slightly at the beginning of exercise.

Although HR and SV vary, depending on the extent of sympathetic activation and venous return, $\dot{Q}$ remains relatively constant in exercise. This discovery was brought out clearly by Ekblom et al.,[30] who related HR to relative oxygen uptake under four different experimental conditions. Subjects performed submaximal and maximal work under the following conditions: (1) control, (2) blockage of sympathetic stimulation to the heart, (3) blockage of parasympathetic impulses to the heart, and (4) blockage of both sympathetic and parasympathetic stimulation to the heart (Fig. 4–17). In the control condition, HR increased steadily from about 60 at rest to 195 at maximum oxygen consumption. When the sympathetic nerves to the heart were prevented from exerting their influence, HR decreased slightly at rest, but the gap widened as work intensity increased. At maximum oxygen consumption, HR was about 160, considerably less than the 195 under control conditions. The inhibiting effect on HR of the parasympathetic nerves to the heart is evident when these nerves are prevented from influencing cardiac function. Even at rest, HR is almost double the control re-

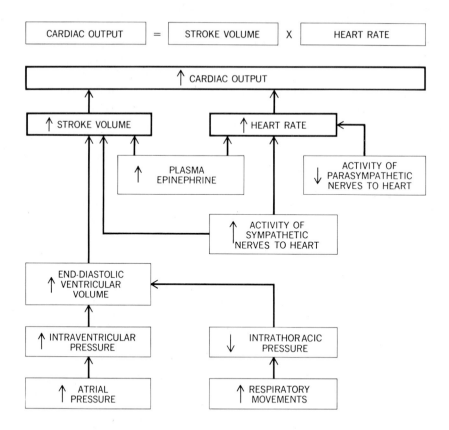

Fig. 4–16.   Major factors determining stroke volume and heart rate in cardiac output. (From Vander, A.J., Sherman, J.H., and Luciano, D.S.: Human Physiology—The Mechanisms of Body Function. New York, McGraw-Hill, Inc., 1975. Used with permission of McGraw-Hill Book Co.)

sponse. Sympathetic stimulation is primarily responsible for this elevation because parasympathetic effects no longer exert a dampening effect on HR. As work intensity increases, parasympathetic inhibition has less of an effect on increasing HR than when inhibition is removed. At maximum oxygen consumption, sympathetic activity does not seem significantly dampened by parasympathetic inhibition because HR is about the same as the HR in the control condition. Removing all autonomic nervous activity to the heart demonstrates the intrinsic control of blood flow on HR when neural, extrinsic control is absent. HR rises at rest, but, as work increases, HR drops below control

levels when oxygen consumption exceeds 50%. The reduction in HR then approaches the values achieved when just the sympathetic nerves were inoperable. However, the work time, when the autonomic nerves are not influencing HR, is significantly less than that under normal conditions. Note that, under all these experimental treatments, $\dot{Q}$ was similar even though HR varied from 160 to 195. This constancy made the achievement of maximum oxygen uptake possible in practically all the treatments. Because $\dot{Q} = SV \times HR$, SV obviously becomes smaller as HR increases and becomes larger as HR decreases. These HR changes under different experi-

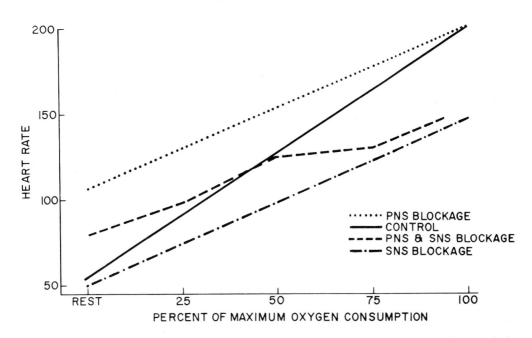

Fig. 4–17. Relationship between heart rate and relative oxygen consumption under normal conditions and when autonomic nervous activity to the heart is partially or completely blocked. (Data from Ekblom B., et al.: Effects of atropine and propranolol on the oxygen transport system during exercise in man. Scand. J. Clin. Lab. Invest., *30*:35, 1972.)

mental treatments involved relatively short work times. But, even in prolonged work when HR and SV are altered, $\dot{Q}$ is still maintained at a relatively constant level (Fig. 4–18).

The early research of Starling and Frank led many investigators to believe that an increase in venous return and in SV were primarily responsible for increases in $\dot{Q}$.[17] However, later research by Rushmer with dogs showed that, in moderate exercise, $\dot{Q}$ is increased primarily by HR with little change in SV.[18] These results were supported by other studies with human subjects when work was mild.[19,31,31a] As the severity of work increases, SV rises to about a work level of 40% $\dot{V}O_2$ max and an HR of 110 (Fig. 4–19). Beyond 40% $\dot{V}O_2$ max, little change in SV occurs, although HR continues to rise. Apparently, in severe work, as well as in moderate work, $\dot{Q}$ is increased more by HR than by SV. The relationship between SV and HR indicates that, even at high levels of

HR, SV is still maintained at maximum levels. However, as was shown with severe work of long duration (see Fig. 4–18), venous pressure, SV, and arterial pressure gradually decrease, whereas $\dot{Q}$ remains relatively constant. The increase in HR indicates an increase in sympathetic stimulation during this phase of heavy work. The causes of these cardiovascular changes probably lie within the peripheral circulation rather than in cardiac fatigue because the drop in SV and venous pressure indicates a reduction in venous return. Apparently, cardiac fatigue is not related because cardiac function among normal people does not seem to lessen, even in severe muscle fatigue. The indefatigability of the heart is exemplified by marathon runners who run for more than 2 hr. at cardiac outputs of 75 to 80% of maximum.[31b] In isolated heart studies, maximum cardiac output was maintained for more than 2 hr. without any apparent damage.[32] Even when myocardial fatigue set in during studies with

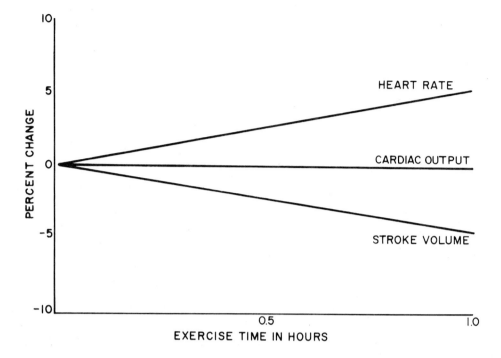

Fig. 4–18.   Changes in heart rate and stroke volume during prolonged work with little change in cardiac output.[9]

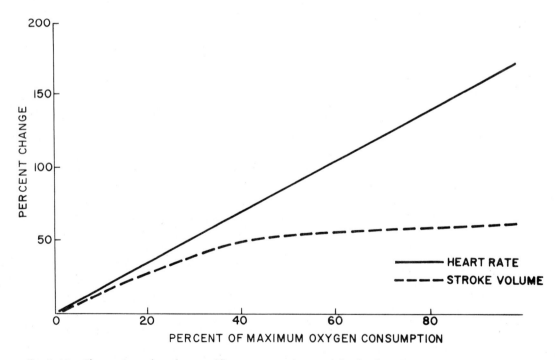

Fig. 4–19.   Changes in stroke volume and heart rate at various work levels of maximum oxygen consumption.[31a]

isolated heart muscle, the damage was repaired after rest.

The relative contributions of SV and HR to Q̇ during severe exercise can be understood by comparing their maximum values. In maximum exercise, HR may increase by 2.5 to 3 times the normal level, whereas SV may be 2 times the resting level.[33] Consequently, if either HR or SV is held constant, Q̇ increases 2 times or 2.5 to 3 times, respectively. However, if both are at maximum values, Q̇ may increase by 5 to 6 times the resting value. This value is found when exercising humans with maximum work loads. Although HR has a greater effect than SV on Q̇, an improvement in Q̇ from training is achieved by increasing SV because HR is not increased by training. In fact, a sedentary individual has a maximum HR similar to that of a trained athlete; however, the resting HR of the sedentary individual may be 50% higher.

Effects of Training on Cardiac Output

Training to improve aerobic capacity is accomplished by exercising relatively large muscle mass. But, the movements must be highly repetitive and prolonged so that the oxygen delivery system is overloaded. Of course, each repetitive muscular contraction is done with a minimal force so that the demands for oxygen by the tissues can be met by the oxygenated blood. The importance of Q̇ in aerobic performance is shown by its relationship with oxygen consumption (Fig. 4–20). Individuals of high Q̇ can consume large quantities of oxygen from the blood. This relationship is understandable because the ability of the heart to pump blood determines the amount of oxygen available to the working muscles. Highly trained athletes can pump about 38 l. of blood through the heart in 1 min. Compare this figure with 20 l. of blood pumped by the average, untrained individual, and one can readily understand why athletes can consume larger amounts of oxygen in heavy work.

The factors that determine Q̇ in maximum work, i.e., SV and HR, do not change in the same way as a result of aerobic training. In fact, maximum HR does not appreciably

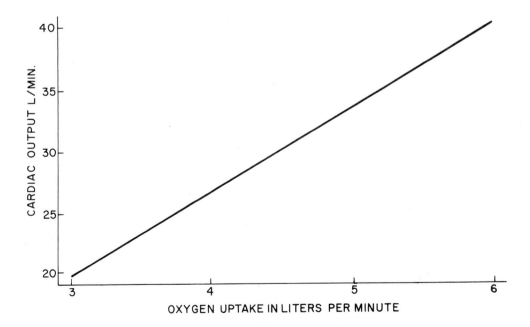

Fig. 4–20. Relationship between oxygen consumption and cardiac output. (Data from Åstrand, P.O., and Rodahl, K.: Textbook of Work Physiology. New York, McGraw-Hill Book Co., 1970.)

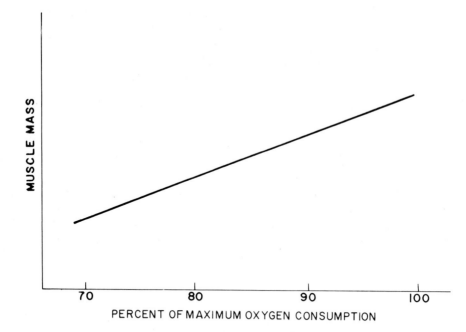

Fig. 4–21.   Muscle mass used in maximum work and corresponding oxygen utilization relative to maximum oxygen consumption. Values are based on arm work at the smallest muscle mass and leg work plus arm work at the largest mass. (Data from Åstrand, P.O., et al.: Intra-arterial blood pressure during exercise with different muscle groups. J. Appl. Physiol., *20*:253, 1965.)

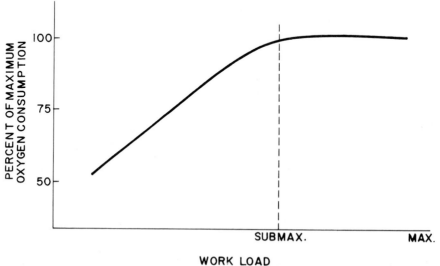

Fig. 4–22.   Maximal oxygen consumption achieved with a submaximal workload. (Data from Pollock, M.L.: Effects of frequency of training on serum lipids, cardiovascular function, and body composition. *In* Exercise and Fitness. Edited by B.D. Franks. Chicago, Athletic Institute, 1969.)

change. The HR curve for maximum values at various ages applies to all individuals regardless of aerobic capacity (see Fig. 4–9). Consequently, training effects in $\dot{Q}$ largely reflect increases in SV. Because of the close relationship between SV and oxygen consumption, activities that improve aerobic capacity also increase SV and $\dot{Q}$.

When large muscle mass contracts in exercise, the demands placed on the oxygen-transportation functions are greater than when smaller mass is worked (Fig. 4–21). Consequently, such activities as cycling and running are excellent for developing aerobic fitness because they place great stress on the heart and circulatory mechanisms. Research evidence has shown that $\dot{Q}$ and SV reach their maximum values when oxygen uptake is maximum. Further evidence has demonstrated that maximum oxygen can be consumed in work of less than maximum (Fig. 4–22).[33a] By training with work loads that elicit 100% $\dot{V}O_2$ max but are less than maximum, athletes can continue work for 5 min. or more. However, maximum work loads that elicit $\dot{V}O_2$ max do not permit as long a work duration because greater involvement of anaerobic metabolism results in excess lactic acid buildup and, consequently, exhaustion. In terms of producing changes in $\dot{Q}$ and SV, training at loads just eliciting $\dot{V}O_2$ max, where the duration of exercise is greatest, has a stronger stimulating effect on the oxygen delivery systems than does training with maximum work loads. An important factor in increasing aerobic capacity is the duration over which a high level of $\dot{Q}$ and SV is maintained. The longer duration is achieved most effectively by training with loads that are less than 100% but more than 80% maximum.[34]

Cardiac Reserve and Adaptation to Work

The cardiovascular system makes adjustments according to the metabolic demands placed on it by the other tissues and organs of the body. Blood is directed to the tissues that need it most and is taken away from tissues whose demand for it is less. During strenuous work, the heart and circulatory system adjust by increasing blood flow from three to five times the resting level. For this increase to happen, a capacity for cardiac function must be kept in reserve to meet extra metabolic demands placed on the system. This reserve is referred to as cardiac reserve.

The best estimate of cardiac reserve is the amount of oxygen that the working muscles can utilize during maximum work ($\dot{V}O_2$max). $\dot{V}O_2$ max is largely based on SV and HR, or on $\dot{Q}$, and ultimately on the ability of the coronary vessels to increase blood flow in response to myocardial oxygen needs. Thus, these factors determine cardiac reserve. The relationships between SV, HR, and $\dot{Q}$ have been discussed and are illustrated in Figures 4–16 and 4–18. The importance of each factor in maximizing blood flow to the working muscles is indicated. However, for optimal cardiac function, the total amount of oxygen available to the myocardium must be adequate to meet all work demands. The achievement of a sufficient oxygen supply depends on the product of coronary blood flow and oxygen content of the arterial blood. As in skeletal muscles and other tissues of the body, blood flow in cardiac tissue is regulated by local control of vasodilatation. When oxygen is low, the coronary vessels dilate to decrease resistance to blood flow and, thereby, enhance flow and the availability of oxygen.

Inadequate coronary flow has often been ascribed to the small cross-sectional area of the coronary artery relative to the mass of muscle supplied with blood. The main reason for a restriction in coronary flow is directly or indirectly related to atherosclerosis, or sometimes called "hardening of the arteries." Atherosclerosis (arteriosclerosis) is a disease characterized by a thickening of the arterial wall with connective tissue and deposits of cholesterol. The exact cause of the disease is not known, but it is no longer considered a degenerative process related to advancing age. Atherosclerosis is considered a metabolic disturbance of lipid metabolism that is, in some unknown way, related to smoking, high-fat diets, nervous tension, and obesity.

ENERGY FOR THE HEART

Cardiac muscle derives its energy from the same substances as do other types of muscle; that is, primarily from the metabolism of glucose, fatty acids, and lactate. During work, lactic acid and pyruvic acid, increased in the blood from the breakdown of glucose for energy, provide proportionately more energy for the heart than during rest if a sufficient supply of oxygen is available. The heart is metabolically similar to the brain because it needs adequate amounts of oxygen to function efficiently. Neither the heart nor the brain has the capacity of skeletal muscle to sustain any oxygen debt. The heart has many more mitochondria than does skeletal muscle to provide large quantities of ATP not only to meet continuous work demands, but also to meet varying work intensities. Energy and oxygen needs of the heart increase as contraction force, speed of contraction, and heart rate increase.

The quantities of substances taken from the blood in the coronary vessels and used for energy by the heart vary between trained and untrained individuals. The extent to which glucose, lactate, and free fatty acids (FFA) are used by the heart at rest, during exercise, and in recovery is shown in Table 4–1. At rest, the trained individuals obtain about half their fuel from FFA, whereas untrained individuals obtain about 38%. When both work at the same work load for 12 min., the substrate used for energy shifts with a reduction in FFA and an increase in lactate. At maximum work, both trained and untrained individuals use similar proportions of each substrate for fuel. During recovery, the trained individuals again receive almost 50% of their fuel from FFA and a lesser amount from glucose and lactate. The untrained individuals rely less on FFA and more on glucose. These figures have several implications in terms of the sparing effect that FFA and lactate have on glucose. Because relatively smaller amounts of glucose are used for energy by the heart at rest, more glucose is available to maintain normal concentrations of plasma glucose, which is essential for the survival of the brain and

Table 4–1.

The Relative Proportion of Fuel Substances Used by the Heart at Rest, During Submaximum and Maximum Work, and in Recovery Among Trained and Untrained Individuals*

		FFA	Lactate	Glucose
Rest	Trained	53	20	27
	Untrained	38	31	31
Same work load (12 min.)	Trained	33	45	22
	Untrained	25	60	15
Maximal work	Trained (18 min.)	20	65	15
	Untrained (12 min.)	25	60	15
Recovery (15 min.)	Trained	48	33	19
	Untrained	33	42	25

*Data estimated from Keul, Doll, and Keppler.[35]

nervous tissue. Whereas virtually all other organs and tissues use the three energy substances, only the nervous system must use glucose on a continuous basis. FFA has the greatest effect in sparing glucose both at rest and during recovery; lactate is of lesser significance. Because the trained heart at rest, during submaximal work up to a point, and in recovery from work uses FFA as its major fuel source, it is assumed that cardiovascular endurance is, thereby, optimized. In the untrained individual, who uses a greater proportion of lactate than of FFA to spare the use of glucose for energy during light work and recovery, the effect is a less efficient achievement of maximum cardiovascular endurance.

THE HEART AT WORK

The immediate response of the heart to the slightest change in metabolic activity of the body makes it an excellent barometer for assessing or predicting physical performance. Because the heart functions in harmony with the circulatory and respiratory systems and because its activity varies in a known and measurable way with these systems, the heart reflects the total response of all the regulating mechanisms involved in meeting the metabolic needs of exercise or work.

The integration of cardiac activity with vascular and respiratory activity occurs in vascular and respiratory control regions located in the brain stem. Nerve impulses are sent from all parts of the body to these regions and are then interpreted. Appropriate responses are made to the input, thereby accomplishing a desired goal. Most often, these events take place at an unconscious level. Because of the intimate and vital relationship between the systems of the body and because the activity of most systems is often difficult to measure without special and expensive laboratory equipment, HR is often used to assess the body's response to work.

Heart Rate as a Measure of Cardiovascular Fitness

The significant relationships between HR and both SV and $\dot{Q}$ and $\dot{V}O_2$ max and the ease of measuring HR without special equipment have made HR a popular measure of cardiovascular fitness. HR is used to measure heart and circulatory fitness in basically two ways: (1) to predict $\dot{V}O_2$ max and (2) to measure work response.

Heart Rate as a Predictor of Maximum Oxygen Consumption

Because $\dot{Q}$ (SV × HR) determines to a large extent the amount of oxygen absorbed by the muscles in exercise, HR relates to oxygen consumption. Tests have been devised to predict $\dot{V}O_2$ max from measures of submaximal HR. Although a direct measurement of $\dot{V}O_2$ max is more accurate and preferred in some circumstances, such as in research, there are some disadvantages to the direct method. Special laboratory equipment is needed and, in the case of older individuals, the physiologic stress on the heart may be inadvisable.

Several methods of predicting $\dot{V}O_2$ max from HR have been determined.[36-38] One method is presented here to assist the reader in understanding the relationship between HR, $\dot{V}O_2$ max, and work loads. Åstrand and Rhyming developed a method to predict aerobic capacity from submaximal HR.[36] A nomogram was constructed for predictive purposes based on data collected from individuals between the ages of 18 and 30 (Fig. 4–23). Work was provided by either a treadmill, a bicycle ergometer, or a 5- to 6-min. step test. Work loads were selected to achieve a steady state in HR between 125 and 170 beats/min. $\dot{V}O_2$ max was estimated from the nomogram by reading horizontally from the "body weight" scale (step test) or "work level" scale (for cycle test) to the oxygen intake scale after alignment with HR. Note that the scale for pulse rate is different for males and females. A female

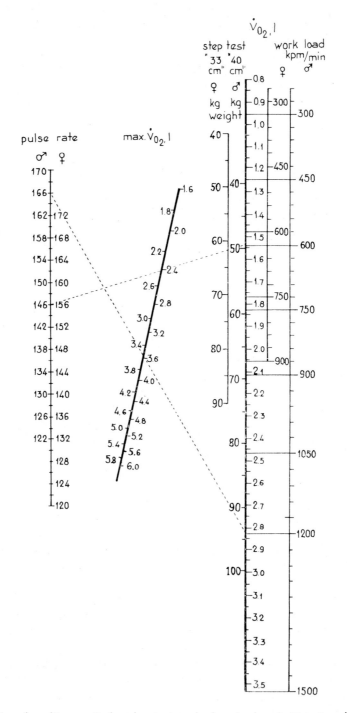

Fig. 4–23. Prediction of aerobic capacity from heart rate and submaximal work. (Data from Åstrand, P.O. and Rhyming, I.: A nomogram for calculation of aerobic capacity (physical fitness) from pulse rate during submaximal work. J. Appl. Physiol., 7:2, 1954.)

can achieve the same $\dot{V}O_2$ max as a male but her HR will be higher than that of the male. The smaller heart volume and, in turn, SV of the female account for these differences in HR. Thus, to achieve the same $\dot{V}O_2$ max as a male (and the same cardiac output), the female with a smaller SV must have a faster HR ($\dot{Q}$ = SV × HR).

Because the basis of all tests that predict $\dot{V}O_2$ max from HR is the relationship between these two variables, the closeness of the relationship determines the validity of the tests. One common flaw in the accuracy of estimating $\dot{V}O_2$ max from HR is caused by the assumption of the tests that the relationship between HR and oxygen uptake is relatively linear. The relationship at submaximal work is linear, but, at maximum or near maximum work, the relationship varies more (Fig. 4–24). In young adults, HR increases steadily with work until it reaches about 180, where it tends to level off. However, oxygen consumption continues to rise. The greatest variations among individuals occur when HR exceeds 180. Because the

prediction of $\dot{V}O_2$ max from submaximal HR does not consider the lack of linearity at the upper levels of performance, there is some error in predicting. Generally, $\dot{V}O_2$ max is underestimated because it increases at a faster rate than does HR at high levels of work. Some indications of the error in predicting $\dot{V}O_2$ max from HR was shown among 80 males between the ages of 20 to 50 years.[38a] After 3 different methods were examined, errors in prediction reached 15%.

Error can also occur when predicting $\dot{V}O_2$ max from HR if age is not considered. Maximum HR declines from about 210 at 10 years of age to 165 at 65 years of age (see Fig. 4–9). A young adult may have an HR of 160 while working at 65% $\dot{V}O_2$ max whereas a 60-year-old man may be working at 95 to 100% $\dot{V}O_2$ max with the same HR. The use of HR alone to compare the fitness levels of the two men would result in gross error. The older male is working much harder at the same HR. But, when both are working at the same proportion of $\dot{V}O_2$ max at similar physiologic stress, the older male may have

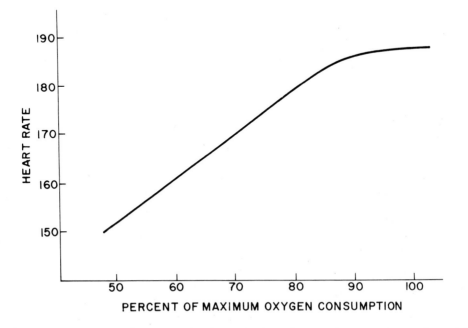

Fig. 4–24.   Relationship between heart rate and work intensity. At maximum work, oxygen consumption tends to rise with little change in heart rate. (Data from Davies, C.T.M.: Limitations to the prediction of maximum oxygen intake from cardiac frequency measurements. J. Appl. Physiol., 24:700, 1968.)

an HR of 110 compared with an HR of 130 in the young male. Even considering the errors in predicting $\dot{V}O_2$ max from HR at submaximal work, some of these tests, used in a classroom situation where all subjects are approximately the same age, can provide valuable information to assess an individual's cardiovascular fitness.

Heart Rate Response to Work as a Measure of Cardiovascular Fitness

When two individuals perform the same amount of work, the individual with better cardiovascular fitness usually shows less increase in HR and a faster recovery after work. An example of an individual's response in HR during and after work is shown in Figure 4–25. The upper curve reflects the period before aerobic training and the bottom curve reflects the time after training. The work effort was the same in both curves but, as a consequence of training, the cardiovascular system found the same amount of work easier to perform. This effect is reflected in a reduced HR. Tests based on this fact have been devised. A test uses as its criterion of fitness either the amount of work completed before reaching a specific HR[39–41] or a combination of both work and recovery HR, expressed as the ratio work/HR recovery.[42] These tests are less valid than tests that measure $\dot{V}O_2$ max, but under certain circumstances they serve a purpose. One test widely used as a measure of cardiovascular efficiency among large numbers of young adults is the Harvard step test or 5- min. step test.[43] In this test, an individual steps up and down on a 20-in. bench at a rate of 30 steps/min. After 5 min. of stepping, pulse counts are taken from 1 to 1.5 min. during recovery. If stepping cannot be continued for 5 min., the amount of time actually stepped is recorded, and recovery HR is taken from 1 to 1.5 min. later. When the individual steps for the entire 5 min., total heart beats of about 100 or more are considered poor; 70 to 99, average; and less than 70, good.[44] The test relates to $\dot{V}O_2$ max ($r = 0.71$) and has an

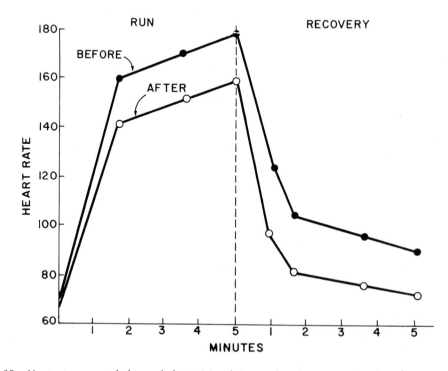

Fig. 4–25.   Heart rate response before and after training during work and recovery. (Data from Åstrand, P.O., and Rodahl, K.: Textbook of Work Physiology. New York, McGraw-Hill Book Co., 1970.)

error potential of up to 27%.[45] Because the test scores are based on young adults whose maximum HRs are higher than those of older adults and who consequently have higher recovery pulse rates for the same work effort, the nomogram must be adjusted for estimating cardiovascular fitness of older individuals.[12]

Another step test that has some advantages over the Harvard step test is the progressive pulse rate test.[2] The work performed is more gradual; the rates of stepping begin at 12 per min. and increase by 6 steps until 36 steps per min. are reached. Stepping up and down occurs on a 17-in. bench for 1 min. at each of the rates. Recovery HR is taken for 2 min. after each 1-min. work bout. The next bout begins after HR drops to within 8 to 12 beats of the standing, normal rate. This test is less strenuous than the Harvard step test and is more appropriate for middle-aged individuals. Norms have been established for both males and females from the ages of 26 to 60[45] and for college males.[46]

Heart Rate as a Training Stimulus

Because HR reflects the metabolic needs of the body during exercise and increases with physiologic stress of work, it may be used in training as a barometer of stress. Before an improvement in cardiovascular fitness can occur, the intensity of stress in training must reach a threshold value. That threshold value is reflected in HR. The threshold value for young, fairly active, adult males is an HR of about 150.[47] Training at values of less than 150 may not improve $\dot{V}O_2$ max. The studies cited were based on prolonged and continuous activity at a given HR.

The threshold value of 150 may be appropriate for young, adult males, but for more sedentary individuals of the same age, HR values of less than 150 can elicit improvement in cardiovascular fitness.[48] Such an improvement was shown in a study where female adults, aged 17 to 20, were trained daily for 15-min. sessions on a treadmill over a period of 4 weeks.[49] Half of the females ran at an HR of 125 and the other half ran at an HR of 145. The subjects were considered sedentary based on their low pretest values for oxygen consumption (26.7 ml./kg./min.). After training, both groups improved significantly in $\dot{V}O_2$ max and neither group differed from the other. When consideration is given to age and initial level of cardiovascular fitness, threshold values for training will

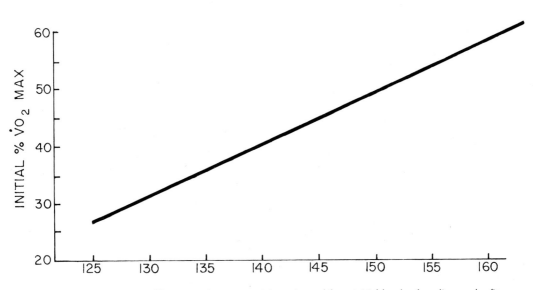

Fig. 4–26. Threshold values of heart rate for young adults estimated from initial levels of cardiovascular fitness.

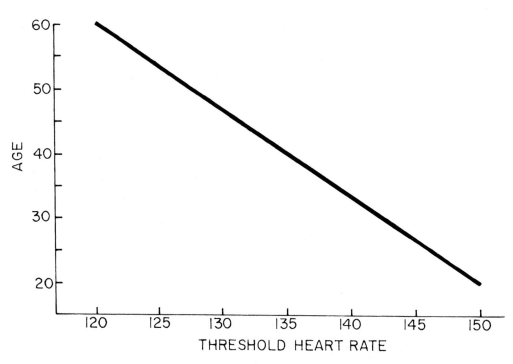

Fig. 4–27.   Threshold heart rates at various ages based on average cardiovascular fitness levels.

vary somewhat, as estimated in Figures 4–26 and 4–27, based on the findings of several studies.[47–51]

Karvonen Method of Predicting Threshold Heart Rate. A method for estimating threshold value of HR for young men was developed by Karvonen.[47] He based his method on the results of training at HRs of 135 and 153 for 30-min. sessions, 5 days a week, for 4 weeks. Improvement was noted only at the HR of 153. Threshold values were estimated to be 60% of the difference between resting HR and maximum HR. That is, if resting HR is 70 and maximum HR is 210, the critical threshold value is 60% × (210 − 70) + 70 = 154. By using Karvonen's method, Costill estimated the threshold values of HR for distance runners and determined the percentages of $\dot{V}O_2$ max corresponding to each HR (Table 4–2).[52] All percentages of $\dot{V}O_2$ max found in the runners exceeded 50%, which is the value considered to be threshold when oxygen consumption is the basis for setting the

training stimulus.[12] Of course, most distance runners in training surpass these values for HR and percentage $\dot{V}O_2$ max and run at levels of 80 to 90% $\dot{V}O_2$ max. In fact, in a marathon race of more than 2 hr., runners may work at 80 to 85% $\dot{V}O_2$ max.

Using percentage HR by the Karvonen method has been a fairly good predictor of the percentage of $\dot{V}O_2$ max at which an indi-

Table 4–2.

Percentage of $\dot{V}O_2$ max Corresponding to Critical Threshold for Heart Rate Among Trained Individuals[52]

Subject	Critical Threshold HR*	% $\dot{V}O_2$ max
S.L.	134	53.2
S.K.	132	59.2
D.K.	132	58.6
K.S.	134	61.1
E.W.	134	57.5

*Calculated as described by Karvonen.[47]

vidual is working, provided certain measuring protocol is followed.[53] Resting HR is determined after 10 min. of standing. The relationship between measured percentages of $\dot{V}O_2$ max (25, 45, 65, and 85%) and the same percentages using the Karvonen method showed that the two were closely correlated (Fig. 4–28). The error in predicting percentage $\dot{V}O_2$ max from HR is, at most, about 12%. Consequently, if 60% of the difference between resting HR and maximum HR is selected in training, the corresponding actual percentage $\dot{V}O_2$ max would probably not exceed the range of 53 to 67% $\dot{V}O_2$ max. Actually, in most instances, the range of variation would fall between 54 and 66% $\dot{V}O_2$ max.

Because the Karvonen method considers maximum HR, a 50-year-old male training at 60% $\dot{V}O_2$ max and an HR of 137 would be working at the same cardiovascular stress as

a 20-year-old male at an HR of 153. For this reason, athletes and nonathletes of all adult ages may use the Karvonen method with similar accuracy as an estimate of percentage $\dot{V}O_2$ max and as a stress barometer in training.

Interval Training and Heart Rate as a Training Stimulus

When intermittent work interspersed by rest periods is done in training, activity is often more intense but of shorter duration each time. In work of this kind, HR exceeds threshold values and may even approach maximum. Of course, activity of such intensity does not permit long and continuous movement. Another term for sporadic work that alternates between highly intense activity and rest is interval training. Overloading is provided by work intensity, length of rest interval, and number of times the work is

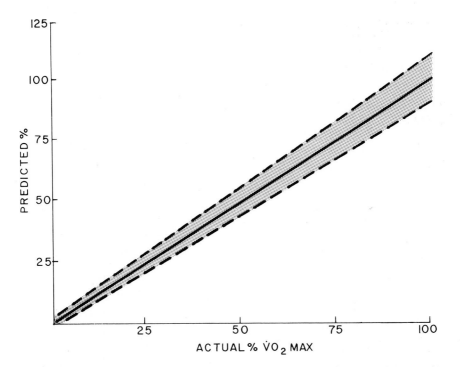

Fig. 4–28. Relationship between predicted and actual percent maximum oxygen consumption using the Karvonen method to predict oxygen consumption. The shaded area indicates the amount of error in prediction. For example, at any predicted value, the corresponding actual value will not exceed about 12% above or below the predicted value based on the research of Davies. (Data from Davis, J.A., and Convertino, V. A.: A comparison of heart rate methods for predicting endurance training intensity. Med. Sci. Sports, 7:295, 1975.)

Table 4–3.

Target Heart Rates During and Between Work Bouts in Interval Training for Various Age Ranges

Age Range	During Work	Between Work Bouts
Under 20	190	150
20–29	180	140
30–39	170	130
40–49	160	120
50–59	150	115
60–69	140	105

repeated.[53a] HR can be used in two ways in interval training: (1) to determine the proper work intensity to ensure that training effects are optimal, and (2) to make sure that the rest period between work bouts is adequate so that the level of fatigue is sufficiently low to permit the next bout to be performed with a predetermined intensity.

An example of how HR can be used in these ways to improve running time in the mile was reported by Wilt.[53b] Training bouts involved a series of 440-yd. runs at relatively high work intensity. Wilt suggested running times of 1 to 4 sec. less than one-fourth the time required to run a mile. If an individual runs a 6-min. mile, each 440 yd. would be run in anywhere from 86 to 89 sec. This work intensity should elicit the desired HR for a given age range (Table 4–3). If the HR is not high enough after a work bout, or if it is too high, an adjustment in running time is made. The other way of using HR is to measure HR after each 440-yd. run. When HR moves down to a particular level (depending on age, as shown in Table 4–3), the next run begins. Ordinarily, 6 to 8 runs of 440 yd. would be performed at each training session. When shorter or longer distances are run in interval training, the specific running times and number of runs are modified.

Electrocardiography in Evaluating the Heart at Work

The electrocardiogram (ECG), which is a recording of all the electrical activity of cardiac fibers during depolarization and repolarization, is an excellent means for detecting abnormalities in heart function (Fig. 4–29). Letters are assigned to various parts of an ECG and these, in turn, correspond to specific functions of the heart. By knowing that the P wave is caused by depolarization of the atria, the QRS interval is caused by depolarization of the ventricles and repolarization of the atria, and the T wave is caused by the repolarization of the ventricles, one can use the ECG to identify the site of abnormal function. ECG recordings from the electrodes attached to the surface of the skin can be made during heavy work and at rest. The characteristic shape of a heartbeat,

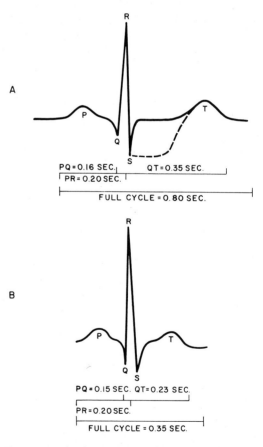

Fig. 4–29.   The shape and cycle length of one heart beat at rest (a) with a heart rate of 75 and in work (b) with a heart rate of 172 as shown on an electrocardiograph. An S–T segment depression is identified by the dotted trace (A).

as registered on an ECG, differs during rest and work. In a normal heart, the general shape of the ECG is the same at rest and work but, because of the increase in heart rate with work, the length of each cycle is shortened. During rest, at a heart rate of 75, the cycle length is about .80 sec.; during work, at a heart rate of 172, the cycle length is only .35 sec. Of course, there are also changes in the P-Q interval and the Q-T interval in work. The change from rest to work in the P-Q interval from .16 sec. to .15 sec. is relatively small compared with the change in the Q-T interval from .35 sec. to .23 sec. These disproportionate changes between P-Q and Q-T intervals indicate that the depolarization and repolarization of the ventricles (Q-T), which represent contraction and relaxation respectively, undergo the greatest variation in heart activity from rest to work.

Abnormalities of heart function also can be detected by the ECG. Changes in depolarization and repolarization that deviate significantly from normal recordings indicate a variety of malfunctions. But, to adequately evaluate cardiac performance, one must work the heart until it calls on its reserves. Any gross limitations in cardiac reserve are reflected in the ECG. For example, a heart with an occluded blood flow in the coronary vessels may show a normal ECG recording under resting conditions. But, when the heart is subjected to work and the demand for oxygen increases, the occlusion is detected by the ECG. A characteristic change in ECG caused by blockage of blood flow in the heart is shown by an S-T segment depression in Figure 4–29. As a consequence of the occlusion, the rate and magnitude of depolarization and repolarization are changed. Other abnormal functions of the heart produce specific and corresponding changes in ECG. These involve abnormalities associated with cardiac rhythm, where the pacemaker of the heart may be at a site other than the SA node in the right atrium, or abnormalities associated with hypertrophy. In any event, these ab-

normalities and others can be recognized by the ECG. Consequently, the ECG is used as one measure in the evaluation and prescription of exercise for adults.

Screening of Adults for Exercise Programs. Although adults of any age can exercise and achieve significant gains in cardiovascular fitness, certain precautions should be taken before beginning a program. Such precautions apply especially to sedentary adults. Before adults begin an exercise program, certain guidelines should be followed in terms of screening and supervising procedures for graded exercise testing. These guidelines are based on age and health status (Table 4–4).[54] The risk factors associated with coronary heart disease are either primary or secondary. Primary risk factors are high blood pressure, high blood lipids, and cigarette smoking. Secondary risk factors are obesity, physical inactivity, family history, diabetes, and high blood glucose.

Certain information about the individual must be known before graded testing can be considered. A comprehensive medical history is obtained to identify possible risk factors, especially secondary factors. The physical examination is concerned with identifying any symptoms indicative of cardiopulmonary disease and other health problems that could contraindicate the need for exercise testing. If a test is needed, the ECG is monitored during work of graded intensity. The response to work in ECG recording provides information to aid in the evaluation of cardiovascular disorders. From this evaluation, exercise programs are prescribed that provide stress appropriate to the physical capacity of the individual.

PRINCIPLES FOR TRAINING

1. Heart rate during and after exercise is a measure of the body's ability to consume oxygen. Although the prediction of $\dot{V}O_2$ max from submaximal or maximal HR is not highly accurate, the 12% error is not high enough to obviate HR as a practical and significant indicator of training effects. If the response of HR to a given work load is re-

Table 4–4.

Screening and Supervisory Procedures for Graded Exercise Testing According to Age and Health Status *

Age	Health status	Screening and supervisory procedures for graded exercise testing
Less than 35 years	No known risk factors or documented coronary artery disease and has had a medical examination in the last 2 years.	No medical clearance is necessary. Test may be administered by a trained exercise technician without presence of physician.
	Suspected or documented coronary artery disease or significant risk factors.	ECG-monitored exercise test administered by an exercise technician with a physician present who is either in visual contact with the subject or is present but not visual, depending on the severity of the symptoms.
35 years or older	No known risk factors or documented coronary artery disease.	ECG-monitored exercise test administered by an exercise technician with a physician present but not necessarily in visual contact with subject.
	Suspected or documented coronary artery disease or significant risk factors.	Same as above but with physician visually present with subject.

* Based on Guidelines for Graded Exercise Testing and Exercise Prescription.[54]

corded both before and after training, the effects of training on oxygen consumption are reflected in the differences in HR response. Work loads may be provided by stepping up and down on a 17-in. or 20-in. bench for several minutes at a given rate, such as 30 steps per min. Running a certain distance, such as 660 yd. or longer, in the same time before and after training and recording the response of HR is another way to assess training effects. Other work loads may be provided by swimming, bicycling, or treadmill running.

2. The effect of training on the capacity of the body to absorb oxygen is indicated by the intensity of training HR, the duration at which an intensity is maintained during each training session, and the frequency of weekly training sessions. Training intensity elicits increases in $\dot{V}O_2$ max when HR is 60% of the way from resting to maximum HR.[47] For the average young adult male, however, an HR of 153 is closer to the criti-

cal threshold value for improving cardiovascular and respiratory capacity. For an adult male who is 65 years old, the threshold value is about 125 HR. Actually, HR intensities beyond this threshold are more effective for increasing endurance,[34] provided the trainee recuperates sufficiently between training sessions. Training for longer durations for each session at the same HR intensities is better for improving endurance.[55] When the frequency of weekly training sessions increases, endurance usually improves,[33a,56] especially when the training period is extended beyond about 15 weeks.[21] Training sessions of 4 days per week increase endurance more effectively than 2 weekly sessions when training programs are continued for 16 and 20 weeks.[33a,56] In general, increasing the intensity, duration, and frequency of training tends to increase the magnitude of improvement.

3. Heart rate can be used as a measure of circulatory and respiratory stress during in-

termittent work as well as during continuous and prolonged work. Endurance is improved when work is of short, but intense, duration. If this intense work is repeated, interspersed by rest periods or low activity, improvements occur in $\dot{V}O_2$ max. Intermittent exercise is referred to as interval training. The advantage of interval training is that more total work can be accomplished at a higher work intensity because of the rest periods. HR is often used to gauge the intensity of the work and the length of the rest interval between work. An athlete may run 440 yd. at a pace that approximates an HR of 180 and then may rest or jog until HR drops to about 140 before beginning another run. There are many variations of interval training and they differ because of the different goals of athletes. A distance runner would train differently from a miler and a football athlete would train differently from a rower.

REFERENCES

1. Morganroth, J., et al.: Comparative left ventricular dimensions in trained athletes. Ann. Intern. Med., 82:521, 1975.
2. Kilbom, A.: Physical training in women. Scand. J. Clin. Lab. Invest., 28:119, 1971.
3. Arcos, J.C, et al.: Changes in ultrastructure and respiratory control in mitochondria of rat heart hypertrophied by exercise. Exp. Mol. Pathol., 8:49, 1968.
4. Oscai, P.A., et al.: Cardiac growth and respiratory enzyme levels in male rats subjected to a running program. Am. J. Physiol., 220:1238, 1971.
5. Eckstein, R.W.: Effect of exercise and coronary artery narrowing on coronary collateral circulation. Circ. Res., 5:230, 1957.
6. Haslam, R.W. and Stull, G.A.: Duration and frequency of training as determinants of coronary tree capacity in the rat. Res. Quart., 45:178, 1974.
7. Nutter, D., et al.: Cardiac hypertrophy in the endurance athletes. Physiologist, 18:336, 1975.
8. Schoop, W.: Bewegungstherapie bei peripheren durchblutungsstorungen. Med. Welt., 10:502, 1964.
9. Terjung, R., and Spear, K.: Effects of exercise training on coronary blood flow in rats. Physiologist, 18:419, 1975.
10. Frick, M., Clovainio, R., and Somer, T.: The mechanism of bradycardia evoked by physical training. Cardiologia, 51:46, 1967.
11. Tipton, C., Barnard, R., and Tcheng, T.: Resting heart rate investigations with trained and nontrained hypophysectomized rats. J. Appl. Physiol., 26:585, 1969.
12. Åstrand, P.O., and Rodahl, K.: Textbook of Work Physiology. New York, McGraw-Hill Book Co., 1970.
13. Åstrand, P.O., and Christiansen, E.H.: Oxygen in the animal organism. In Aerobic Work Capacity. Edited by F. Dickens, E. Neil, and W.F. Widdas. New York, Pergamon Press, 1964.
14. Hollmann, H.: Hochst—und dauerleistungsfahegheit des sportlers. Munich, Johann Ambrosiu Barth, 1963.
15. Rowell, L.B., et al.: Splanchnic removal of lactate and pyruvate during prolonged exercise in man. J. Appl. Physiol., 21:1773, 1966.
16. Mellander, S.: Comparative studies on the adrenergic neurohumoral control of resistance and capacitance blood vessels in the cat. Acta Physiol. Scand., 176:1, 1960.
17. Patterson, S.W., Piper, H., and Starling, E.H.: The regulation of the heart beat. J. Physiol., 48:465, 1914.
18. Rushmer, R.F., Smith, O., and Franklin, D.: Mechanisms of cardiac control in exercise. Circ. Res., 7:602, 1959.
19. Rushmer, R.F.: Constancy of stroke volume in ventricular responses to exertion. Am. J. Physiol., 196:745, 1959.
20. Smith, E.E., et al.: Integrated mechanisms of cardiovascular response and control during exercise in the normal human. Prog. Cardiovasc. Dis.,28:421, 1976.
20a.Ehrlich, W., et al.: The effect of beta-blockade on coronary and systemic circulation in dogs at rest and during adaptation to exercise. Arch. Int. Pharmacodyn. Ther., 204:213, 1973.
21. Bassenge E., et al.: Effect of chemical sympathectomy on coronary flow and cardiovascular adjustment to exercise in dogs. Pfluegers Arch.,341:285, 1973.
22. Ceretelli, P.: Kinetics of adaptation of cardiac output in exercise. In Physical Activity in Health and Disease. Edited by K. Evang, and K.L. Anderson. Baltimore, The Williams & Wilkins Co., 1966.
23. Pickering, T.G., et al.: Effects of autonomic blockade on the baro-reflex in man at rest and during exercise. Circ. Res., 30:177, 1972.
23a.Edis, A.J., Donald, D.E., and Shepherd, J.T.: Cardiovascular reflexes from stretch of pulmonary vein-atrial junction in the dog. Circ. Res.,27:1091, 1970.
24. Cureton, T.K.: The nature of cardiovascular condition in normal humans. J. Assoc. Phys. Ment. Rehabil., 12:41, 1958.
25. Coleridge, H.M., and Coleridge, J.C.G.: Cardiovascular receptors. Mod. Trends in Physiol., 1:245, 1972.
26. Sleight, P., and Widdicombe, J.G.: Action potentials in fibers from receptors in the epicardium and myocardium of the dog's left ventricle. J. Physiol., 181:235, 1965.
27. Coote, J.H.: Physiological significance of somatic afferent pathways from skeletal muscle and joints with reflex effects on the heart and circulation. Brain Res., 87:139, 1975.
28. McCloskey, D.J., Matthews, P.B.C., and Mitchell, J.H.: Absence of appreciable cardiovascular and

respiratory responses to muscle vibration. J. Appl. Physiol., *33*:623, 1972.

29. Mohrman, D.E., and Sparks, H.V.: Resistance and venous oxygen dynamics during sinusoidal exercise of dog skeletal muscle. Circ. Res., *33*:337, 1973.

30. Ekblom, B., et al.: Effects of atropine and propranolol on the oxygen transport system during exercise in man. Scand. J. Clin. Lab. Invest., *30*:35, 1972.

31. Olsson, K.E., and Saltin, B.: Diet and fluids in training and competition. Scand. J. Rehabil. Med., *3*:31, 1971.

31a. Saltin, B., and Stenberg, J.: Circulatory response to prolonged severe exercise. J. Appl. Physiol., *19*:833, 1964.

31b. Fox, E.L., and Costill, D.L.: Estimated cardiorespiratory response during marathon running. Arch. Environ. Health, *24*:316, 1972.

32. Sugimoto, T., Allison, J.L., and Guyton, A.C.: Effect of maximal work load on cardiac function. Jpn. Heart J., *14*:146, 1973.

33. Braunwald, E., et al.: An analysis of the cardiac response to exercise. Circ. Res., *20*:44, 1967.

33a. Pollock, M.L.: Effects of frequency of training on serum lipids, cardiovascular function, and body composition. *In* Exercise and Fitness. Edited by B.D. Franks. Chicago, Athletic Institute, 1969.

34. Sharkey, B.J., and Holleman, J.P.: Cardiorespiratory adaptations to training at specified intensities. Res. Q., *38*:698, 1967.

35. Keul, J., Doll, E., and Kepplon, D.: Energy Metabolism of Human Muscle. Baltimore: University Park Press, 1972.

36. Åstrand, P.O., and Rhyming, I.: A nomogram for calculation of aerobic capacity (physical fitness) from pulse rate during submaximal work. J. Appl. Physiol., *7*:2, 1954.

37. Margaria, R., Aghemo, P., and Rovelli, E.: Indirect determination of maximum O_2 consumption in man. J. Appl. Physiol., *20*:1070, 1965.

38. Martiz, J.S., et al.: A practical method of estimating an individual's maximal oxygen intake. Ergonomics, *4*:97, 1961.

38a. Davies, C.T.M.: Limitations to the prediction of maximum oxygen intake from cardiac frequency measurements. J. Appl. Physiol., *24*:700, 1968.

39. Balke, B.: Correlation of static and physical endurance. I. A test of physical performance based on the cardiovascular and respiratory responses to gradually increased work. USAF School of Aviation Medicine, Project No. 21-32-004, Report No. 1, Randolph AFB, Texas, April, 1952.

40. Balke, B.: Work capacity at altitude. *In* Science and Medicine of Exercise and Sports. Edited by W.R. Johnson. New York, Harper & Row, 1960.

41. Sjostrand, T.: Changes in the respiratory organs of workmen at an ore melting works. Acta Med. Scand. [Suppl.], *196*:687, 1947.

42. Johnson, R.E., Brouha, L., and Darling, R.C.: A test of physical fiitness for strenuous exertion. Rev. Can. Biol., *1*:491, 1942.

43. Brouha, L., Graybiel, A., and Heath, C.W.: The step test. A simple method of measuring physical fitness for hard muscular work in adult man. Rev. Can. Biol., *2*:86, 1943.

44. deVries, H.A.: Fitness after fifty. Englewood Cliffs, N.J., Prentice-Hall, 1974.

45. deVries, H.A., and Klafs, C.E.: Prediction of maximal O_2 intake from submaximal tests. J. Sports Med. Phys. Fitness, *5*:207, 1965.

46. deVries, H.A.: Laboratory Experiments in Physiology of Exercise. Dubuque, Wm. C. Brown Co., Publishers, 1971.

47. Karvonen, M.J.: Effects of vigorous exercise on the heart. *In* Work and the Heart. Edited by F.F. Rosenbaum, and E. L. Balknap. New York, Paul B. Hoeler, 1959.

48. Kilbom, A.: Effect on women of physical training with low intensities. Scand. J. Clin. Lab. Invest., *28*:345, 1971.

49. Edwards, M.A.: The effects of training at predetermined heart rate levels for sedentary college women. Med. Sci. Sports, *6*:14, 1974.

50. Durnin, J.F.G.A., Brockway, J.M., and Whitcher, H.N.: Effects of a short period of training of varying severity on some measurement of physical fitness. J. Appl. Physiol., *15*:161, 1960.

51. Hollman, W., and Venrath, H.: Die Beeinflussung von herzgrosse, maximaler O_2—aufnahme und ausdauergrenze durch ein ausdauer-training mettlerer und hoher intensitat. Der Sportarzt, *14*:189, 1963.

52. Costill, D.L.: What research tells the coach about distance running. AAHPER, Washington, D.C., 1968.

53. Davis, J.A., and Convertino, V.A.: A comparison of heart rate methods for predicting endurance training intensity. Med. Sci. Sports, *7*:295, 1975.

53a. Fox, E., and Mathews, D.: Interval Training: Conditioning for Sports and General Fitness. Philadelphia, W.B. Saunders Co., 1974.

53b. Wilt, F.: Training for competitive running. *In* Exercise Physiology. Edited by H. Falls. New York, Academic Press, 1968.

54. Guidelines for Graded Excercise Testing and Exercise Prescription. American College of Sports Medicine, Philadelphia, Lea & Febiger, 1975.

55. Yeager, S.A., and Brynteson, P.: Effects of varying training periods on the development of cardiovascular efficiency of college women. Res. Q., *41*:589, 1970.

56. Pollock, M.L., Cureton, T.K., and Greninger, L.: Effects of frequency of training on working capacity, cardiovascular function, and body composition of adult men. Med. Sci. Sports, *1*:70, 1969.

57. Saltin, B.: Oxygen transport by the circulatory system during exercise in man. *In* Limiting Factors of Physical Performance. Edited by J. Keul. Stuttgart, Georg Thieme, 1973.

CHAPTER 5

The Circulatory System in Work and Exercise

Cells in the body can survive only if their internal environment remains constant. Thus, the fluids bathing the cells must not vary greatly in either temperature or concentrations of oxygen, carbon dioxide, nutrients, and inorganic ions. Practically every activity of the body contributes in some way to maintaining the integrity of the cells: the liver stores and metabolizes carbohydrates, fats, and proteins; the lungs take in oxygen and eliminate carbon dioxide; the kidneys eliminate wastes, water, and salts; the gastrointestinal tract conveys body water, nutrients, and salts into the body; and other organs contribute in other ways. But, for these activities to take place, there must be a system to transport materials among all the tissues and organs in the body. This function is performed by the circulatory system, which is comprised of the blood and the apparatus moving the blood, the cardiovascular system. Because the heart and its functions were presented in Chapter 4, the focus in this chapter is on the vascular system.

THE BLOOD

The blood is involved directly or indirectly in practically all body activities because of its transport function. It carries nutrients and other chemical substances to the interstitial fluids bathing the cells. When the cells take what they need, their metabolic waste products are carried back to the interstitial fluids and then to the blood. The body contains approximately five quarts of blood, which is composed of plasma and specialized cells. Plasma is a liquid solution that makes up about 7% of the total body fluid. It is colorless and contains proteins and smaller amounts of salts, glucose, amino acids, and other substances. The proteins in plasma are important because they help to keep the fluids within the blood vessels, thereby preventing excess fluid from escaping from the blood. Fibrinogen, one of the plasma proteins, is involved in blood clotting when it combines with platelets, red cells, and white cells. (White cells are specialized cells distinct from, but suspended in, plasma.) Normally, plasma proteins are not taken from the blood to be used as an energy source by other tissues; blood glucose, however, is used in this way. Before any protein can be metabolized for energy, it must first be changed to acetyl-CoA and then moved into the Krebs' cycle, where the oxidation process begins (see Chap. 2). The specialized cells making up the rest of the blood, in addition to plasma, are red cells, or erythrocytes; white cells, or leukocytes; and platelets. Red cells receive their color from hemoglobin, a protein that carries oxygen. The major function of these cells is to transport oxygenated hemoglobin from the lungs to the body tissues and to carry carbon dioxide in the other direction. White cells combat infectious agents that enter the body either by destroying them directly or by first forming antibodies that then destroy the infectious agent.

WATER AND ELECTROLYTES IN PHYSIOLOGIC FUNCTION

The regulation of the internal environment of the cell requires a continuous supply of nutrients and the elimination of metabolic end products. For this internal regulation to happen, the balance between the chemical substances in the intracellular fluid and the extracellular fluid must be stable. In addition, the concentrations of water in the cell and in its surrounding fluid must be balanced. Such balances are provided by sodium, potassium, calcium, and hydrogen ion. These chemical substances reside in and are transported by water. The abundant supply of water in the body comprises from 45 to 75% of body weight and acts as a large reservoir to provide the kind of internal environment essential to maintaining the life of body tissues. The large component of water in the blood plasma and in the extracellular fluids plays a major role in delivering nutrients to the cell and in eliminating metabolic by-products.

At rest and during light work, adequate amounts of liquids are consumed to maintain the integrity of the internal environment. But, in heavy and prolonged work during which sweating is profuse, the quantities of water lost by the body may pose difficulties for the adaptive processes. Excessive water loss may upset the balance between the intracellular and extracellular fluids. To understand how this imbalance occurs, one must first know about the roles of water and certain chemical substances in the body.

Water Balance in the Body

The proper balance of water between the intracellular fluid and the extracellular fluid is accomplished by balancing intake and output. Some average values for sources of intake and output of water are presented in Table 5–1. About half of the intake comes from drinking liquids, whereas the other half comes from food and from the breakdown of foods used for energy. Much of the metabolically produced water comes from the oxida-

Table 5–1.

Sources of Water Intake and Output in Adults

		Milliliters Per Day
Intake:		
Drink		1,200
Food		1,100
Metabolically produced		300
	Total	2,600
Output:		
Insensible loss		
Skin		300
Lungs		700
Sweat		100
Feces		100
Urine		1,400
	Total	2,600

tion of carbohydrates, whose end-products are CO_2 and H_2O. Water is lost through four sites: skin, lungs, gastrointestinal tract, and kidneys. Water loss from the skin and lungs is referred to as insensible loss because a person is unaware of its occurrence. Additional losses from the skin occur during heavy work and may amount to as much as 1.8 l./hr. in heat-acclimatized men. If water loss is not partially replaced while working and sweating profusely, the balance between the intracellular and extracellular fluids may be upset. A chain of physiologic events occurs as a consequence and can lead to such injury as heat stroke or heat exhaustion.

The loss of water from the lungs under normal conditions amounts to approximately 15 ml./hr., but may reach 130 ml./hr. or more during heavy work. Water loss from the urine is also affected by prolonged work. When sweating is excessive, the volume of urine may decrease to 5 or 10 ml./hr. from the normal values of 30 to 60 ml./hr. This reduction in urine water as a result of extensive work indicates an adaptation to excessive water loss from sweating and conserves more water.

Water balance is primarily controlled by voluntary intake (thirst) and urinary loss.

Although the other processes provide some control, they are not primarily oriented toward water balance. For example, in the catabolism of carbohydrates, which provides the major source of water from oxidation, control is held by mechanisms directed toward regulation of energy balance. In sweat production, control is held by the mechanisms directed toward temperature regulation. Loss of water by the skin and lungs is really uncontrollable, and fecal water is usually small.

Of the two primary mechanisms that control water balance, thirst and urination, the major automatic mechanism by which body water is regulated is urination. Control by thirst is certainly less automatic and is conditioned somewhat by psychologic factors. Whereas thirst may be prolonged or even forgotten for a long time, this is not the case with the desire to urinate. There is a time interval between water loss and thirst in man. This time lapse does not occur with some animals, such as dogs, who drink sufficient amounts of water in several minutes to equal the amount depleted. Human beings may maintain a water deficit amounting to 4% of body weight for hours after dehydration.[1] Even though thirst responds slowly to water loss, it eventually achieves a balance within 1% of normal.

The concentrations of certain chemical substances in the extracellular fluid are also associated with a proper water balance in the body. These substances are vital to life processes.

Regulation of Water Volume in Extracellular and Intracellular Fluids

The volume of water inside and outside cells is maintained within narrow limits primarily by the concentrations of sodium in the fluids. The measure of the concentration of sodium, or any other substance dissolved in a fluid, is the osmolarity of a fluid. The higher the osmolarity (or sodium dissolved in water), the lower the water concentration. Because all cell membranes are freely permeable to water, a permanent difference

between extracellular and intracellular water cannot exist. Consequently, when water concentration decreases because of increased osmolarity in the extracellular fluid, water in greater concentrations in the intracellular fluid leaves the cell until a new equilibrium is reached. Correspondingly, there is also an equilibrium in osmolarity between the two fluids. Because osmolarity is an inverse measure of water concentration, the movement of water between intracellular and extracellular fluids can be explained on the basis of osmolarity or sodium concentration in the fluids. Any difference in the osmolarity across cell membranes causes movement of water from low osmolarity (high water concentration) to high osmolarity (low water concentration) until equilibrium is reached. For example, when several pints of pure water are ingested, water is absorbed from the gastrointestinal tract into the blood, where it moves rapidly throughout the extracellular fluid, thereby making its osmolarity lower (higher water concentration) than that of the cells. As a result, water diffuses into the cells until the osmolarities are again equal. If the water ingested had exactly the same osmolarity as the extracellular fluid, the water would not pass into cells because the force needed to move it across cell membranes would not exist. As long as the osmolarity remains the same outside and inside the cells, regardless of the greater volume of water on one side, shifting of water does not take place. Thus, the volume of water in the extracellular fluid depends primarily on the quantity of extracellular sodium. Because sodium does not pass easily into cells, the osmolarity of extracellular fluids determines the movement and volume of water in the cells.

Sodium in extracellular fluids is balanced so that normal quantities of water are present in cells. Any excess sodium draws water out of the cells, and insufficient quantities move water into the cells. Several mechanisms remove excessive amounts of sodium from the extracellular fluids. One such mechanism is a relatively slow process involving the storage of excess sodium in bone tissue, whereas the other process is more rapid and involves the excretion of sodium largely from the urine. When extracellular volume is decreased, bone can liberate sodium into the extracellular fluid to increase osmolarity and to draw water out of the cells. But, a more long-term regulator of extracellular volume must control total body sodium and water by balancing intake and excretion. Such regulation is accomplished by food intake of salt and the excretion of sodium in sweat, feces, and urine.

The most important mechanism for the regulation of extracellular volume and osmolarity involves the kidney and the factors controlling its function. The excretory rates of sodium and water can be varied over a wide range depending on water intake and excretion. In a normal kidney, sodium excretion may be regulated for intakes of sodium chloride varying from 25 g. to as low as 50 mg. Similarly, water excretion in urine can be varied by the kidney from approximately 400 ml. per day to 25 l. per day. During prolonged and severe exercise in the heat, when sweating rate is high, the excretion of water by the kidneys is relatively low. However, when large amounts of fluid are ingested, excretion is high. The kidney responds in function to the amount of extracellular volume. To prevent a deficit, the excretion of sodium and water is held to a minimum. Conversely, an increased extracellular volume is prevented by excess secretion of sodium and water.

Electrolytes in Physiologic Functions

Chemical substances that dissociate into electrically charged particles, called ions, when placed in water are called electrolytes. For example, when sodium chloride (NaCl) is placed in water, the sodium breaks away from the chlorine. The result is a positively charged sodium ion (cation), or Na^+, and a negatively charged chloride ion (anion), or Cl^-. The electrolytes in the body are potassium, magnesium, phosphate, sodium, calcium, and chloride. The distribution of these ions in the intracellular and extracellular fluids is such that relatively more positive ions (cations) are outside the cell and more negative ions (anions) are inside. The main electrolytes in the extracellular fluid are sodium and chloride. Potassium is the main electrolyte in the intracellular fluid. The negative electrochemical force inside the cell (negative charge of about -85 millivolts) tends to attract the positive ions on the outside and, at the same time, tends to move the negative ions from the inside to the outside. The rapid shifting of positive and negative ions across cell membranes in muscle fibers occurs in the propagation of an impulse and is referred to as depolarization (see Fig. 1–8). But, for this shifting to happen, the cell membrane must first become permeable so that the ions can pass back and forth. The acetylcholine, secreted by an axon of a motor neuron at the neuromuscular junction, initiates the events leading to an increased membrane permeability in the muscle fiber (see Fig. 1–7). The increased permeability is primarily due to the main electrolytes, sodium chloride and potassium. The shifting of these electrolytes is responsible for depolarization, repolarization, and polarization. In the process of repolarization, sodium and chloride are moved out of and potassium is moved into the cell to result in more positive ions outside and more negative ions inside the cell. The specific mechanisms involved in moving sodium out and potassium in are not known. However, it is believed that a carrier molecule attaches to potassium ions and passes across the membrane into a cell. Inside the cell, the potassium ions are released and the same number of sodium ions are attached to the carrier molecule and passed to the outside of the cell. This process requires energy because the carrier molecule carries these ions against their electrochemical gradients. In other words, each ion is carried from a more concentrated area to a less concentrated area. Moving ions or molecules from a less dense area to a more dense area is akin to rowing upstream in a boat; it takes more energy. The difference in this analogy is that, in the case of a river, there is not an electrochemical gradient but an energy gradient in that the water upstream has a greater potential energy than does the water downstream.

A proper balance of electrolytes between the intracellular and extracellular fluids not only ensures normal nerve conduction, but also ensures neuromuscular irritability to stimuli, muscle contractility, energy metabolism, cardiac conduction of impulses, bone growth, regulation of blood volume, and normal kidney functions.

THE CIRCULATORY SYSTEM

The circulatory system is divided into the systemic circulation and the pulmonary circulation (Fig. 5–1). The systemic circulation is the circuit through which the blood is pumped from the left half of the heart to the right half of the heart. Blood pumped from

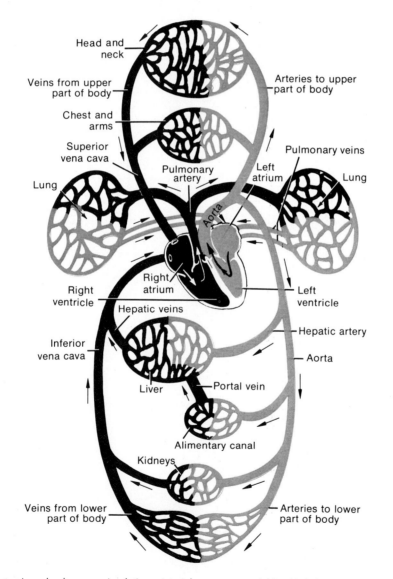

Fig. 5–1. Systemic and pulmonary circulations. Arterial, or oxygenated, blood is light; venous blood is dark. (From Schottelius, B.A., and Schottelius, D.D.: Textbook of Physiology. 18th Edition. St. Louis, The C. V. Mosby Co., 1978.)

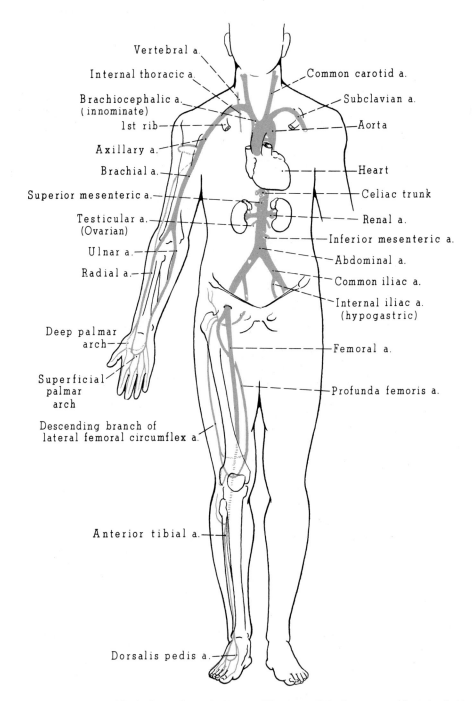

Vertebral a.
Internal thoracic a.
Brachiocephalic a.
(innominate)
1st rib
Axillary a.
Brachial a.
Superior mesenteric a.
Testicular a.
(Ovarian)
Ulnar a.
Radial a.
Deep palmar arch
Superficial palmar arch
Descending branch of lateral femoral circumflex a.
Anterior tibial a.
Dorsalis pedis a.

Common carotid a.
Subclavian a.
Aorta
Heart
Celiac trunk
Renal a.
Inferior mesenteric a.
Abdominal a.
Common iliac a.
Internal iliac a.
(hypogastric)
Femoral a.
Profunda femoris a.

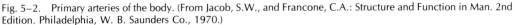

Fig. 5–2.   Primary arteries of the body. (From Jacob, S.W., and Francone, C.A.: Structure and Function in Man. 2nd Edition. Philadelphia, W. B. Saunders Co., 1970.)

the right half of the heart through the lungs and back to the left half of the heart travels through the pulmonary circulation. Both circuits are made of blood vessels of different sizes and functions. Vessels leaving the heart are large and taper in diameter as they branch off to various organs and tissues. Vessels returning to the heart enlarge as the branches lead into larger vessels that feed into the heart. The sequence of blood flow from the heart begins with the arteries and leads to the arterioles, capillaries, venules, veins, and back to the heart.

Arteries

The largest vessels are called arteries, and they transport blood from the heart under high pressure (Fig. 5–2). The walls of arteries are especially strong to tolerate the high pressure and the rapid flow of blood. Blood pressures in the arteries of the systemic circulation drop from an average of about 100 mm Hg at the aorta coming off the heart to 0 to .5 mm Hg in the large veins feeding into the right atrium. Arteries consist of three coats: an inner coat (tunica intima vasorum), a middle coat (tunica media vasorum), and an outer coat (tunica adventitia) (Fig. 5–3). The inner coat consists of primarily endothelial cells and connective and elastic tissues; the middle coat consists mostly of smooth muscle and elastic tissue; and the outer coat contains connective and elastic tissues.

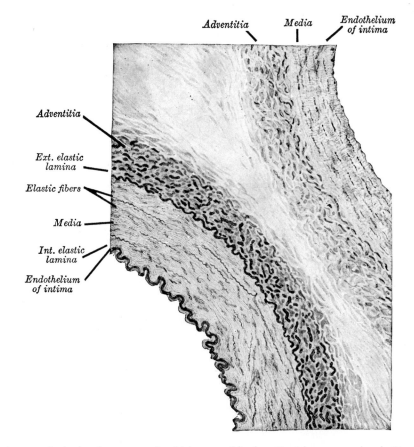

Fig. 5–3.   Artery and vein showing comparative thicknesses of the three tissue layers around each. Muscle and outer tissues of the arteries are larger than those in the veins. (From Gray's Anatomy of the Human Body. 29th Edition. Revised and edited by Charles M. Goss. Philadelphia, Lea & Febiger, 1973.)

Arterioles

The next smaller branches of the arterial system are the arterioles, which play the largest part in controlling the flow of blood to the capillaries. An arteriole contains smooth muscle that can either constrict and close off blood flow completely or relax and permit a sevenfold increase in flow. The large diameters of arteries and veins provide little resistance to flow. Consequently, the control of blood pressure in the total circulation is mainly determined by the resistance at the arteriolar level.

Capillaries

Following the arterioles in size are the capillaries, where the exchange of fluid and nutrients takes place between the blood and the interstitial spaces in the systemic circulation. The necessary nutrients and chemicals are taken from the interstitial fluid by the cells in exchange for the end products of metabolism. In the lungs, the exchange at the site of the capillaries is between gases in the alveoli of the lungs and in the blood. Exchanges occur in the thin capillary walls, which are permeable to small molecular substances. Their permeability varies throughout the body; the liver capillaries have the largest openings and the brain capillaries have the smallest. No capillary is large enough, however, to allow the passage of red cells. Capillaries do not have elastic tissue, connective tissue, or smooth muscle to impede the passage of substances through

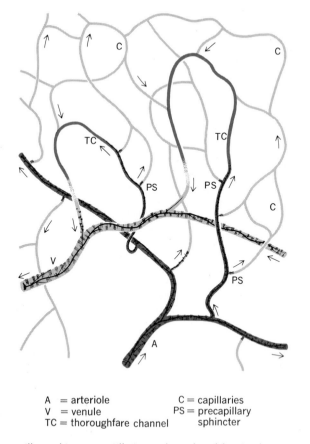

A = arteriole   C = capillaries
V = venule   PS = precapillary
TC = thoroughfare channel   sphincter

Fig. 5–4.   Arterioles, precapillary sphincters, capillaries, and venules of the circulatory system. (From Vander, A.J., Sherman, H.H., and Luciano, D.S.: Human Physiology—The Mechanisms of Body Function. New York, McGraw-Hill, Inc., 1975. Used with permission of McGraw-Hill Book Co.)

their walls. The network of capillaries is so profuse in the body and their cross-sectional area is so large that, if all the capillaries were filled, they would hold about eight quarts of blood, more than could fit in the whole body. But at rest, only about 5% of the total circulating blood flows through the capillaries. During heavy exercise, more than five times as many capillaries may be open in a muscle to meet cellular needs. Blood enters the capillaries from the arterioles only when the precapillary sphincters open. These sphincters are located at the entrances to the capillaries and contain a ring of smooth muscle (Fig. 5–4). Blood flow through any capillary is usually intermittent because its precapillary sphincter opens and closes periodically. The sphincters function in a coordinated fashion with arteriolar smooth muscle to regulate both the flow of blood through the capillaries and the number of functioning capillaries. Their smooth muscle is stimulated to constrict or to relax by local chemical factors and only to a limited degree by nerve activity.

Venules and Veins

Blood is transported from the capillaries into small vessels, called venules, and then into veins (Figs. 5–4 and 5–5). By the time blood passes through the arterioles and capillaries, most of the pressure imparted to the blood by the heart is lost. Therefore, pressure in the venules is only about 15% of the pressure in the arteries. Even though the pressure in the veins is small, the large diameter of the veins permits great quantities of blood to flow to the heart.

The veins perform an important function by controlling the amount of blood circulating through the heart and circulatory systems. This control in exercise is provided by the sympathetic nerves to veins, which cause vasoconstriction, and by mechanical factors involving muscular contractions. Blood flow to working muscles is enhanced by the movement by vasoconstriction of large amounts of blood from the reservoirs in the veins of the viscera to the heart, where

it is pumped to skeletal muscles. At rest, the veins contain about 65 to 70% of the total blood volume, whereas the arteries hold less than 15%. During strenuous exercise, most of the venous blood is pumped to the working muscles. In fact, total blood flow through the circulatory system increases fivefold or more during heavy work. This increase occurs because of the greater availability of venous blood to the muscles and the increased cardiac output.

The mechanical factors operating on the veins to control blood flow through the circulatory system produce an increase in venous pressure and facilitate venous return to the heart. These factors involve the skeletal muscle ''pump'' of working muscle and the movement of breathing. A contracting skeletal muscle applies pressure to the veins within it, thus pushing blood toward the heart. The one-way valves in the vessels prevent the blood from moving away from the heart. When a muscle alternately contracts and relaxes, a ''pumping'' action squeezes the venous blood along its way. The breathing mechanism also moves venous blood, but does so only on specific veins. During inspiration, the descent of the diaphragm pushes on the large veins in the abdomen and thoracic cavity. At the same time, the inferior vena cava is shortened, thus reducing its volume and increasing pressure to expedite blood flow. Consequently, the movement of blood to the heart is facilitated.

CONTROL OF BLOOD FLOW IN ARTERIOLES

Blood flow in the vessels is primarily controlled by the resistances in the arterioles. When the vessels dilate, resistance is reduced and flow is increased; when the vessels constrict, the opposite actions occur. Caliber size in the blood vessels is mainly controlled by the degree of contraction of smooth muscle around the vessels. Smooth muscle responds to a great variety of inhibitory and excitatory stimuli, such as chemicals at the ends of motor nerves to

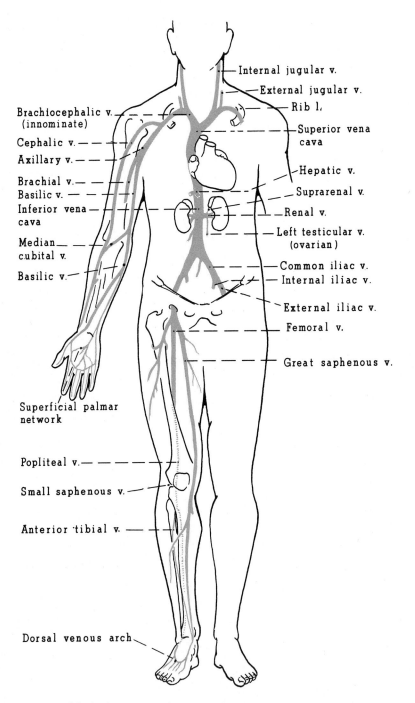

Fig. 5–5. Primary veins of the body. (From Jacob, S.W., and Francone, C.A.: Structure and Function in Man. 2nd Edition. Philadelphia, W. B. Saunders Co., 1970.)

the vessel (sometimes called vasomotor nerves), certain substances from metabolism of the tissue cells surrounding the vessels, changes in the blood entering the vessels (e.g., hormones, carbon dioxide, oxygen, pH), and changes in temperature. The response of smooth muscle to these stimuli varies depending on the location of the vessels in the body. For example, smooth muscle of the arterioles in the brain is sensitive to carbon dioxide and either contracts or relaxes when carbon dioxide is present. However, when the muscle is stimulated by motor nerves, it barely responds. The arterioles in the skin overlying the skull are hardly activated by carbon dioxide, but are greatly affected by their vasomotor nerves.

The total effect of all the stimuli activating smooth muscle at the arteriolar level in controlling blood flow can be expressed in terms of resistance to blood flow. Resistance to blood flow in the entire body is referred to as total peripheral resistance. Arteriolar constriction and dilatation, which determine total peripheral resistance, are controlled by two mechanisms: (1) local controls that serve the metabolic needs of the tissue, and (2) reflex controls that coordinate the needs of the entire body. These mechanisms are illustrated in Figure 5–6.

Local Control of Flow

Some organs and tissues, such as the heart and skeletal muscles, experience an increase in blood flow whenever their metabolic activity is increased. In fact, the blood flow to the exercising skeletal muscle is directly proportional to the increased activity of the muscle. Increased flow is a direct result of arteriolar dilatation within the active tissue. This vasodilatation is not a result of nerves or hormones inhibiting the contraction of smooth muscle of the arterioles, but is a locally initiated response. The exact cause of the metabolic vasodilatation in contracting muscle is not known. However, it is believed that the lack of oxygen in the muscle either initiates vasodilatation or directly relates to another metabolite that has such an effect. Some of the metabolites and chemicals that may directly regulate blood flow are potassium ions, hydrogen ions, and lactate.

Blood flow to an active muscle during exercise may increase 15 times the normal blood flow, mostly because of local control. The decrease in vascular resistance permits an increase of oxygen and metabolic foodstuffs to the working muscles. The effects of local vasodilatation are not limited to the working muscle; there are also secondary effects in the entire circulation. Vasodilatation in the muscle is associated with lowered resistance to flow in the veins so that venous return to the heart is increased. In fact, local vasodilatation alone plays a significant role in increasing cardiac output by enhancing venous return. When sympathetic stimulation is added to local vasodila-

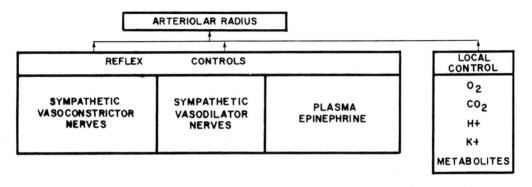

Fig. 5–6.   Control of blood flow in arterioles by local controls and reflex controls.

tation, a further enhancement in blood flow occurs.

Reflex Control of Flow

The sympathetic nerves of the autonomic nervous system supply many fibers to most arterioles and veins in the body. A majority of these nerves releases norepinephrine which causes smooth muscle to contract around vessels, thus restricting blood flow. The only arterioles not constricted by these sympathetic fibers are located in the brain and the heart.

In addition to sympathetic-constrictor fibers supplying the arterioles in skeletal muscle, sympathetic fibers to these arterioles also dilate the arterioles. For dilatation to occur, the nerve fibers must release acetylcholine instead of norepinephrine. These dilator fibers increase blood flow to skeletal muscle before exercise actually begins. For such an increase to occur, impulses are sent to the sympathetic-dilator fibers of skeletal muscle via the higher brain centers of the cerebral cortex.

Because the dilatation and constriction of arteriolar smooth muscle are controlled by sympathetic nerve fibers, the extent to which the nerves are stimulated determines the caliber of the arterioles. A good example of this relationship is the control of the skin arterioles by the sympathetic fibers. Skin arterioles are greatly stimulated to constrict by sympathetic discharge. When these arterioles are further stimulated by fear or cold, their increased constriction caused by reflex action inhibits blood flow and pales the skin. In contrast, when one is embarrassed or when body temperature increases, the reflex inhibits the sympathetic nerves to the skin, causing the arterioles to dilate and the skin to flush. When body temperature increases during exercise, the increased quantities of blood in the dilated arteries allow the body to release more heat through the blood.

The constrictor effect on arterioles by the sympathetic nerves reduces the blood flow to organs not directly involved in exercise, such as the gastrointestinal tract and kidneys, and increases blood flow to the heart and skeletal muscles. This effect occurs even before exercise commences. In addition, blood to the skeletal muscles is increased by the vasodilator effects of sympathetic stimulation on the arterioles. The activation of vasodilator fibers of the sympathetic nerves supplying the arterioles of skeletal muscle is of short duration (about 10 sec. into exercise).[6] After this activation, the vessels in the muscles directly involved in the exercise remain open in proportion to metabolic rate at the local level. The vessels of nonworking muscles constrict by the dominance of sympathetic vasoconstrictor fibers.

Parasympathetic nerves of the autonomic nervous system supply some blood vessels in the genital tract only. Consequently, the parasympathetic nerves have no direct effect on modifying the caliber of arterioles. However, they do increase blood flow in certain glands, but primarily by increasing the glands' metabolic activity. In exercise, as the sympathetic system is stimulated to move blood from internal organs to the working muscles, the activity of the parasympathetic system is curtailed. Thus, blood flow to the exercising muscle increases.

The most important hormone causing dilatation of arterial smooth muscle is epinephrine. This hormone is released from the adrenal medulla gland by direct activation of sympathetic nerve fibers to this organ. In addition to epinephrine, the adrenal gland secretes norepinephrine, which also circulates in the blood to other tissues. Total adrenal secretions are comprised of 80% epinephrine and 20% norepinephrine. Both increase heart rate and dilate coronary vessels, but epinephrine dilates and norepinephrine constricts the arterioles in skeletal muscle. Before exercise, activation of the adrenal medulla and secretion of epinephrine readies the body. But, shortly after exercise begins, the effects of the circulating epinephrine on the arterioles are probably minimal when compared with the effects exerted by norepinephrine, which is released at the endings of sympathetic nerve fibers.

REGULATION OF SYSTEMIC ARTERIAL PRESSURE

Blood flow through the circulation is maintained by a continuous pressure exerted on the blood. Reflex activity of the blood vessels and local metabolic needs of skeletal muscle modify circulatory resistance and the activity of the heart (see Fig. 5–6). As total peripheral resistance in the blood vessels increases, cardiac output ($\dot{Q}$ = stroke volume × heart rate) must increase to maintain an adequate flow. Conversely, as resistance in the vessels decreases to improve flow, cardiac output decreases. These relationships are illustrated in Figure 5–7. To maintain an adequate blood flow to the tissues and organs, arterial blood pressure must remain relatively constant. During exercise, when large quantities of blood are sent to the dilated vessels of working skeletal muscle, pressure tends to fall. To prevent this decrease, either cardiac output, the caliber of other arteriolar vascular beds, or both must be changed. Usually, arterial pressure in exercise is maintained or increased by elevation of cardiac ouput.

Vasomotor Region in Controlling Blood Pressure

Reflex control of blood flow by the sympathetic nerves occurs via the vasomotor region in the medulla of the brain stem (see Fig. 3–10). Three major regions in the medulla control reflex functions: vasomotor, cardiac, and respiratory. Information to these regions comes from a variety of afferent receptors. The motor response to the information travels via the autonomic nervous system (Fig. 5–8). The functional relationships between the vasomotor and cardiac regions are primarily responsible for

the regulation of blood pressure. Input from a variety of afferent receptors is continually conveyed to, and interpreted by, the three regions. Information comes from arterial receptors that are stimulated by stretch (baroreceptors) or by concentrations of oxygen, carbon dioxide, and hydrogen ions (chemoreceptors). Other receptors are located in the periphery and respond to cold, pain, heat, pressure, or movement in the joints. Afferent receptors that are close to these regions, located in the hypothalamus or center of the brain, are activated by specific gases and temperature changes in the fluid bathing these tissues. The response to input, in the regulation of blood pressure, occurs largely through the autonomic nervous system.

Afferent Receptors and the Autonomic Nervous System in Regulating Blood Pressure

Afferent receptors, when activated, initiate a chain of events that results in a reflex response evoked by the autonomic nervous system. The same response occurs every time a specific receptor is stimulated. This consistency indicates that the neural pathway between the afferent and the efferent fibers is not randomly determined. All afferent input goes to the central nervous system, but the output by way of the autonomic system is unique to the receptor initiating the response. Sometimes the receptor primarily responsible for a specific response is difficult to determine because all receptors play some part in the effect. In other instances, this is not a problem because a specific effector response is more clearly identified with a particular afferent receptor.

Regulation of blood pressure occurs by the interacting relationship between cardiac function and arteriolar resistance to blood flow. The factors influencing heart activity and vascular resistance, illustrated in Figure 5–7, show the importance of the autonomic nervous system, and particularly of sympathetic activity, in regulating blood pressure. The large role played by the sympathetic

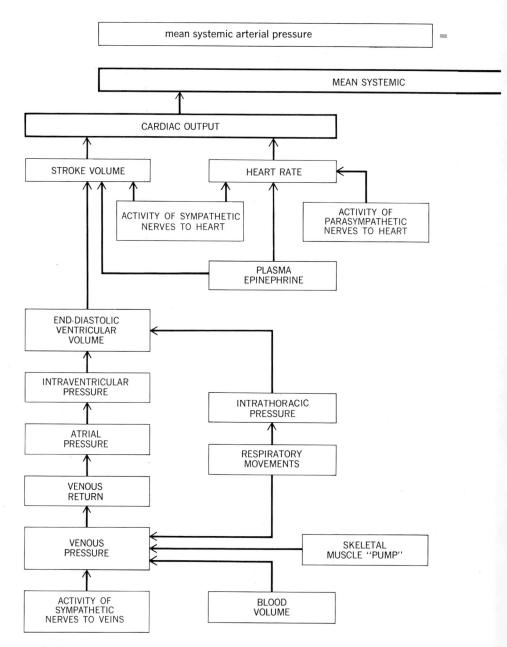

Fig. 5–7.   Factors affecting cardiac output and total peripheral resistance in systemic arterial blood pressure. (From Vander, A.J., Sherman, J.H., and Luciano, D.S.: Human Physiology—The Mechanisms of Body Function. New York, McGraw-Hill, Inc., 1975. Used with permission of McGraw-Hill Book Co.)

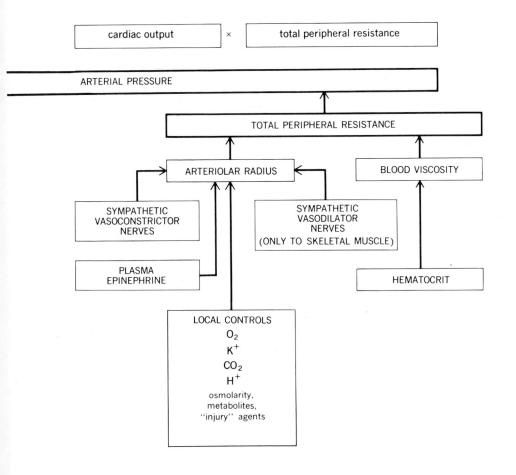

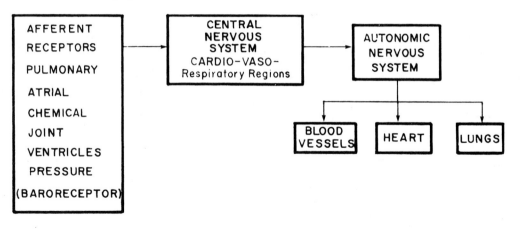

Fig. 5–8.   Sources of afferent input to the cardio-vaso-respiratory regions in the central nervous system and sources of output via the autonomic nervous system in regulating blood flow and pressure by reflex activity.

nerves in controlling blood pressure is understandable—the sympathetic nerves are in a better anatomic position than are the parasympathetic nerves. Practically all the blood vessels of the body, except the capillaries, are supplied with sympathetic fibers. Such is not the case with parasympathetic fibers.

The most important receptors bringing information to the vasomotor and cardiac regions for the control of blood pressure are the arterial stretch receptors (baroreceptors) and the chemoreceptors (Fig. 5–9). These receptors lie close to each other where the two major arteries (carotid) supplying the brain each divide into two smaller arteries. The afferent nerves for the baroreceptors and for the chemoreceptors are located at this bifurcation. Similar receptors are found in the arch of the aorta as it leaves the top of the heart and descends into the lower portions of the body. The areas on the carotid arteries and on the aorta containing the baroreceptors are called carotid sinuses and aortic sinuses, respectively. Chemoreceptors located nearby are referred to as carotid bodies and aortic bodies. Baroreceptors in the aortic sinus control the general blood pressure throughout the body, whereas those in the carotid sinuses control blood pressure in the brain.

Arterial baroreceptors are stimulated by mean arterial pressure and by pulse pressure. When an increase in pressure occurs, the rate of discharge of the carotid and aortic sinuses increases. These impulses are sent

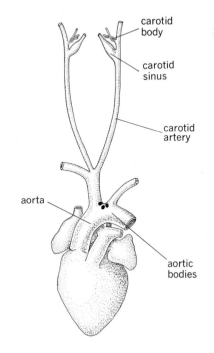

Fig. 5–9.   Location of the carotid and aortic bodies and sinuses. (From Vander, A.J., Sherman, J.H., and Luciano, D.S.: Human Physiology—The Mechanisms of Body Function. New York, McGraw-Hill, Inc., 1975. Used with permission of McGraw-Hill Book Co.)

by the afferent nerves to the vasomotor and cardiac regions to induce (1) slowing of the heart by increased parasympathetic discharge and decreased sympathetic discharge; (2) reduction of the force of cardiac contraction by a lowering of sympathetic activity; (3) dilatation of arteries as a result of inhibition of sympathetic discharge to arteriolar smooth muscle; and (4) dilatation of veins as a result of a decrease in sympathetic discharage to venous smooth muscle. Consequently, blood pressure is reduced by decreasing cardiac output (decreased heart rate and stroke volume) and by peripheral resistance. When pressure at the baroreceptors drops excessively, the reduced rate of discharge is conveyed to the vasomotor and cardiac regions via afferent nerves. Sympathetic discharge to the heart and blood increases heart rate and force and general vasoconstriction, thus increasing cardiac output and peripheral resistance to elevate blood pressure.

When exercise begins, vasodilatation in the working muscles decreases total peripheral resistance. As arterial pressure begins to fall, the baroreceptors are stimulated. Sensory nerves from the receptors convey information to the vasomotor region where the sympathetic nerves to the vascular system and heart are stimulated. The result is vasoconstriction in the nonworking muscles and viscera and increased heart activity to elevate blood pressure. However, when blood pressure is raised during work, the increased stimulation of the baroreceptors is not sufficient to reduce pressure. Excessive stress on the baroreceptors by high blood pressure in exercise eventually reduces activation of the sympathetic nerves to the blood vessels and heart, tending to lower blood pressure. But, because the other factors of cardiac output (stroke volume and heart rate) have a greater effect on increasing blood pressure than the sympathetics have on reducing blood pressure, it remains elevated in exercise.

The role of the chemoreceptors in controlling blood pressure is not as important as the role of the baroreceptors; however, the chemoreceptors have some effect. When arterial oxygen is low, stimulation of the chemoreceptors and, in turn, the cardiovascular regions results in an elevation of blood pressure. This elevation occurs by greater stimulation of the sympathetic nerves to the heart and to blood vessels in nonworking tissues. As a result, cardiac force in systole and vasoconstriction in nonworking muscles are enhanced.[3]

Other afferent receptors influence blood pressure by their effects on cardiac function and vasodilatation. Atrial receptors, located at both junctions where the veins meet the atria, are stimulated by pressure or increased blood volume. When this stimulation happens, heart rate is increased by sympathetic stimulation, but sympathetic fibers to the working muscles are inhibited, resulting in greater vasodilatation.[4,5] Thus, heart rate adjusts to venous return. Similar reflex responses occur when the pulmonary receptors, located in the lungs, are stretched during heavy breathing in exercise.[6] Heart rate increases and vasodilatation occurs in the exercised muscles. Even movements of skeletal joints during exercise affect blood pressure. The joint proprioceptors are stimulated by muscle action and reflexly increase heart rate and vasoconstriction in nonworking tissues.[7,8] As a result, blood pressure increases.

BLOOD PRESSURE AT REST AND WORK

As blood is pumped from the heart through the aorta to the other vessels of the circulation, arterial pressure gradually decreases. Blood-pressure changes in the different portions of the systemic and pulmonary circulatory systems are shown in Figure 5–10. For example, when blood leaves the left ventricle and passes into the systemic system, the pressure of about 100 mm Hg at rest in the contracting ventricle is conveyed to most of the aorta. Immediately before entering the arterioles, the pressure drops to about 85 mm Hg. The blood pressure of 100 mm Hg in the aorta is based on

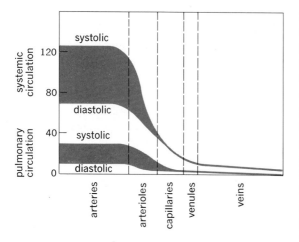

Fig. 5–10.   Changes in blood pressure in the systemic and pulmonary circulations. (From Vander, A.J., Sherman, J.H., and Luciano, D.S.: Human Physiology—The Mechanisms of Body Function. New York, McGraw-Hill, Inc., 1975. Used with permission of McGraw-Hill Book Co.)

the average values for diastolic and systolic blood pressures, which are 100 and 120 mm Hg, respectively. Systolic pressure is measured at the brachial artery, which passes through the upper arm. The amount of pressure required to permit blood flow through the artery is diastolic pressure. Blood pressure is measured by the height in millimeters to which mercury (Hg) is raised or lowered in a hollow tube. The instrument used to measure blood pressure is called a sphygmomanometer. Resistance to blood flow is greatest in the arterioles, where about one half of all the resistance is found. Therefore, by the time the blood reaches the capillaries, the pressure has dropped from about 55 mm Hg in the arterioles to about 30 mm Hg just before entering the capillaries. The pressure in the capillaries drops from 30 mm Hg to 10 mm Hg just before entering the venules. The pressure then decreases to about 0 to 0.5 mm Hg at the right atrium of the heart.

During heavy work, systolic and diastolic pressures may reach 175 and 110 mm Hg, respectively.[9] During moderate to strenuous exercise, systolic pressure increases to 160 mm Hg but diastolic pressure barely

changes.[10] When large muscle groups are exercised continuously by cycling, running, or walking to achieve blood pressures of 160 to 175 mm Hg, and additional muscles involving smaller muscle mass are also worked, blood pressure exceeds the expected level. When work is performed by walking on a treadmill, blood pressure increases beyond the expected level if a handgrip is also held at 50% of maximum force for 60 sec.[11] Systolic pressure rises by 45 mm Hg and diastolic pressure rises by 40 mm Hg. Work performed by the arms results in a greater arterial pressure than does work done by the legs at a given cardiac output (Fig. 5–11). Consequently, a larger contraction force in the heart is required to overcome the increased pressure in the aorta. The higher aortic pressure in exercise with small muscle groups is probably caused by the increased vasoconstriction in inactive muscles. Contrast this effect to the greater amount of vasodilatation occurring in large muscle groups during exercise. Increased vasodilatation tends to lower blood pressure, whereas vasoconstriction increases blood pressure.

The large increase in blood pressure resulting from work performed with small muscle groups has implications for individuals with suspected or known coronary heart disease. The excess pressure placed on the heart to maintain blood flow against a large vascular resistance may exceed the cardiac reserve capacity of the individual. If so, the abnormally functioning heart may further reduce its capacity for work and/or experience a failure. Activities to be discouraged when cardiac reserve is at a low level are those that elicit maximum or near-maximum contractions of relatively small muscle groups and even of large muscles if the effort is sustained. Weight training lifts and certain calisthenic exercises fall into this category, as do certain gymnastic stunts on parallel bars or rings. To work well within cardiac reserve, individuals should participate in activities that involve large muscle groups and relatively small forces of contraction to be

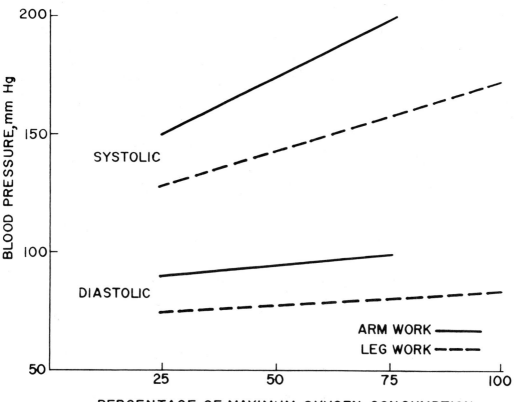

Fig. 5–11.   Changes in systolic and diastolic blood pressures in arm work and leg work. Arm work did not result in maximum oxygen consumption. (Data from Åstrand, P.O., et al.: Intra-arterial blood pressure during exercise with different muscle groups. J. Appl. Physiol., *20:*253, 1965.)

sustained for about 5 min. or longer. Of course, individuals who are 35 years old or older without previous history or symptoms of coronary heart disease and individuals who are younger but have symptoms or high risk factors should follow the guidelines in Table 4–4 before beginning an exercise program.

When exercise involves strong muscular contractions and the holding of one's breath, pressure in the thoracic cavity may more than double. Consequently, pressure on the veins leading to the heart increases, thereby restricting blood flow. When this happens, both systolic and diastolic pressures increase sharply. The drop in venous return to the right atrium reduces blood flow to the brain. A small drop in blood oxygen to the brain can cause dizziness or fainting. The result, which is initiated by pressure of the thorax on the intrathoracic veins, is called Valsalva's maneuver. It most often occurs when lifting a heavy load while holding the breath (glottis closed) for several seconds. Dizziness in weight training usually occurs during the performance of a lift involving large muscle groups when the effort is sustained while holding the breath. To prevent Valsalva's maneuver, the athlete should inhale while lifting. Inhalation increases intrathoracic pressure, thereby helping to move the blood in the abdominal and thoracic veins to the heart, provided the breath is not held too long.

BLOOD DISTRIBUTION AND VOLUME IN EXERCISE

The redistribution of blood in the body during exercise provides an internal environment that optimizes physical performance. Blood shifts from the viscera into the circulation to increase plasma volume and cardiac output (see Fig. 4–12). The availability of more oxygenated blood to the working muscle results in greater endurance. If endurance training is continued on a regular basis, an increased amount of circulating blood can be a permanent result. In terms of performance, the larger quantity of blood volume enhances cardiac ouput and endurance.

Blood Volume and Training

Cardiac output is increased when the amount of blood in the circulatory system is enlarged. As more oxygenated blood reaches the working muscles, oxygen consumption at the cellular level and performance increase. One of the important training effects of endurance activities is the increased blood volume made available during work. Increases varying from 10 to 25% have been reported.[12,13] A corresponding increase in hemoglobin occurs with greater blood volume and further enhances the ability of the body to utilize more oxygen.[12,13a] A large blood volume indicates that the adjustment to heat stress should be more effective. Because much of the blood goes to the skin to cool the body when exercising in hot temperatures, less blood is available to the systemic circulation. Consequently, cardiac output decreases and performance is impaired. When blood volume is enhanced as a training effect, adaptation to heat stress is more effective.

Blood Plasma Changes in Exercise

As blood volume in the systemic circulation increases during exercise as a result of vasoconstriction of nonworking tissues (see Fig. 4–13), plasma volume into the interstitial fluid surrounding the working muscle

decreases.[14,15] The decrease in plasma, which occurs during the first 10 to 15 min., is a result of fluid leaving the capillaries almost immediately after exercise begins. The total decrease in plasma volume varies between 10 and 15%. The reason for the initial loss of plasma volume is explained by cardiovascular mechanisms. As exercise begins, both cardiac output and arterial pressure increase and resistance to blood flow in the working muscles decreases. As a result of the increased pressure in the capillaries and the reduced resistance to flow in the working muscles, more fluid is pushed into the interstitial fluid, which bathes the muscle fibers. After about 10 to 15 min., fluid stops filtering out through the capillaries in excessive amounts because of the build-up of pressure in the interstitial fluid. The pressure in the fluid counteracts the pressure in the capillaries. Eventually, equilibrium is reached and plasma volume becomes stable.

Blood Doping and Endurance

By increasing the blood's capacity for carrying oxygen, it may be possible to improve work endurance in activities requiring high oxygen uptake. Although other factors contribute to $\dot{V}O_2$ max, such as the respiration between the tissues in the lungs and the capillary blood and between the capillaries in the working muscles and the cells, the amount of oxygen carried in the blood is crucial to the achievement of high endurance. Of course, if cardiac output is maximal, additional oxygen can be transported to the muscles only by increasing the concentrations of blood hemoglobin.

Attempts have been made to determine whether increasing the number of red blood cells by infusion into the circulation is beneficial to runners in endurance activities. A special concern was voiced during the 1976 Olympics about the use of injected blood to improve performance in endurance events. Some believe that this practice is unethical and should be prohibited because it may give undue advantages to certain athletes. The term used to describe the infusion of blood into the athlete just before competition is blood doping. Research on blood doping and performance has uncovered conflicting results. Although some studies have shown an improvement in work capacity,[16,16a] others have shown varying results[16] or no changes.[17] Further research is needed before definite conclusions can be made about the effects of blood doping on endurance performance.

THE CIRCULATION IN BODY TEMPERATURE CONTROL

One important function of the circulation is to cool or heat various tissues as needed and to carry excess heat from the interior of the body to the exterior surface or skin. The purpose of controlling body temperature is to keep certain tissues, such as the brain, heart, and intestines, at a relatively constant temperature. The blood effectively controls temperature because it has a high heat capacity. Thus, the blood can carry a lot of heat with only a moderate increase in temperature. At rest, the temperature of the "core" of the body is about 100.4°F (38°C) and the "shell" (the skin) is about 96.2°F (34°C). But, within the core, temperature varies from one tissue to another. Even skin temperature can vary by as much as five times between the cooler skin of the head and the warmer skin of the trunk. Oral temperature is about 1.0°F (35°C) less than rectal temperature, and both vary according to work, emotions, and the waking and sleeping states.

Maintaining a constant body temperature within relatively narrow limits requires precise physiologic control to achieve a balance between heat production and heat loss. This control is brought about by balancing metabolic rate to the external environment.

Regulation of Temperature by Heat Loss or Gain

Loss or gain of heat from the body occurs mainly through the skin, but also partly through the respiratory tract and the lungs. Heat loss is determined by the temperatures of the skin and the surroundings, by the movement of air over the skin and respiratory surfaces, and by the amount of water vapor in the air. In fact, these mechanisms can maintain the core temperature of a nude man within a range of about 1°F (.35°C) in environmental temperatures ranging from about 30°F (−1°C) to 170°F (77°C).

The temperature of the skin depends on the rate at which blood passes through the vessels in the skin. During heavy exercise, when heat increases in the body, blood flow through the dilated vessels of the skin carries excessive heat from the core to the body surface. Blood vessels in the skin are primarily controlled by the sympathetic nerves either by their stimulation to produce vasoconstriction or by inhibition. From the skin, the heat in the blood transfers to the environment by conduction, convection, radiation, or evaporation.

Conduction is the process whereby heat is transferred from a substance of high temperature to a substance of lower temperature. In the body, heat is transferred from the skin to the external environment—a solid substance (cold bench), liquid (water), or gas (air). Heat can also be transferred by convection, which is a process that involves conduction of body heat to a moving fluid (liquid gas). When cooling off in front of a fan, the moving air passing over the skin receives the heat by conduction and carries it away by convection. The moving air is then replaced by cooler air and the process is repeated. Heat may be transferred from the body by the process of radiation during which electromagnetic waves pass from a warm object to a cooler object without warming the air through which they pass. The sun heats the body in this way, and the warm body may heat a cooler object nearby, such as a chair.

The amount of heat loss or gain by the body depends on the difference in temperature between the core and the external environment (temperature gradient). When environmental temperature is low, the skin increases its insulating capacity by vasoconstriction to retain body heat. Even then, if the environmental temperature drops farther, the gradient increases and excessive heat is lost by the skin. To control core temperature, the body must increase its heat production by the amount of combustion occurring in the tissues. At rest or under basal conditions, the intestines, spleen, liver, kidneys, brain, and cardiac muscle produce 62.8% of the metabolic heat generated. But, in moderate exercise, when total heat production may rise to three times the resting level, 75 to 80% of the heat is generated in the skeletal muscles. Even when shivering, the skeletal muscles can double the total heat production. In the cold, the normally sustained muscle "tone" of skeletal muscles, which is maintained by low-frequency discharges over motor nerves, is increased to produce heat even before shivering occurs.

Although most metabolic heat comes from muscular "tensing" during exposure to cold, some heat is produced by the action of several glands that increase metabolic rate. The thyroid gland and the adrenal medulla (epinephrine secretion) increase metabolism of many tissues and organs by the actions of their hormonal secretions, but the extent to which they contribute is not clear. In any event, hormonal factors are considered of secondary importance in temperature regulation. High environmental temperatures reverse the temperature gradient between the skin and the core. To keep core temperatures within normal limits, body heat is released at the skin by vasodilatation. But, at extremely high temperatures, vasodilatation is not sufficient to maintain core temperature. To further remove excess heat on the body surface, water in sweat is evaporated.

Temperature Control through Sweating

In physical work, when core temperatures tend to rise, sweating is important for maintaining a relatively constant internal temperature. Sweating occurs by the active secretion of fluid by sweat glands into ducts that carry it to the skin's surface. The production and delivery of sweat to the skin's surface is stimulated by the sympathetic nerves via the hypothalamus. Sweat is a dilute solution containing primarily sodium chloride or salt. During severe sweating, the human body may lose more than four quarts of water in an hour. Although an individual at rest may lose 40% of his heat by convection (includes conduction), 40% by radiation, and 20% by evaporation, heat loss by evaporation plays a much larger role during heavy exercise. Evaporation as a means to eliminate heat from the body is important during work because of the large increase in metabolic activity. The other means of cooling the body, convection and radiation, are not rapid enough to sustain a high work level. Even when environmental temperature exceeded skin temperature, the body would absorb heat if it were not for evaporation because convection and radiation only cool the skin when the external temperature is less than skin temperature.

There is a limit to the rate at which the body can lose heat by sweating, and this limit depends on the air temperature and humidity. If the air is completely dry and the convection air currents are sufficient to permit rapid evaporation from the body, an individual can tolerate air temperatures of 200°F (93°C) without ill effects. However, if the humidity is 100% with no air flow, air temperatures of around 94°F can be harmful. Basal metabolism increases about 6% for each degree of temperature rise above 94°F (34°C) because of the intrinsic effects that heat has on the rate of chemical reactions. In fact, when body temperature rises to approximately 110°F (43°C), the rate of metabolism doubles.

Nervous Regulation of Temperature

The effector mechanisms that regulate body temperature by vasoconstriction or vasodilatation of skin vessels, skeletal muscular contractions, and glandular activity receive their innervation from the hypothalamus in the brain stem (Fig. 5–12).

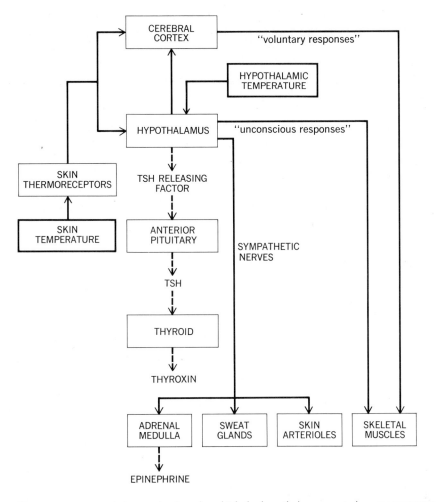

Fig. 5–12. The temperature-regulating mechanisms by which the hypothalamus controls core temperature. (From Vander, A.J., Sherman, J.H., and Luciano, D.S.: Human Physiology—The Mechanisms of Body Function. New York, McGraw-Hill, Inc., 1975. Used with permission of McGraw-Hill Book Co.)

The afferent input to the hypothalamus comes from the thermoreceptors in the skin and in the hypothalamus itself.

In the hypothalamus, thermoreceptors are stimulated by temperature changes in arterial blood. Because the hypothalamus regulates core temperature rather than skin temperature, the hypothalamic thermoreceptors have a greater regulating effect on the former than on the latter. Skin receptors transmit information via afferent nerves and ascending pathways to the hypothalamus. When cold receptors are stimulated, efferent output stimulates heat-producing mechanisms. Stimulation of warmth receptors activates cold-producing mechanisms. In the cold, adaptations that minimize heat loss and maximize heat production occur. To conserve heat, the sympathetic nerves to the skin are activated and cause vasoconstriction of the arterioles. At the same time, the sympathetic fibers to the sweat glands are inhibited. The hypothalamus stimulates the efferent somatic nervous system, causing skeletal muscles to contract and, thereby, increasing heat by metabolic processes. This reflex shivering can be partly suppressed by voluntary and conscious control via the cerebral cortex. In addition, the sympathetic nerves to the adrenal medulla cause the secretion of epinephrine, primarily, and of smaller amounts of norepinephrine. Thus, metabolic rate and, consequently, heat production rise.

When the thermoreceptors are stimulated by excessive heat, sympathetic activity produces vasodilatation of the skin arterioles, increases contraction of the smooth muscle around sweat glands, decreases muscle tone by inhibition of motor neurons of the somatic efferent system, and reduces epinephrine from the adrenal medulla.

HEAT IN EXERCISE AND WORK

Heat is always present in the body because energy is constantly produced to sustain life. When the activity of any tissue or organ in the body is increased, there is a

corresponding increase in heat. The greater temperatures in the muscles are associated with changes in function so that the muscle can contract faster and with more force. Problems arise in the adaptation of the thermoregulatory mechanisms to increased work and/or environmental temperatures when heat becomes excessive. When work continues beyond the ability of the thermoregulatory mechanisms to adapt, injury occurs. The physical symptoms preceding an injury should be recognized so that preventive measures may be taken.

Exercise and Body Temperatures

During rest, muscle contributes about 20% of the total heat of the body although it represents about 50% of body mass. But, in exercise, working muscle can increase body heat tenfold. The severity of work and the increase in core and muscle temperatures

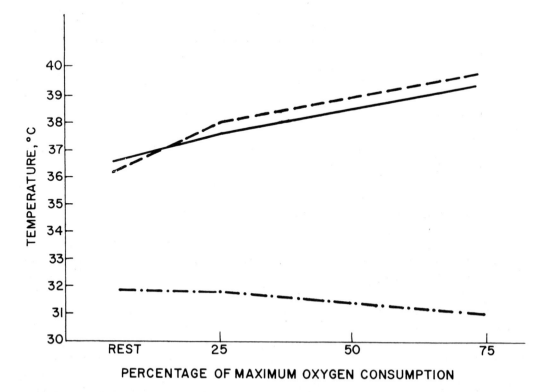

Fig. 5–13.   Changes in core (— — — —), muscle (————), and skin (— · — · —) temperatures with increases in work effort. (Data from Saltin, B., and Hermansen, L.: Esophageal, rectal and muscle temperature during exercise. J. Appl. Physiol., *21:*1757, 1966.)

are directly related (Fig. 5–13). Core temperatures rise from about 98.6°F (37°C) at rest to about 100.2°F (39°C) at a work load of 75% $\dot{V}O_2$ max.[18] The core temperature increases steadily with work intensity, but levels off after reaching maximal values of around 104°F (40°C). In attempting to continue to work at such a high temperature, greater stress is placed on the cardiovascular and the thermoregulatory systems. As expected, muscle increases in temperature and corresponds to temperature changes in the core. However, because of the cooling effect of evaporation on the skin, the temperature of the skin decreases during exercise.

Heat Stress in Exercise and Work

Stress on the cardiovascular system during work of short duration is affected by local vasodilatation and sympathetic vasoconstriction in nonworking muscles. When blood flow in the working muscles is enhanced by vasodilatation and even more blood is made available to the muscles by constriction of vessels in nonworking tissues, endurance is likely to be optimal. However, in exercise of long duration, another factor places additional stress on the cardiovascular system. This factor is heat, which accumulates as work continues. In time, the added burden of removing excessive heat from the body produces functional changes in the cardiovascular system.

The effect of prolonged work and heat accumulation is noticeable in the central circulation, where venous pressure and stroke volume diminish while cardiac output remains relatively constant. This is a response to the competition between local vasodilatation, which maximizes blood flow to the working muscles, and sympathetic stimulation, which constricts blood flow to the viscera and dilates vessels in the skin to increase blood flow and heat loss. During near maximal work and cardiac output, the increase in blood at the skin is subtracted from the flow of blood in the working muscles, thus diminishing endurance perform-

ance. The general increase in sympathetic outflow increases heart rate. The decrease in stroke volume occurs because heart rate increases while venous return and cardiac output remain about the same (see Fig. 4–19).

It may be difficult to understand how venous return and cardiac output can remain the same when so much blood is diverted from the central circulation to the peripheral circulation of the skin to remove heat, especially when the shifting of blood to the skin reduces venous pressure. Also, the resistance to venous return probably decreases because of the shifting of blood to the skin. But, because mean blood pressure also decreases, this phenomenon can be logically explained by the following formula:

$$\text{Venous return} = \frac{\text{Mean blood pressure}}{\text{Resistance to venous return}}$$

The decrease in mean blood pressure tends to reduce venous return, whereas the decrease in resistance tends to increase venous return. The relative changes in these parameters have a balancing effect resulting in a constant venous return. But, even though cardiac output remains the same, the endurance of the muscles diminishes because blood flow to the working muscle is curtailed by the greater shifts of blood to the skin.

Dehydration, Performance, and Heat Injuries

In prolonged and severe exercise, when the body becomes dehydrated because of water loss through sweating, the intracellular fluid volume is significantly reduced but blood volume remains the same. In fact, a water deficit of about 4 L still may not reduce blood volume.[19] In addition to a loss of intracellular fluid, there is also a reduction of interstitial fluid. These reductions in fluid occur because of the need to maintain blood volume, which depends on the other fluid compartments. When sweating is impaired because of excessive dehydration, internal core temperature rises. The high temperature in the fluids surrounding the hypothalamus in the brain stem depresses its regulation over the sympathetic nerves controlling vasodilatation in the skin and sweating. As sweating decreases, body heat increases, further compounding the problem. When temperatures rise above 107 to 110°F (41.7 to 43.3°C), the heat regulating mechanisms can no longer rid the body of excess heat. High temperatures may cause a degeneration of body cells as they become dehydrated. Other effects may include hot, flushed, and dry skin. When such symptoms are present, an individual has heat stroke.

Whereas dehydration from severe and continued work results not in a loss of plasma volume but in a reduction of intracellular fluids, such is not the case when dehydration occurs from a hot, external environment. A 25% loss in plasma volume may be caused by thermal dehydration of about 5% in body weight with no significant loss in fluids of the cells or surrounding tissues.[19] The effect on cardiovascular function is deleterious as stroke volume and blood pressure decrease, signaling a failure of the system. When these conditions are associated with a rapid and weak pulse, and when the skin is cool and moist, heat exhaustion is present. The difference between heat stroke and heat exhaustion is the mechanisms that fail. During heat stroke, the thermoregulatory center in the hypothalamus fails, whereas during heat exhaustion the cardiovascular system fails. In both conditions, core temperatures rise significantly.

When exercise places great stress on the cardiovascular system over a prolonged period of time, such as when running or cycling long distances, and when the work is performed in a hot environment, regulating heat gain with heat loss becomes more of a problem. Because heat loss by sweating involves water taken from blood plasma, interstitial fluid, and intracellular fluid, there is a more rapid depletion of water and eventually a dangerous rise in core temperature. Stress on both the circulatory and thermoregulatory mechanisms as a consequence of a water loss of only 2% can impair their functions. Often in athletics, participants are exposed to prolonged work in hot temperatures. As body temperatures increase from activity and sweating becomes profuse to cool the body, liquids must be replaced, even if only partially, because performance becomes adversely affected and injury may occur in the form of heat stroke or exhaustion (Table 5–2).

Dehydration and Performance. In such sports as wrestling and weight lifting, athletes lose weight to have an advantage over their opponents. Usually weight is reduced by sweating and water deprivation. The methods most often used to stimulate

Table 5–2.

Changes in Fluid Volumes From Heat and Exercise and Associated Heat Injuries[24]*

Condition	Stroke volume	Heart rate	Cardiac output	Blood volume	Interstitial volume	Intra-cellular volume	Symptoms	Cardiovascular failure	Thermoregulation failure
Heat exhaustion at rest or in mild activity	↓	↑	↓	↓	↓	↔	Moist skin. Rapid, weak, pulse.	X	
Heat stroke in exercise	↓	↑	↔	↔	↓	↓	Dry, hot skin. Flushed.		X
Exercise in heat	↓	↑	↓	↓	↓	↓	Depends on failure.	X or	X

*Arrows indicate an increase (↑), decrease (↓), or no change (↔).

sweating are exercise and environmental heat in a sauna bath or steam room. If too much weight is lost by dehydration, performance may be less than expected.

In sport activities that last more than a few minutes, the circulatory systems are important for achieving endurance. Nutrients must be available to the active muscles and heat must be dissipated during any endurance work, and these functions are performed by the circulatory systems. If the extracellular fluids (blood and interstitial fluid) decrease from dehydration, the ability of the circulatory systems to perform these functions may be seriously impaired.[20] A loss of 5.2% of body weight caused by exposure to a hot external environment may result in a 25% reduction in plasma volume.[21] As a consequence, stroke volume decreases and heart rate increases to maintain cardiac output during submaximal work.[22] Even in maximum work, cardiac output and oxygen consumption are maintained at a level achieved prior to dehydration. However, the ability to sustain hard work decreases significantly.[23,24]

In addition to the alterations in circulatory function during dehydration, there is an inability to rid the body of heat. As water is lost, core temperatures rise. In fact, for each percent body weight lost through sweating, there is an increase of 0.35°F (.13°C) to 0.55°F (.20°C) in core temperatures.[25] However, the increase in core temperatures with water loss is apparently not caused solely by a reduction in the cooling effect of sweat evaporation because sweat rates and skin blood flow may not be altered significantly during dehydration.[26,27] The reasons for the increase in core temperatures with water loss are not clear but, nevertheless, dehydration may impair performance as a consequence of the inability of the body to dissipate heat.

The effect of rapid dehydration on other kinds of performances, such as strength, speed, and reaction time, has been studied. Varying results were found; some studies indicated that dehydration has an adverse effect on strength[28] and others revealed no effect on strength.[29-32] Dehydration showed no detrimental effects on speed or reaction time.[24,31]

Hyperhydration and Performance. The ingestion of extra water prior to competition may improve performance in races stressing the cardiovascular system during prolonged work. Apparently, the extra weight or feeling of distention in the stomach during short races does not adversely affect performance,[33,34] even when 1.5 l. of water are taken 5 min. before the race.[35] Consequently, any physical discomfort from water ingestion should not impair performance in long races. In fact, the increased performance from water intake more than offsets the possible adverse effects of physical discomfort. Intakes of up to 2 l. before prolonged work increased running time[36] and resulted in less stress on the thermoregulatory mechanisms, as indicated by reduced heart rate and rectal temperature[37,38] and increased sweating.[38]

Avoiding Heat Injuries by Water and Salt Intake During Exercise. To avoid excessive body heat during exercise, the athlete must consume adequate amounts of water. In this way, the cooling effect of evaporation is maintained over a longer period of time. Otherwise, core temperatures rise and place an added burden on the circulatory and thermoregulatory functions. Because a water deficit during exercise appears primarily in intracellular space, the fluids surrounding the cells cannot efficiently serve the metabolic needs of the cells. This effect is observed in a reduced endurance capacity. In addition to water loss in exercise, salt and other electrolytes are lost from the body. These losses also contribute to performance decrement.[21,39]

The importance of ingesting fluid while exercising is shown in Figure 5–14.[34] When cold fluids are consumed, core temperature levels off after about 45 min. and rises only slightly after 120 min. When fluids are not taken, core temperature rises continuously during the entire running time. Similar re-

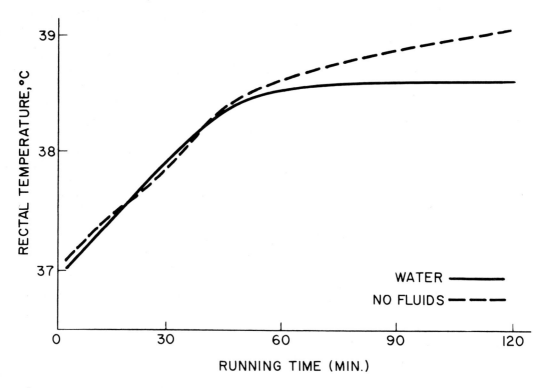

Fig. 5–14.   The effects of fluid intake on rectal temperatures during prolonged running. (Data from Coote, J.H.: Physiological significance of somatic afferent pathways from skeletal muscle and joints with reflex effects on the heart and circulation. Brain Res., *87*:139, 1975.)

sults occur when walking 5 or more hr. in a 100°F (38°C) temperature at 35 to 45% relative humidity under different conditions of water consumption (Fig. 5–15).[40]

When the water lost from sweating was not replaced, rectal temperatures rose steadily after 3 hr. to dangerous levels approaching exhaustion. Consuming water to satisfy thirst during the walk resulted in an increase in rectal temperature and a subsequent leveling off until about 4.5 hr. Afterward, temperatures climbed to exhaustion levels. When water was ingested to balance water loss, which meant drinking beyond the point of satisfying thirst, body temperature remained relatively low throughout the walk.

Even though optimal performances are only achieved when water is consumed during an endurance event, the water lost from sweating during a race cannot be completely replaced. In moderate to heavy exercise, the ability of the stomach and small intestine to empty is inhibited. In a 2-hr. run, a water loss of 1.67 l./hr. can be replaced by only about 0.82 l./hr. from oral ingestion of water.[34] Nevertheless, replacing water during work minimizes the drop in performance and reduces the probability of heat injury.

The American College of Sports Medicine presented a position statement on the prevention of heat injuries during distance running.[41] Their statement can be applied to any athletic endurance event provided that the expenditure of energy during the contest is comparable to a distance run of 10 miles or more. Some of their position statements have been paraphrased as follows:

1. Distance races of 10 miles or more should not be conducted when the wet-bulb temperature (air temperature allowing for the cooling effect of vaporization) exceeds 82.4°F (28°C).[42,43] This temperature is simi-

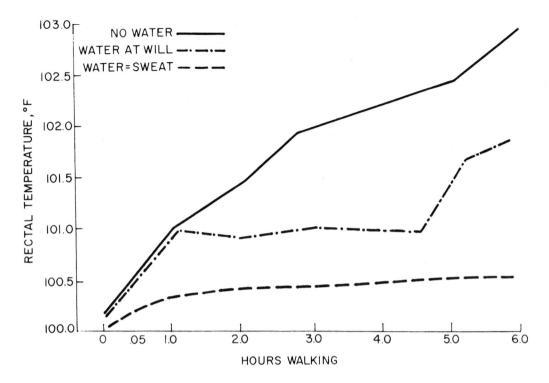

Fig. 5–15. The effects of water intake on rectal temperatures during prolonged walking. (Data from Moroff, S.V., and Bass, D.E.: Effects of overhydration on man's physiological responses to work in the heat. J. Appl. Physiol., *20*:267, 1965.)

lar to dry-bulb temperatures ranging from 98.6°F (37°C) down to 87°F (30.5°C) for corresponding relative humidities ranging from 50 to 80%. The higher the humidity, the smaller the "safe" temperature, and vice versa. Figure 5–16 indicates the dry-bulb temperatures at each relative humidity above which a wet-bulb temperature of 82.4°F (28°C) is exceeded. Any dry temperatures above the curve contraindicate distance races of 10 miles (16 km.) or more.

2. Even though a wet-bulb temperature of 82.4°F (28°C) is the absolute maximum temperature for conducting a distance race, lower temperatures are preferred. When daylight dry-bulb temperature exceeds 80°F (27°C), races should be conducted before 9 a.m. or after 4 p.m.[44,45]

3. Fluids that supply small amounts of sugar (less than about 6 level teaspoons per quart of water or 2.5 g. of glucose per 100 ml.

of water) and electrolytes (less than 10 mEq. sodium and 5 mEq. potassium per liter of solution) should be provided.[39,46] Excessive sugar intake with water may impair the emptying rate of the intestines and can lead to gastric discomfort or a feeling of fullness. As a result, a runner consumes less liquid, thereby jeopardizing performance.[22,46]

4. Athletes should consume fluids frequently while running and should ingest about 1.5 to 2 cups of fluid before competition.[22,46]

5. Runners should be able to recognize the early warning symptoms of heat injury. These symptoms are piloerection ("goose flesh") on chest and arms, chilling, throbbing pressure in the head, unsteadiness, nausea, and dry skin.[41,47]

Warm-Up Effects on Performance. Increased physical activity just prior to a race better prepares the body for the impend-

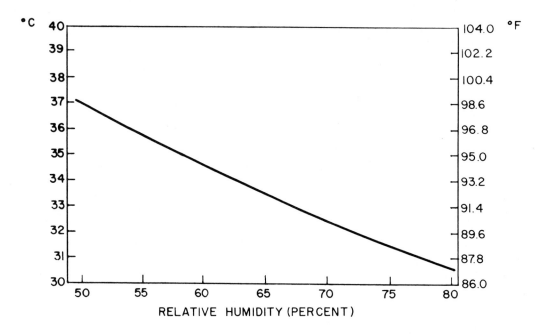

Fig. 5–16.   Dry bulb temperatures in °F and °C corresponding to specific relative humidities to achieve a wet bulb temperature of 82.4°F or 28°C. Dry bulb temperatures and humidities resulting in wet bulb temperatures exceeding 82.4°F or 28°C on the day of a scheduled long distance race (10 miles or 16 km.) contraindicate the conduction of the race. (Data from Buskirk, E.R., and Grasley, W.C.: Heat injury and conduct of athletics. *In* Science and Medicine of Exercise and Sport. 2nd Edition. New York, Harper and Row, 1974; and Ladell, W.D.S.: The Physiology of Human Survival. New York, Academic Press, 1965.)

ing event. Warming up increases muscle temperature, activates energy sources in muscle, stimulates hormones, activates the nervous system, and increases core temperature. When muscle temperature and/or core temperature are increased, faster times can be achieved in sprint cycling[48] and swimming 40 to 220 yd.[49] Studies have shown that warming up improves running speed,[50-52] arm speed,[53] muscle force,[53,54] muscle endurance,[53,55] power,[55] and cardiovascular endurance.[55] Some research studies have shown no significant improvement in performance from warming up, but these studies are in the minority.[56] The general consensus is that warming up is beneficial, especially in activities involving explosive movements.

Actually the initiation of the warm-up process occurs at the cortical level before any increased work is evident. Just anticipating exercise stimulates sympathetic activity and causes vasodilatation in all skeletal muscles. Of course, when exercise begins, vasoconstriction occurs in the non-working muscles, and vasodilatation occurs in the exercised muscles.

An added advantage of warming up is the prevention of muscle injury, although the evidence supporting this advantage is sparse because of the hesitancy to subject individuals to possible injury during a research study. An indication of the effects of warming up on muscle soreness was inadvertently determined in a study of metabolic efficiency.[10] When four subjects ran without warming up, two developed muscle soreness that could have been severe had not preventive measures been taken.

Generally, the best kind of warm-up is related to the actual athletic activity. A sprinter should warm up and stretch the hip and leg muscles; the football player should run short dashes and do calisthenic exercises to activate the muscles involved in the game; the basketball player should run and shoot baskets; and the swimmer should swim. The exact amount of warm-up is an individual matter; however, sweating should occur.

When muscle and general body temperature (measured best by rectal temperature) both increase, the warm-up has approached optimal conditions. The exact intensity and duration of warm-ups not only vary among different activities but also among individuals in the same activity. Some may warm up for 30 min. whereas others find that 5 min. is sufficient. For a warm-up to be beneficial, the time between the warm-up and the activity should not normally exceed 45 min. unless warm clothing is worn until the start of the activity.[57]

Acclimatization to Hot and Cold Environments

Continuous and prolonged exposure to heat causes a gradual adjustment or acclimatization to heat stress. In fact, acclimatization occurs after a few days of exposure. Tolerance to heat is associated with an increase in sweating and a consequent lowering of skin temperature by evaporation. Thus, body temperature is also lowered by the cooling of blood flowing through the skin. With a reduction in the amount of blood needed to cool the body after acclimatization, more blood can be available to the working muscles during exercise. Within four to seven days of exposure to working in a hot environment, rectal temperature and heart rate decrease to a more normal level and sweat losses increase.[57a] After about 12 to 14 days, the acclimatization to heat is complete.

To achieve optimal adjustment to a hot environment, an athlete must be physically trained.[58] During this period, fluid and salt losses must be replaced. Although the well-conditioned individual adjusts better than the individual in poor condition to heat, training alone is not sufficient to produce complete acclimatization.[59] When preparing for competition in a hot climate, an athlete performs better by training for 12 to 14 days in that climate or by exercising in an artificially heated room. Heat acclimatization may last for several weeks following heat exposure, although some tolerance is lost after a few days.[60]

Acclimatization to cold is usually not as difficult as acclimatization to heat. In cold, the amount and kind of clothing worn can be modified so that comfortable temperatures are maintained; in extreme environmental heat, dressing to achieve agreeable body temperatures is limited. Two noticeable effects of acclimatization to cold are an elevation in metabolism and a decrease in shivering when exposed nude to the cold.[61] But, at normal room temperature, metabolic rate is unchanged. The exact mechanisms involved in physiologic acclimatization to cold in human beings is difficult to ascertain. Some investigators have shown lowered skin temperatures whereas others have found unchanged or elevated temperatures among cold-acclimatized individuals.[62] The adaptation of an athlete to cold has little practical significance in terms of safety in performance or of actual competitive performance. The advantage held by a cold-acclimatized athlete when competing in a cold environment is practically nonexistent unless, perhaps, the game is played in the nude.

PRINCIPLES FOR TRAINING

1. Inhaling while lifting a heavy weight prevents dizziness, provided the breath is not held for more than 2 to 3 sec. The pumping action of breathing on the large veins in the thoracic cavity moves blood into the veins leading to the heart. When the breath is held for an extended time, there is no pumping action and venous return is reduced. Consequently, the oxygenated blood to the brain is diminished and fainting or dizziness results. By inhaling as the weight is lifted and forcing blood out of the chest cavity, venous return is ensured, provided

the cycle of inspiration and expiration is continued without too much interruption.

2. If a concern in exercise is to minimize the increase in blood pressure, large muscle activity is preferable to exercise that involves relatively smaller muscle groups.[9] The higher arterial blood pressure in arm exercise than in leg exercise at the same cardiac output ($\dot{Q}$ = HR × SV) means that the contraction force of the heart increases. The greater blood pressure resulting from work with the arms is probably caused by the vasoconstriction of more inactive muscles. Higher peripheral resistance results in increased blood pressure at the same cardiac output because arterial blood pressure (BP) is the product of cardiac output ($\dot{Q}$) and peripheral resistance (R), or BP = $\dot{Q}$ × R. Older individuals and heart patients should receive approval from their physicians before doing strenuous lifting exercises involving small muscle groups.

3. Injuries caused by excessive heat can be avoided by recognizing the symptoms of heat exhaustion: a rapid and weak pulse and cold and usually moist skin. These symptoms reflect a failure of the cardiovascular system. Treatment involves rest and fluid intake. A failure in the heat regulatory system induces heat stroke, whose symptoms are: a hot and flushed skin, usually dry; high body temperature; and possibly delirium. If the condition is not severe, resting while cooling off and liquid intake are sufficient for recovery. In severe cases, immersion in an ice-cold bath may be necessary. Quick medical attention is needed.

If salt is not taken regularly, excessive sweating can cause heat cramps in the skeletal muscles. When cramps occur, rest is needed and adequate amounts of salt and fluid should be consumed.

4. To maximize performance in a hot environment, the total amount of water expected to be lost during competition should be consumed preferably before the contest, but at least during the game.[37,38] The liquid consumed should contain about 6 level tea-spoons of sugar[30,46] and about one-half teaspoon of salt per quart of water.[46]

Performance is less likely to decrease if water volume is maintained during the activity. By doing so, core temperature may remain stable. Sugar added to the fluids taken during the competition aids in providing additional energy, and salt helps to maintain the electrolyte balance, so necessary for muscle function. An athlete should weigh-in before competition and attempt to drink enough fluids to maintain that weight during the contest.

5. Warming up is more likely to improve athletic performance and reduce sore muscles or injury when it involves activities that are specific to the sport and when it results in sweating. Warming the specific muscles by the exact movements used in the athletic event gives the best results. In this way, much of the blood from the inactive muscles is shunted to the working muscles. If the exact movement of the performance cannot be duplicated, the movements should be as similar as possible. Sweating while warming up indicates that both the temperature of the muscles and the temperature of the internal body are sufficiently high to improve performance.

6. Warming up is most effective when it is soon followed by the performance or game; otherwise, the benefits of warming up may be lost after 45 min.[51]

Because the effectiveness of a warm-up depends on the increase in temperature of the working muscles and of the internal body, any cooling off may diminish the force and endurance capacity of the muscles and the ability of the muscles to avoid soreness. If competition occurs 45 min. or less after warming up, performance will probably be enhanced, provided clothes retain body heat.

7. Acclimatization to heat is best achieved by a systematic exercise program in a heated environment rather than by exposure to the heat during inactivity.[32] With exercise, acclimatization is almost complete

in 4 to 7 days and is complete in about 12 to 14 days.[3] After training in a hot environment, rectal temperature drops noticeably after several days. This drop in temperature indicates that the body's cooling mechanisms are functioning more effectively. A corresponding drop in heart rate at the same work load also indicates a reduction in heat stress. The large increase in sweat loss over the same period contributes to this adjustment by increasing the evaporative and cooling effect on the skin surface.

REFERENCES

1. Greenleaf, J.E., and Sargent, F.: Voluntary dehydration in man. J. Appl. Physiol., *20:*719, 1965.
2. Bevegard, B.S., and Shepherd, J.T.: Regulation of the circulation during exercise in man. Physiol. Rev., *47:*178, 1967.
3. Kirihheim, H.R.: Systemic arterial baroreceptor reflexes. Physiol. Rev., *56:*100, 1976.
4. Edis, A.J., Donald, D.E., and Shepherd, J.T.: Cardiovascular reflexes from stretch of pulmonary vein-atrial junction in the dog. Circ. Res., *27:*1091, 1970.
5. Pelletier, C.L., and Shepherd, J.T.: Circulatory reflexes from mechanoreceptors in the cardioaortic area. Circ. Res., *33:*131, 1973.
6. Daly, M.deB., Hazzledine, J.L., and Ungar, A.: The reflex effects of alterations in lung volume on systemic vascular resistance in the dog. J. Physiol., *195:*387, 1968.
7. Coote, J.H.: Physiological significance of somatic afferent pathways from skeletal muscle and joints with reflex effects on the heart and circulation. Brain Res., *87:*139, 1975.
8. McCloskey, D.J., Matthews, P.R.C., and Mitchell, J.H.: Absence of appreciable cardiovascular and respiratory responses to muscle vibration. J. Appl. Physiol., *33:*623, 1972.
9. Åstrand, P.O., et al.: Intra-arterial blood pressure during exercise with different muscle groups. J. Appl. Physiol., *20:*253, 1965.
10. de Vries, H.A.: Physiology of Exercise. 2nd Edition. Iowa, Wm. C. Brown Co., 1974.
11. Lind, A.R., and McNicol, G.W.: Muscular factors which determine the cardiovascular responses to sustained and rhythmic exercise. Can. Med. Assoc. J., *96:*706, 1967.
12. Kjellberg, S.R., Rudhe, V., and Sjostrand, T.: Increase of the amount of hemoglobin and blood volume in connection with physical training. Acta Physiol. Scand., *19:*146, 1949.
13. Saltin, B., et al.: Response to submaximal and maximal exercise after bed rest and training. Circulation [Suppl. 7], *38:*1, 1968.
13a. Åstrand, P.O., et al.: Girl swimmers. Acta Paediat. [Suppl. 147]: 1, 1963.
14. Costill, D.L., and Finks, W.J.: Plasma volume changes following exercise and thermal dehydration. J. Appl. Physiol., *37:*521, 1974.
15. Gill, D.B., and Costill, D.L.: Calculation of percentage changes in volumes of blood and red cells in dehydration. J. Appl. Physiol., *37:*277, 1973.
16. Ekblom, B., Goldbarg, A.N., and Gullbring, B.: Response to exercise after blood loss and reinfusion. J. Appl. Physiol., *33:*175, 1972.
16a. Gullbring, B., et al.: The effect of blood volume variations on the pulse rate in supine and upright positions and during exercise. Acta Physiol. Scand., *50:*62, 1960.
17. Williams, M.H., et al.: Effect of blood reinjection upon endurance capacity and heart rate. Med. Sci. Sports, *5:*181, 1973.
18. Olsson, K.E., and Saltin, B.: Diet and fluid in training and competition. Scand. J. Rehabil. Med., *3:*32, 1971.
19. Åstrand, P.O., and Saltin, B.: Plasma and red cell volume after prolonged severe exercise. J. Appl. Physiol., *19:*829, 1964.
20. Koslowski, S., and Saltin, B.: Effect of sweat loss on body fluids. J. Appl. Physiol., *19:*1119, 1964.
21. Saltin, B.: Circulatory response to submaximal and maximal exercise after thermal dehydration. J. Appl. Physiol., *19:*1125, 1964.
22. Saltin, B.: Aerobic work capacity and circulation at exercise in man. Acta Physiol. Scand. [Suppl.], *62:*1, 1964.
23. Block, W., Fox, E.L., and Bowers, R.: The effects of acute dehydration upon cardio-respiratory endurance. J. Sports Med. Phys. Fitness, *7:*67, 1967.
24. Nichols, H.: The effects of rapid weight loss on selected physiologic responses of wrestlers. Doctoral dissertation. University of Michigan, Ann Arbor, 1957.
25. Adolph, E.F.: Physiology of Man in the Desert. New York, John Wiley & Sons, 1947.
26. Hertzman, A.B., and Ferguson, J.D.: Failure in temperature regulation during progressive dehydration. U. S. Armed Forces Med. J., *11:*542, 1960.
27. Senay, L.C., and Christensen, H.L.: Cutaneous circulation during dehydration and heat stress. J. Appl. Physiol., *20:*278, 1965.
28. Bosco, J.S., Terjung, R.L., and Greenleaf, J.E.: Effects of progressive hypohydration on maximal isometric muscular strength. J. Sports Med. Phys. Fitness, *8:*81, 1968.
29. Doscher, N.: The effects of rapid weight loss upon the performance of wrestlers and boxers, and upon the physical proficiency of college students. Res. Q., *15:*317, 1944.
30. Edwards, J.B.: The effect of semi-starvation and dehydration on strength and endurance with reference to college wrestling. Master's thesis, University of North Carolina, Charlotte, 1951.
31. Elfenbaum, L.: The physiological effects of rapid weight loss among wrestlers. Doctoral dissertation. Ohio State University, Columbus, 1966.
32. Singer, R.N., and Weiss, S.A.: Effects of weight reduction on selected anthropometric, physical, and performance measures of wrestlers. Res. Q., *39:*361, 1968.

33. Blank, L.B.: An experimental study of the effect of water ingestion upon athletic performance. Res. Q., *30:*131, 1959.

34. Costill, D.L., Kammer, W.F., and Fisher, A.: Fluid ingestion during distance running. Arch. Environ. Health, *21:*520, 1970.

35. Little, C.C., Strayhorn, H., and Miller, A.T.: Effect of water ingestion on capacity for exercise. Res. Q., *20:*298, 1949.

36. Blyth, C.S., and Burt, J.J.: Effect of water balance on ability to perform in high ambient temperatures. Res. Q., *32:*301, 1961.

37. Ladell, W.D.S.: The Physiology of Human Survival. New York, Academic Press, 1965.

38. Moroff, S.V., and Bass, D.E.: Effects of overhydration on man's physiological responses to work in the heat. J. Appl. Physiol., *20:*267, 1965.

39. Fordtran, J.A., and Saltin, B.: Gastric emptying and intestinal absorption during prolonged severe exercise. J. Appl. Physiol., *23:*331, 1967.

40. Pitts, G., Johnson, R., and Consolazio, F.: Work in the heat as affected by intake of water, salt, and glucose. Am. J. Physiol., *142:*253, 1944.

41. The American College of Sports Medicine: Position statement on prevention of heat injuries during distance running. Med. Sci. Sports, *7:*vii, 1975.

42. Buskirk, E.R., and Grasley, W.C.: Heat injury and conduct of athletics. *In* Science and Medicine of Exercise and Sport. 2nd Edition. Edited by W. R. Johnson, and E. R. Buskirk. New York, Harper & Row, 1974.

43. Londeree, B.R., Updyke, W.F., and Burt, J.J.: Water replacement schedules in heat stress. Res. Q., *40:*725, 1969.

44. Pugh, L.G., Corbett, J.I., and Johnson, R.H.: Rectal temperatures, weight losses and sweating rates in marathon running. J. Appl. Physiol., *23:*347, 1967.

45. Wyndham, C.H., and Strydom, N.B.: The danger of an inadequate water intake during marathon running. S. Afr. Med. J., *43:*893, 1969.

46. Costill, D.L., and Saltin, B.: Factors limiting gastric emptying during rest and exercise. J. Appl. Physiol., *37:*679, 1974.

47. Buskirk, E.R., Iampetro, P.E., and Bass, E.E.: Work performance after dehydration: effects of physical conditioning and heat acclimatization. J. Appl. Physiol., *12:*189, 1958.

48. Asmusen, E., and Boje, O.: Body temperature and capacity for work. Acta Physiol., *10:*1, 1945.

49. Muido, L.: The influence of body temperature on performance in swimming. Acta Physiol. Scand., *12:*102, 1946.

50. Blank, L.B.: Effects of warm-up on speed. Athletic J., *10:*45, 1955.

51. Grodjinovsky, A., and Magel, J.R.: Effect of warm-up on running performance. Res. Q., *41:*116, 1970.

52. Thompson, H.: Effect of warm-up upon physical performance in selected activities. Res. Q., *29:*231, 1958.

53. Phillips, W.H.: Influences of fatiguing warm-up exercises on speed of movement and reaction latency. Res. Q., *34:*370, 1963.

54. Burke, R.K.: Relationship between physical performance and warm-up procedures of varying intensity and duration. Doctoral dissertation. University of Southern California, 1957.

55. Carlile, F.: Effect of preliminary passive warming on swimming performance. Res. Q., *27:*143, 1956.

56. Franks, B.D.: Physical warm-up. *In* Ergogenic Aids and Muscular Performance. Edited by W. P. Morgan. New York, Academic Press, 1972.

57. Hogberg, P., and Ljunggren, O.: Uppvarmingens inverkan pa lopprestationerna, Svensk Idrott, *40:*688, 1947.

57a. Lind, A.R., and Bass, D.E.: Optimal exposure time for development of acclimatization to heat. Fed. Proc., *22:*204, 1963.

58. Wyndham, C.H.: Heat reactions of caucasians in temperate, in hot dry, and hot humid climates. J. Appl. Physiol., *19:*607, 1964.

59. Strydom, N.B., et al.: Acclimatization to humid heat and the role of physical conditioning. J. Appl. Physiol., *21:*636, 1966.

60. Williams, C.G., Wyndham, C.H., and Morrison, J.F.: Rate of loss of acclimatization in summer and winter. J. Appl. Physiol., *22:*21, 1967.

61. Wyndham, C.H., et al.: Physiological reactions to cold of Bushman, Bontu and Caucasian males. J. Appl. Physiol., *19:*8, 1964.

62. Burton, A.C.: The pattern of responses to cold in animals and the evolution of homeothermy. *In* Temperature: Its Measurement and Control in Science and Industry. Edited by J. D. Hardy. New York, Reinhold Book Corp., 1963.

6 The Respiratory System in Work and Exercise

Most cells in the body derive their energy from chemical reactions involving oxygen. The major end product of these oxidations is carbon dioxide, which must be removed from the cells. Specialized systems in the body supply oxygen to the tissues and remove carbon dioxide to the external environment. The organs of gas exchange with the external environment in man are the lungs. Also, specialized blood components transport large quantities of oxygen and carbon dioxide between the lungs and all tissue cells. During rest, the body's cells consume about 250 ml. of oxygen per minute. But, in heavy exercise, the rate of oxygen consumption may be 30 times more, with proportionately more carbon dioxide produced. To meet the body's changing needs for oxygen, mechanisms coordinate breathing with the metabolic needs of the tissue cells.

There are actually two different aspects of respiration: (1) the metabolic reaction of oxygen with foodstuffs at the cellular level (see Chap. 2), and (2) the exchange of gases between the cells and the external environment. The concern in this chapter is with the second aspect of respiration and deals with external respiration and internal respiration. External respiration is the exchange of air between the atmosphere and the lungs. This process includes the movement of air in and out of the lungs and the distribution of air within the lungs. The whole process is called ventilation. Internal respiration deals with three processes that are involved in moving air back and forth between the cells and lungs: (1) the exchange of oxygen and car-

bon dioxide between the alveoli of the lungs and lung capillaries, (2) the transportation of oxygen and carbon dioxide by the blood, and (3) the exchange of oxygen and carbon dioxide between the blood and tissue cells of the body. The respiratory system, which consists of the lungs, the passageways leading to the lungs, and the chest structures involved in the movement of air in and out of the lungs, is presented first.

ANATOMY OF THE RESPIRATORY SYSTEM

Air reaches the lungs through a series of air passages (Fig. 6–1). Beginning at the nasal passages, air flows past the larynx into the trachea. The trachea is a long tube that branches into two bronchi; one bronchus enters each lung. Branching continues from the bronchi into smaller vessels, called bronchioles. and then to the alveolar ducts through which air passes into the alveoli. The alveoli are tiny sacs, numbering about 300 million, where the actual exchange between the gases and the blood takes place. The lungs are encased by a thin membrane called the pleura, which allows the lungs to move freely and without friction inside the thoracic cavity. The pleura has two layers: an outer layer (parietal pleura) that lines the rib cage and intercostal muscles and an inner layer (visceral pleura) that covers the two lungs. Between the two pleurae is a thin layer of intrapleural fluid, which plays a significant role in breathing. Smooth muscle that is sensitive to certain circulating hormones, such as epinephrine, lines the respiratory passages. The contraction of these

205

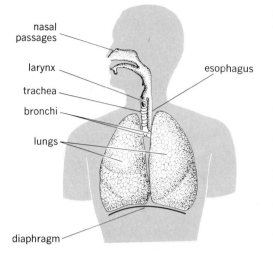

nasal passages

larynx

trachea

bronchi

lungs

esophagus

diaphragm

Fig. 6–1. Anatomy of the respiratory system. (From Vander, A.J., Sherman, J.H., and Luciano, D.S.: Human Physiology—The Mechanisms of Body Function. New York, McGraw-Hill, Inc., 1975. Used with permission of McGraw-Hill Book Co.)

muscles, especially in the bronchioles, alters resistance to airflow into the lungs. All the air passageways and alveoli receive blood by way of the pulmonary artery from the heart. The pulmonary artery branches into arterioles and then into capillaries that lie adjacent to the alveoli. Carbon dioxide passes from the blood into the lungs while oxygen flows in the opposite direction into the blood. The oxygenated blood returns to the heart by way of the venules and the pulmonary veins.

Between the air passageways and blood vessels in the thoracic cavity are large quantities of elastic connective tissue. The lungs are also elastic and, therefore, can expand or decrease in volume depending on the quantity of airflow. The lungs fill and partially empty by the contraction and relaxation of the diaphragm (the muscle separating the thoracic and abdominal cavities) and the muscles of the ribs. The respiratory muscles control lung volume and air pressure in the lungs. The total area of gas exchange in the hollow sacs of the alveoli, in contact with capillaries, is 70 square meters in man. This area permits a rapid exchange of large

amounts of oxygen and carbon dioxide between the blood and lungs.

EXCHANGE OF AIR IN LUNGS

Air moves into the alveoli of the lungs by pressure differences between the atmosphere and the alveoli. When atmospheric pressure (760 mm Hg at sea level) exceeds the pressure within the alveoli, air rushes into the lungs (inspiration). The opposite pressure relationship causes the air to pass out of the lungs (expiration). This exchange of air between the atmosphere and alveoli is called ventilation and is the process of external respiration.

Inspiration

The reduction of air pressure in the lungs, which causes atmospheric air to move into the alveoli, is caused by an enlargement of the thoracic cage. When thoracic volume is increased, the pressure inside decreases and literally sucks in the outside air. The thoracic cage is a closed compartment surrounded at the neck by muscles and connective tissue. It is separated from the abdomen by a large dome-shaped sheet of skeletal muscle called the diaphragm. The outer walls of the thoracic cage are shaped by the breast bone (sternum), 12 pairs of ribs, and the intercostal muscles lying between the ribs. The walls of the thoracic cage contain much elastic connective tissue.

Inspiration is initiated by the contraction of the diaphragm and intercostal muscles. Contraction of the diaphragm moves the muscle downward into the abdomen while the intercostal muscles, which attach to the ribs, contract and lift the ribs upward and outward. These movements enlarge the thoracic cage. In quiet respiration, the diaphragm descends about 0.6 in. but, during heavy exercise, it descends about 2.5 to 4.0 in.[1] During heavy exercise, when greater pulmonary ventilation is needed, the muscles around the neck (scalenus and sternomastoid) contract and help to lift the ribs, thereby increasing chest volume. During inspiration, the alveolar duct leading to the alveoli, and the alveoli themselves increase in volume by twofold.

Expiration

The elastic tissues in the lungs and thoracic wall stretch during inspiration. At the completion of inspiration, the muscles relax and the stretched tissues recoil to their original length. With the reduced volume in the chest cavity and lungs, the air pressure in the alveolar air increases beyond the atmospheric pressure, and air is expelled in expiration. Under normal conditions, expiration is passive, depending only on the alternating contraction and relaxation of inspiratory muscles. During exercise, when ventilation increases to meet the needs of muscle cells for more oxygen, the abdominal and oblique muscles aid in expiration by pushing up on the diaphragm and compressing the rib cage.

Pressure in the Lungs and Thorax

When the thorax is expanded by the chest muscles, the outer layer of the pleura, which is attached to the rib cage and to the intercostal muscles, also expands. The increase in volume of the intrapleural fluid reduces its pressure from about −4 to −6 mm Hg, and the inner layer of the pleura, adjacent to the lungs, transmits this reduction to the intrathoracic fluid surrounding the lungs, heart, and other structures in the cavity (Fig. 6–2). Consequently, intrathoracic pressure drops. During normal breathing at rest, when about 500 ml. of air moves into the lungs, intrathoracic pressure is about −5 mm Hg (relative to atmospheric pressure of 760 mm Hg at sea level). At the same time, the pressure in the air passages and alveoli in the lungs (intrapulmonary pressure) is about −3 mm Hg. Intrathoracic pressure (−5 mm Hg) is always less than intrapulmonary pressure (−3 mm Hg), thereby preventing the lungs from collapsing. The 500 ml. of air is blown out of the lungs at rest by the relaxation of the chest muscles, which decreases lung volume and, in turn, increases intrapulmonary pressure to about +3 mm Hg.

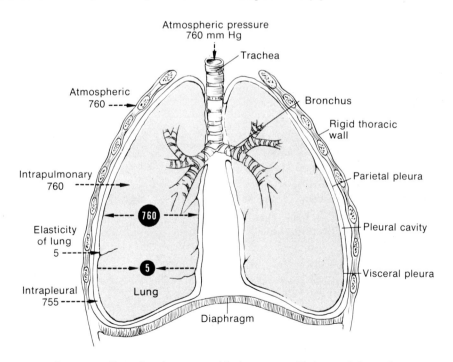

Fig. 6–2. Intrapulmonary and intrapleural pressures of the lungs at rest. During work, intrapulmonary pressure may be 790 mm Hg in inspiration and 740 mm Hg in expiration. (From Schottelius, B.A., and Schottelius, D.D.: Textbook of Physiology. 18th Edition. St. Louis, The C. V. Mosby Co., 1978.)

During strenuous exercise, intrapulmonary pressures may vary from −20 mm Hg during inspiration to +30 mm Hg during expiration because of the effect of strong muscular contractions. If intrapulmonary pressure is held too long at a high level, intrathoracic pressure on the large veins increases and impedes blood flow to the heart. Thus, oxygen supply to the brain is reduced, and dizziness or fainting occurs (Valsalva's maneuver).

Local Control of Pulmonary Ventilation

As the volume of air moving in and out of the lungs increases, the resistance to airflow increases. Resistance to airflow is provided by mostly elastic lung tissue and by airway resistance. Increased flow causes turbulence in the trachea and the main bronchi, resulting in high resistance. This turbulence decreases as the air passes into the finer air tubes, where the large cross-sectional area of the lung tissue disperses the resistance over a much greater area. Of the total pulmonary resistance, about 20% comes from tissue resistance and 80% from airway resistance.[2]

Because the respiratory muscles primarily work to overcome airway resistance and the resistances provided by the chest wall and pulmonary tissue and because increased flow enhances airway resistance in particular, the muscles must work harder in exercise. Ventilation may increase airflow from about 6 l./min. during rest to 150 l./min. or more during heavy work. At rest, the oxygen cost for ventilation is, at the most, about 2% of total oxygen consumption. In strenuous exercise, up to 10% of the total oxygen consumed is used by the respiratory muscles for ventilation. In fact, the additional amount of oxygen needed increases at a faster rate for ventilation than for working muscles. The large demands for oxygen during hard work are primarily the result of greater effort made by respiratory muscles to overcome the resistances of elastic tissue and airway passages.

Factors other than increased air flow affect airway resistance. These factors oper-ate at a local level either to dilate or to constrict bronchioles. The bronchioles contain smooth muscle that is highly responsive to the concentration of carbon dioxide in the lungs. A high level of carbon dioxide in the lungs causes bronchodilatation, while low concentrations cause bronchoconstriction. These effects occur without pulmonary control by nerves or hormones. This bronchial response to carbon dioxide matches the right proportion of alveolar air to a given quantity of capillary blood in the alveoli of the lungs. For example, if a particular alveolus has a small blood supply, but a large amount of airflow, the concentration of carbon dioxide in the alveolus is low. Consequently, the bronchioles constrict to reduce airflow to the alveolus to match the blood supply. Conversely, another alveolus may have a high blood flow and a low

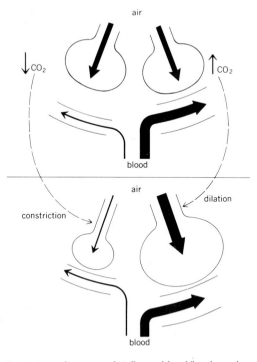

Fig. 6–3.   Adjustment of air flow to blood flow by carbon dioxide which affects bronchiolar constriction and dilation. Top panel shows the initial state, and the lower panel is after adjustment. (From Vander, A.J., Sherman, J.H., and Luciano, D.S.: Human Physiology—The Mechanisms of Body Function. New York, McGraw-Hill, Inc., 1975. Used with permission of McGraw-Hill Book Co.)

airflow, which would increase the concentration of carbon dioxide in the alveolus leading to the bronchioles. Consequently, the bronchioles would dilate to increase airflow (Fig. 6–3). In this way, alveoli needing either more or less airflow, depending on the amount of blood flow reaching their capillaries, are accommodated by the dilation or constriction of the bronchioles supplying them.

A second factor has a local chemical control at the alveolar site that balances blood flow to airflow. The concentration of oxygen in the alveolar air stimulates the lung arterioles either to constrict or to dilate (Fig. 6–4). The difference between carbon dioxide and oxygen is that carbon dioxide modifies airflow to meet a given amount of blood flow to the alveoli, whereas oxygen

changes blood flow to match a given airflow. When oxygenated airflow is high, but blood flow is low, oxygen stimulates the smooth muscle of the pulmonary arterioles to dilate and to increase capillary blood flow to the alveoli. The result is balanced blood flow and airflow in the capillaries. If airflow is small, concentration of oxygen is low, and blood flow is high, alveolar oxygen stimulates the lung arterioles to constrict and to reduce blood flow to match airflow. Of course, the controlling effects of carbon dioxide and oxygen operate simultaneously so that both airflow and blood flow are continually changing to maintain a balance. Note that the effects of carbon dioxide and oxygen on smooth muscle in the lung are opposite to their effects on blood vessels in skeletal muscle.

Volume of Air in the Lungs

The total amount of air in the lungs, total lung capacity, is made up of four different volumes: tidal volume, inspiratory reserve volume, expiratory reserve volume, and residual volume. If the lungs are visualized as an air-filled balloon, the different volumes can be illustrated, as in Figure 6–5. The volume of air leaving or entering the lungs in a single breath is called tidal volume. Under resting conditions, this volume is approximately 500 ml. The volume expired beyond

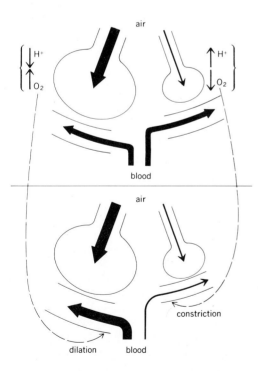

Fig. 6–4.   Adjustment of blood flow to air flow by oxygen which affects arteriolar constriction and dilation. Top panel shows the initial state, and the lower panel is after adjustment. (From Vander, A.J., Sherman, J.H., and Luciano, D.S.: Human Physiology—The Mechanisms of Body Function. New York, McGraw-Hill, Inc., 1975. Used with permission of McGraw-Hill Book Co.)

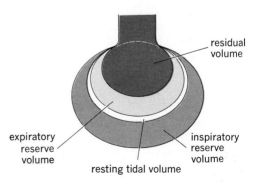

Fig. 6–5.   The volumes of air in the lungs at rest. (From Vander, A.J., Sherman, J.H., and Luciano, D.S.: Human Physiology—The Mechanisms of Body Function. New York, McGraw-Hill, Inc., 1975. Used with permission of McGraw-Hill Book Co.)

tidal volume is called the expiratory reserve volume and amounts to about 1,000 ml. The amount of air inhaled beyond tidal volume and the expiratory reserve volume is called the inspiratory reserve volume and amounts to about 2,500 to 3,500 ml. The volume of air that can be moved out of the lungs after a maximum inspiration is called vital capacity. It comprises tidal volume, inspiratory reserve volume, and expiratory reserve volume. Thus, vital capacity equals 500 ml. (tidal volume) plus 1,000 ml. (expiratory reserve volume) plus approximately 3,000 ml. (inspiratory reserve volume) for a total of 4,500 ml. or 4.5 l. Even after a maximal expiration, some air still remains in the lungs and is called the residual volume (approximately 1,000 ml.). During heavy exercise, an individual uses part of the expiratory and inspiratory reserve volumes as tidal volume to meet the increased needs of the cells for more oxygen and the removal of excessive carbon dioxide. Tidal volume seldom approaches vital capacity because excessively deep breaths rapidly exhaust the inspiratory and expiratory muscles. On the average, maximum work in 5 min. results in a tidal volume of 50 to 55% of vital capacity or about 2,500 ml.[3]

Vital capacity has been used in the past as a measure of physical fitness because it is related to $\dot{V}O_2$ max. When $\dot{V}O_2$ max was related to vital capacity among 190 individuals from the ages of 7 to 30 years, there was a relatively linear relationship.[3] This occurred because vital capacity is highly related to body size and age,[4] and both are related to $\dot{V}O_2$ max. When vital capacity is expressed per unit of body weight, no apparent relationship exists between vital capacity and cardiovascular efficiency.[5] Consequently, vital capacity adds little to the assessment of physical fitness.

ALVEOLAR VENTILATION

The exchange of gases between the air and the blood takes place only in the alveoli.

Consequently, the crucial determinant of respiratory efficiency is the volume of fresh air reaching the alveoli, or alveolar ventilation. To understand how alveolar ventilation is determined, one must know how the air is distributed in the lungs. During expiration at rest, approximately 500 ml. of air is forced out of the alveoli and through the airway passages. But, only 350 ml. of this air actually leaves at the nose or mouth. The remainder, 150 ml., remains in the airways after expiration. When the next inspiration occurs, 500 ml. of air flows into the alveoli, but the first 150 ml. entering the alveoli is not atmospheric air, but is the 150 ml. of air left behind after the previous expiration. Consequently, only 350 ml. of new atmospheric air enters the alveoli during inspiration. At the end of inspiration, 150 ml. of fresh atmospheric air is left in the conduction airways and is pushed out during expiration. Another 150 ml. of old alveolar air takes its place. The cycle is continued over and over.

The space within the airways where the gases do not exchange with the blood is called anatomic dead space. The volume of fresh air entering the alveoli in each breath is equal to:

tidal volume	500 ml.
anatomic dead space	− 150 ml.
fresh air entering alveoli	350 ml.

This total of 350 ml. is the alveolar ventilation.

The most efficient way to enhance alveolar ventilation is to increase tidal volume to an extent greater than respiratory frequency. Table 6–1 demonstrates the effects of frequency of breaths on alveolar ventilation. Subject A achieves a smaller alveolar ventilation than does subject B, even though both have the same pulmonary ventilation of 6,000 ml./min. This difference occurs because the larger respiratory rate of subject A results in a greater ventilation of dead space. Thus, subject A receives 4,200 ml. of air per min. (6,000 ml. − 1,800 ml.) in the alveoli

Table 6–1.
Effect of Respiratory Rate on Alveolar Ventilation

Subject	Tidal volume ml./breath	×	Respiratory rate breaths/min.	=	Total pulmonary ventilation ml./min.	−	Dead space ventilation ml./min.	Alveolar ventilation ml./min.
A	500		12		6,000		150 × 12 = 1,800	4,200
B	1,000		6		6,000		150 × 6 = 900	5,100

and subject B receives 5,100 ml. per min. (6,000 ml. − 900 ml.).

PULMONARY VENTILATION

The amount of respiratory activity reflects the metabolic needs of the body. As work increases and oxygen demands by the tissues increase, pulmonary ventilation is elevated to supply sufficient quantities of oxygen and to remove carbon dioxide. Pulmonary ventilation is determined by tidal volume and respiratory rate. The average person at rest has a total minute pulmonary ventilation of 500 ml. (average tidal volume) × 10 (average respiratory rate), or 5,000 ml./min. During light physical work, tidal volume may increase, but respiratory rate may not change. As work becomes heavy, respiratory rate may increase to 40 to 45 per min. for 25-year-old males, 55 per min. for 12-year-old males, and 70 per min. for 5-year-old males.[6] The increased tidal volume of about 2,500 ml. comes from the inspiratory and expiratory reserve volumes. There is indication that an individual naturally balances tidal volume and respiratory frequency to achieve optimal efficiency.[7–9] If so, an individual working or exercising should breath naturally without necessarily being conscious of a particular respiratory pattern. Of course, if an individual is hyperventilating because of emotional factors, a conscious effort should be made to correct the condition.

Pulmonary Ventilation and Metabolic Needs

At rest, pulmonary ventilation sufficiently meets all the needs for oxygen by the tissues and, at the same time, removes carbon dioxide from the lungs. As metabolic needs of the tissues increase, as occurs in work or exercise, pulmonary ventilation also increases, but not necessarily in direct proportion. In fact, ventilation not only varies with the amount of work being done, but also varies before and after work. The physiologic responses in ventilation during rest and work are shown in Table 6–2. Responses in other physiologic parameters are also indicated. Ventilation rises even before work or exercise begins. This rise is probably caused by stimulation of the respiratory centers by the cerebral cortex in anticipation of work. When work begins, there is a sharp rise in ventilation that is not indicative of a corresponding increase in metabolism (Fig. 6–6). If the work is submaximal, ventilation levels off. This leveling off occurs in primarily aerobic metabolism. But, if work is maximal, ventilation continues to climb until the end of work. At the completion of work, ventilation declines rapidly. The extent of decline depends on the severity of work. In heavy work, the decrease of ventilation is slower while oxygen debt is paid back after exercise.

The rise in ventilation during exercise is a better indicator of oxygen needs by the muscles than are the changes in ventilation just

Table 6–2.
Physiologic Responses Associated With Respiration at Rest and Work

Parameter	Rest	Work
O_2 consumption	200 ml./min.	4,000 ml./min.
Descent of diaphragm	.6 in.	2.4–4 in.
Intrapulmonary pressure	757–763 mm Hg	740–790 mm Hg
Air flow	5 l./min.	100 l./min.
O_2 cost for ventilation	2% of total O_2	10% of total O_2
Total minute pulmonary ventilation (Tidal vol. × respiration rate)	600 ml. × 10 = 6 l./min.	3,000 ml. × 40 = 120 l./min.
Hemoglobin saturation at tissue level	75%	1.4% (working muscle)
Hemoglobin saturation in venous blood	75%	20%
PO_2 in venous blood	40 mm Hg	15 mm Hg
Affinity of hemoglobin for oxygen	high	low
Arterial PO_2	95–100 mm Hg	85–90 mm Hg
PCO_2	40 mm Hg	35 mm Hg or less
H ions	—	increase

before and after exercise. Generally, the steeper the rate of incline in ventilation, the greater the metabolic needs of the tissues and the consumption of oxygen. The positive relationship between ventilation and oxygen consumption permits an estimation of $\dot{V}O_2$ max from liters of air moved in or out of the lungs (Fig. 6–7).[10,11] However, at maximum work, when ventilation increases at a much faster rate than oxygen consumption, the predication of $\dot{V}O_2$ max from ventilation would obviously be in error. Apparently, the proportionately larger rise in ventilation than in oxygen consumption reflects the greater demands placed on the anaerobic mechanisms in maximum work.

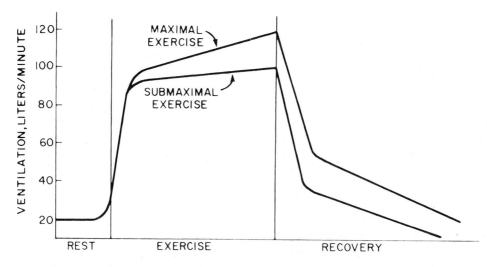

Fig. 6–6.   Changes in pulmonary ventilation before, during, and after exercise at submaximal and maximal work loads. (Data from Comroe, J.J., Jr.: The lung. Sci. Am., *214*(2):56, 1966; and Holmgren, A., and Åstrand, C.O.: DL and the dimensions and functional capacity of the O_2 transport system on humans. J. Appl. Physiol., *21*:1463, 1966.)

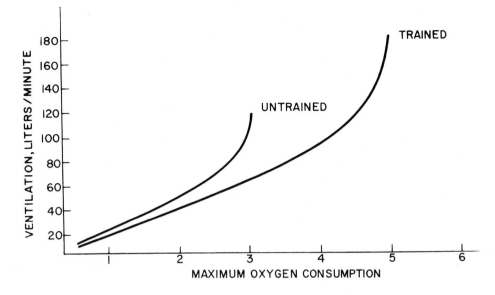

Fig. 6–7.　Relationship between pulmonary ventilation and maximal oxygen consumption in trained and untrained individuals. (Data from Saltin, B., and Åstrand, C.O.: Maximal oxygen uptake in athletes. J. Appl. Physiol., *23*:353, 1967.)

Because anaerobic metabolism provides energy without oxygen and simultaneously increases carbon dioxide at a faster rate than does aerobic metabolism, the stimulating effect of CO_2 on respiration results in a proportionately greater increase in ventilation than in oxygen consumption.

The two curves in Figure 6–7 for trained and untrained individuals point out that there are training effects on pulmonary function. When both groups work at the same load, more of the total oxygen consumed is available to the working muscles in the trained individual because less is used for ventilation. The untrained individuals use proportionately more oxygen for breathing than do the trained individuals when working at the same submaximal load. Apparently, the respiratory muscles of trained individuals have a greater capacity to utilize oxygen and, therefore, can accomplish a given amount of work with less oxygen. The increased endurance of the trained muscle is partly the result of enzymatic and mitochondrial changes at the cellular level. Other changes in the elasticity of the tissues

in the lungs and thoracic wall as a result of training probably contribute to the accomplishment of more work with less oxygen by the trained individuals. Perhaps the increased elasticity of the tissues provides less resistance to the respiratory muscles in work; therefore, less oxygen is needed.

Factors Affecting Pulmonary Ventilation

Pulmonary ventilation varies with work intensity not only within the same individual but also among individuals because of other factors. These factors relate to body size, age, and sex. In addition, factors evident during exercise, such as a "pain in the side" and "second wind," influence pulmonary ventilation. Even before exercise begins, the inhalation of certain substances, such as cigarette smoke, may adversely affect ventilation at rest and, subsequently, affect work performance.

AGE. Pulmonary ventilation reaches a peak value at about 15 years of age for females and 25 years of age for males. It then decreases until old age when it is less than one-half the peak value.[3,12] The relationship between ventilation and age is shown in Figure 6–8. Increases in ventilation from young age to adulthood are primarily caused by physical maturation. Beyond the young-adult age, the drop is caused by a decrease in the inspiratory volumes, the expiratory volumes, and the vital capacity as a consequence of inactivity,[13] and by a reduction of elastic components in the wall of the thoracic cage.[14,15]

SEX. The greater pulmonary ventilation in males compared to females after about the age of 14 is primarily the result of body size (see Fig. 6–8).[4,15a,15b] During the adolescent period, when the male hormone, testosterone, is secreted in large quantities, the skeleton and muscle mass of males develop rapidly. As the rib cage enlarges, the thoracic cavity can accommodate larger quantities of air. Consequently, pulmonary ventilation is enhanced.

BODY SIZE. As children grow in weight and particularly in height, total lung capacity and pulmonary ventilation increase accordingly.[4,15c,15d] However, adults over 25 years of age, who have reached full physical growth, experience reduced ventilation even though body size remains the same or increases.[3,12]

PAIN IN THE SIDE. Occasionally, an individual experiences a pain or a "stitch" in the side while running. This pain is probably brought about by lack of oxygen in the intercostal muscles of the chest or in the diaphragm muscles. During strenuous exercise there is a time lag between the outset of exercise and the most efficient regulation of respiratory muscles. The muscles may be working anaerobically at the beginning of exercise until the blood circulation catches up. The pain often subsides while running. However, if the pain persists the runner has difficulty maintaining an adequate pulmonary ventilation.

SECOND WIND. At the beginning of aerobic exercise, metabolites accumulate in the tissues and blood because oxygen transport to the muscles has not caught up to the metabolic demands. When blood flow to the muscles matches metabolic needs, aerobic metabolism takes over. At this point, breathing is controlled and regulated, and the work stress initially encountered is reduced.

SMOKING. Inhalation of cigarette smoke causes a two- to threefold increase in airway resistance after several seconds. The resistance lasts for 10 to 30 min.[16] Small particles stimulate the bronchioles to constrict. Al-

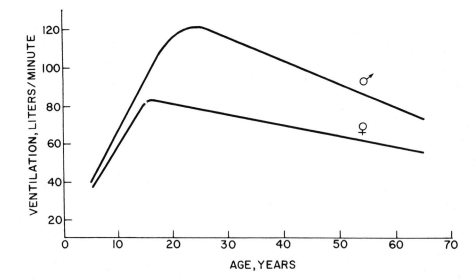

Fig. 6–8.   Relationship between pulmonary ventilation and age among males and females. (Data from Åstrand[2] and Åstrand.[5])

though the effect may not be observable during rest, pulmonary ventilation is noticeably more labored when exercising. As a result, more oxygen is needed by the respiratory muscles to maintain a given pulmonary ventilation. In chronic smokers, the oxygen cost of ventilation is about twice that of nonsmokers during heavy exercise.[17,18] Even when only a few cigarettes are smoked within one hour before exercise, the same results occur. When smokers abstain for 24 hr. prior to exercise, the oxygen cost of ventilation is about 25% lower, but is still about 50% higher than that in nonsmokers. If smoking occurs just prior to exercise, less hemoglobin is available to carry oxygen because hemoglobin prefers to carry the carbon monoxide in cigarette smoke instead of oxygen.

Hyperventilation

When the ventilation rate exceeds the metabolic needs of the body, hyperventilation results. It can be initiated consciously or unconsciously. Hyperventilation causes an individual to expire more carbon dioxide than is produced, thus lowering blood CO_2. If an athlete is overemotional in competition, unconscious hyperventilation can restrict venous return and reduce oxygenated blood flow to the brain, thus causing dizziness or fainting. Sometimes, holding the breath for a long time enhances athletic performance. Hyperventilating just before holding the breath allows a longer holding time. In sprint swimming, less water resistance is encountered when the athlete can avoid turning the head to breathe. Hyperventilating just before a short race reduces the urge to breathe and allows the face to be submerged for the entire race.

EXCHANGE OF GASES IN THE LUNGS

Pulmonary ventilation or external respiration provides alveoli with oxygenated air. The next step in the respiratory process moves oxygen from the air into the blood capillaries and, at the same time, removes

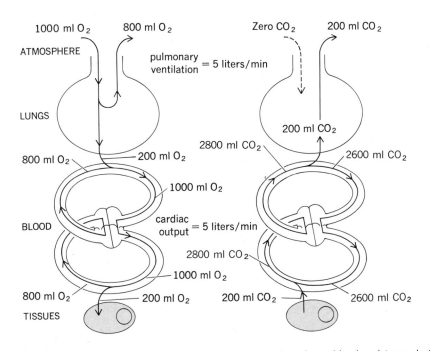

Fig. 6–9. Exchanges of oxygen and carbon dioxide between the atmosphere, lungs, blood, and tissues during 1 min. RQ is assumed to be 1. (From Vander, A.J., Sherman, J.H., and Luciano, D.S.: Human Physiology—The Mechanisms of Body Function. New York, McGraw-Hill, Inc., 1975. Used with permission of McGraw-Hill Book Co.)

carbon dioxide from the blood into the alveoli. This step is the first stage of internal respiration. At rest, approximately 200 ml. of oxygen each minute pass from the alveoli into the pulmonary capillaries to be used by the body cells while the same amount of carbon dioxide passes from the blood into the alveoli, provided that only glucose is utilized for energy so that the RQ = 1 (Fig. 6–9). Because about 5 l./min. of air pass in and out of the lungs during pulmonary ventilation at rest and because about 20% of atmospheric air is oxygen (the remainder is nitrogen), the amount of oxygen inspired each minute is 20% × 5 l./min., or 1 l./min. If the amount of oxygen taken into the lungs is 1 l./min., but the amount actually absorbed is one-fifth that amount, or 200 ml., the pulmonary capillaries that carry venous blood must be highly saturated with oxygen at rest. In fact, the blood in the capillaries is about 80% saturated. Each minute, about 5 l. of blood (cardiac output) pass through the pulmonary capillaries carrying 800 ml. of oxygenated blood, During that time, 200 ml. is added to the 800 ml. so that the arterial blood then contains 1,000 ml. of O_2. As oxygen moves into the blood, carbon dioxide moves out. About 200 ml. of CO_2 per minute pass from the arterial blood through the pulmonary capillaries into the alveoli. This quantity of carbon dioxide represents only a portion of the total amount of carbon dioxide in the blood.

During exercise and work, when the need for oxygen by the tissues increases and more carbon dioxide is produced, a relatively smaller amount of oxygen and more carbon dioxide are present in the blood of the pulmonary capillaries. Consequently, more oxygen diffuses from the alveoli into the blood, and more carbon dioxide diffuses from the blood to the alveoli.

Transport of Oxygen and Carbon Dioxide Across Cell Membranes at Rest and Work

The behavior of gases moving by diffusion from the alveolar air to the pulmonary capillary blood and vice versa is explained in terms of pressure differences, or pressure gradients, rather than in terms of differences in gas concentrations. The concept of individual gas pressures in a mixture of several gases is important in understanding the diffusion of oxygen and carbon dioxide across cell membranes. The weight of the atmosphere exerts a pressure on all substances on and above earth. This pressure varies according to the quantities of air above a body. At sea level, atmospheric pressure or barometric pressure is 760 mm Hg, but at higher altitudes this pressure decreases (Fig. 6–10). The total pressure of a mixture of gases at sea level, such as oxygen, carbon dioxide, and nitrogen, is equal to the atmospheric pressure of 760 mm Hg. However, their individual pressures are related to their concentrations in the air. Because the concentration of oxygen in the atmosphere is 20.93%, its individual pressure is equal to 20.93% × 760 mm Hg, or 159 mm Hg. The individual pressures of carbon dioxide and nitrogen are calculated in the same manner. Carbon dioxide, comprising 0.04% of the air, has an individual gas pressure of .04% × 760 mm Hg, or 0.3 mm Hg. Because nitrogen

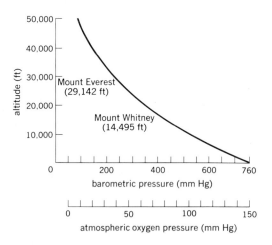

Fig. 6–10.   Relationship between altitude and barometric pressure. The PO_2 is always approximately 20% of the barometric pressure regardless of altitude. (From Vander, A.J., Sherman, J.H., and Luciano, D.S.: Human Physiology—The Mechanisms of Body Function. New York, McGraw-Hill, Inc., 1975. Used with permission of McGraw-Hill Book Co.)

makes up 78.62% of the air, its pressure is 78.62% × 760 mm Hg, or 600.7 mm Hg. Of course, the sum of these individual gas pressures is equal to the atmospheric pressure at sea level, which is 760 mm Hg (159 + 0.3 + 600.7 = 760 mm Hg). (Figure 6–11 presents a summary of carbon dioxide and oxygen pressure in the inspired and expired air and in various places within the body at rest and during work.) Therefore, pressures in a mixture of different gases are expressed as partial pressures. These pressures are denoted by a P placed in front of the symbol for the gases: the partial pressure for oxygen is written PO_2 and for carbon dioxide, PCO_2. Oxygen passes from the alveolar air to the pulmonary capillaries by diffusion because the quantity of PO_2 is greater in the air than in the blood. In the same way, PCO_2 in the alveolar blood is greater than that in air and results in diffusion of carbon dioxide from the blood to the air.

Inspired air has a PO_2 of 159 mm Hg; however, by the time it reaches the alveoli, the PO_2 is 104 mm Hg at rest. This decrease occurs for several reasons. When atmospheric air enters the respiratory passages, it is exposed to the fluids covering the respiratory surfaces and becomes totally humidified. This water vapor expands the volume of the inspired air and dilutes oxygen to a PO_2 of 149.3 mm Hg. In addition, atmospheric oxygen is further diluted because the inspired air mixes with three sources of air in the lungs: (1) the air remaining in the lungs after the end of expiration (expiratory reserve volume), (2) the air in the lungs after the most forceful expiration (residual volume), and (3) the air remaining in the passages after expiration (dead air space). Consequently, the amount of alveolar air replaced by the new atmospheric air with each breath is only about one seventh of the total, resulting in an alveolar PO_2 of 104 mm Hg. The relatively slow replacement of alveolar air is important in the prevention of sudden changes in gaseous concentrations in the blood. Consequently, when respiration is temporarily interrupted, excessive increases or decreases in tissue oxygenation, carbon dioxide concentration, or pH are prevented, thus maintaining the stability of respiratory control.

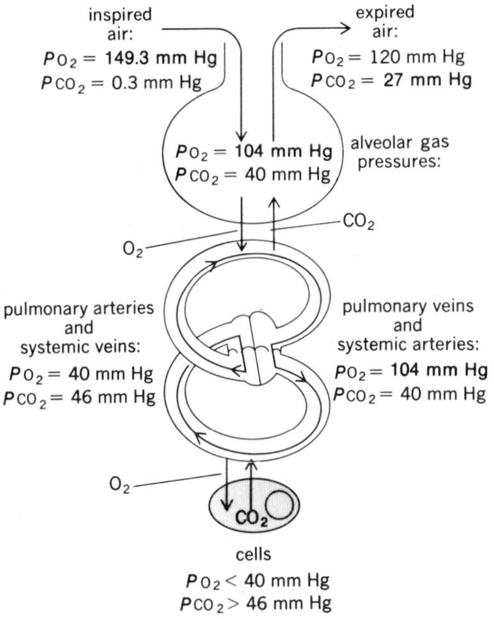

Expired air (see Fig. 6–11) contains more PO_2 (120 mm Hg) and less PCO_2 (27 mm Hg) than does the alveolar air ($PO_2 = 104$ mm Hg and $PCO_2 = 40$ mm Hg, respectively) because, during expiration, the alveolar air mixes with the approximately 150 ml. of air in the dead space. Because this 150 ml. of air was left over from the previous inspiration and never reached the alveoli, it contains a relatively high level of oxygen ($PO_2 = 149.3$ mm Hg). Consequently, when the lower PO_2 and the higher PCO_2 in the alveoli are expired, the partial pressures in the expired air fall between these values.

The blood entering the pulmonary capillaries is venous blood pumped to the lungs

Fig. 6–11. Partial pressures of oxygen and carbon dioxide in inspired and expired air and in different sites within the body during rest at sea level. Blood flow forms a loop from the alveoli to the pulmonary veins, heart, systemic circulation, back to the heart and out the pulmonary arteries. (From Vander, A.J., Sherman, J.H., and Luciano, D.S.: Human Physiology—The Mechanisms of Body Function. New York, McGraw-Hill, Inc., 1975. Used with permission of McGraw-Hill Book Co.)

via the pulmonary arteries. Because it comes from the tissues, it has a high PCO_2 (46 mm Hg) and a low PO_2 (40 mm Hg). As it flows through the pulmonary capillaries, it releases carbon dioxide and receives oxygen through an extremely thin layer of tissue. The diffusion of these gases ceases when the alveolar and capillary partial pressures become equal. As a result, the blood in the pulmonary veins leading back to the heart and in the systemic arteries leading from the heart have the same partial pressures as the alveoli, i.e., $PO_2 = 104$ mm Hg and $PCO_2 = 40$ mm Hg. When the arterial blood reaches the tissue capillaries throughout the body, diffusion of oxygen into the interstitial fluid bathing the cells and then into the cells themselves provides the oxygen needed for aerobic metabolism. Excessive carbon dioxide in the cells takes the same path back to the capillaries. At the end of the capillaries, equilibrium of the gases in the capillaries and in the tissue cells has been reached

and accounts for the values of $PO_2 = 40$ mm Hg. and $PCO_2 = 46$ mm Hg in the venous blood.

The partial pressures of the gases in maximum work are different from the partial pressures at rest. The increased metabolic needs of the working muscles for oxygen and the removal of metabolites, especially carbon dioxide, result in a shifting of the partial pressures of these gases in the alveolar air, arterial blood, and venous blood. These changes in partial pressures of oxygen and carbon dioxide from rest to maximum work are gradual and are related to work intensity (Fig. 6–12). As work severity increases to about 50% $\dot{V}O_2$ max, a level considered close to the threshold for producing a training effect, alveolar PO_2 climbs slightly higher than the drop in alveolar PCO_2. With more work, the gap between the alveolar pressures of the gases widens. These changes with work intensity indicate an effective exchange of gases in the lungs. As a

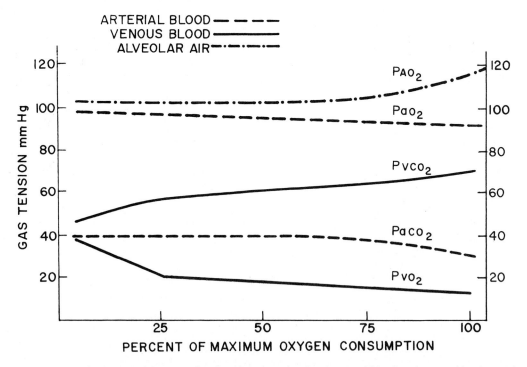

Fig. 6–12.   Partial pressures of oxygen and carbon dioxide in the alveoli, arterial blood, and venous blood at work levels of various percentages of maximum oxygen consumption. (Data from Åstrand, P.O., and Rodahl, G.K.: Textbook of Work Physiology, New York, McGraw-Hill Book Co., 1977.)

result of the increasing oxygen tension in the alveoli with work intensity, arterial PO_2 does not appreciably change from work to rest (a drop from 97 mm Hg to about 92 mm Hg). The drop in venous oxygen tension corresponding to the increase in venous carbon dioxide tension with work is expected because more oxygen is extracted from the blood and more carbon dioxide is produced. The efficiency of the gas-exchange systems can be appreciated when one realizes that cardiac output increases about 5 times (5 l./min to 25 l./min), oxygen consumption increases 20 times (.2 l./min. to 4 l./min.), and pulmonary ventilation also increases 20 times (6 l./min. to 120 l./min.).

Diffusing Capacity in Exercise

At rest, the equilibrium of PO_2 and PCO_2 in the pulmonary capillaries occurs in about 0.75 sec. Therefore, the blood in the pulmonary veins returning to the heart contains about the same carbon dioxide and oxygen as does the alveolar air. Even during strenuous work, when capillary blood flow increases 5 times or more, a gaseous equilib-

rium occurs in only 0.5 sec. or less. The greater diffusion of gases between the alveoli and capillaries in exercise is probably caused by the increased number of pulmonary capillaries opened to the alveoli.[19] Diffusing capacity increases while exercising until about 40% $\dot{V}O_2$ max and levels off beyond that value. Physical training improves diffusion both at rest[20] and at work (Fig. 6–13).[21,22] In highly trained marathon runners, diffusion capacity at rest is almost twice that of untrained men working maximally.[20] Trained athletes have demonstrated better pulmonary diffusion both in submaximal work[23] and in maximal work.[22] Apparently, greater diffusion from training is attributable to the larger lung volumes that increase the surface area between the alveoli and the capillaries.[24,25]

TRANSPORT OF OXYGEN IN BLOOD TO TISSUES

The cardiovascular system moves blood to the various tissues of the body; the amount of blood moved depends on the metabolic activity of the muscles. When

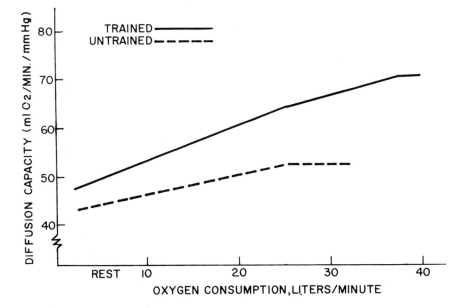

Fig. 6–13. Changes in pulmonary diffusing capacity with exercise between trained and untrained at submaximal and maximal work loads. (Data from Bannister, R.G., et. al.: Pulmonary diffusing capacity on exercise in athletes and non-athletic subjects. J. Physiol., *152*:66, 1960.)

metabolism is high in a particular organ or tissue, more oxygen is supplied by the increased blood flow to that site. The amount of oxygen available to the tissues depends on the quantity of oxygen contained within the blood plasma and within the hemoglobin of the red cells. About 1.5% of the total oxygen in the arterial blood is physically dissolved in the plasma and 98.5% is chemically bound to hemoglobin. When expressed in terms of 1 l. of arterial blood, which contains 200 ml. of oxygen, 3 ml. of oxygen are carried in the plasma and 197 ml. are chemically bound to hemoglobin to form oxyhemoglobin. The oxygen dissolved in the plasma is free in solution; the oxygen combined to hemoglobin is not. Gases chemically bound to another substance, such as oxyhemoglobin, are not free in solution and, therefore, cannot provide pressure on the container in which they lie. As a result, only the oxygen in the plasma can exert pressure on the blood vessels. This pressure causes oxygen to diffuse out of the capillaries into the interstitial fluid surrounding the cells.

Effect of PO_2 on the Oxygen Content of Hemoglobin

By raising the concentration of oxygen in the blood plasma, which increases PO_2, one can determine the amount of oxygen that combines with hemoglobin. Although oxyhemoglobin does not contribute to the PO_2 in the blood because the oxygen is not free in solution, hemoglobin is important in determining the amount of oxygen that diffuses in and out of the blood. For example, the hemoglobin in the blood of the pulmonary capillaries contributes to the low PO_2 and causes more alveolar oxygen to diffuse into the capillary blood. By taking oxygen out of the plasma to form more oxyhemoglobin, the hemoglobin reduces the PO_2 and, thereby, increases the pressure gradient for oxygen. Consequently, more oxygen diffuses from the lungs into the blood. At the end of the pulmonary capillaries, hemoglobin and plasma are almost completely saturated with oxygen. The oxygenated blood

leaving the lungs and passing to the other tissues via the heart has a larger PO_2 at the capillaries than does the interstitial fluid. As a result, oxygen diffuses across the capillary membranes into the interstitial fluid and then into the cells. As plasma PO_2 is reduced, oxygen dissociates from hemoglobin and diffuses into the plasma where it passes out of the capillaries to provide additional oxygen to the cells.

Even after the blood leaves the tissues and returns to the heart, its PO_2 of 40 mm Hg (a drop from 104 mm Hg in arterial blood) leaves the hemoglobin saturated at 75% (down from about 100% in arterial blood) under resting conditions. During strenuous exercise, active muscles may use practically all the oxygen from the capillary blood. Venous blood from these muscles may have a PO_2 of only 12 mm Hg and an actual volume of oxygen of 1.4%.[26] However, this blood is still above the critical level of about 7 mm Hg PO_2, which is necessary for the continued life of the cells.[27]

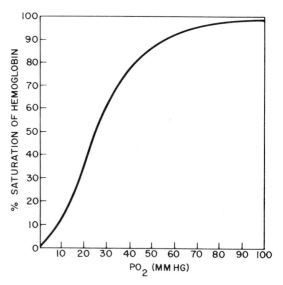

Fig. 6–14. Hemoglobin-oxygen dissociation curve. Note how a drop from 100 mm Hg PO_2 to 40 mm Hg only reduces hemoglobin saturation from 98% to 75%. (From Vander, A.J., Sherman, J.H., and Luciano, D.S.: Human Physiology—The Mechanisms of Body Function. New York: McGraw-Hill, Inc., 1975. Used with permission of McGraw-Hill Book Co.)

Because the concentration of oxygen in the physically dissolved state in blood plasma, or PO_2, determines the extent to which hemoglobin is saturated with oxygen, the relationship between the two can be illustrated (Fig. 6–14). The curve is called an oxyhemoglobin dissociation curve. Generally, as PO_2 increases, oxyhemoglobin increases. The greater the absorption of oxygen by the blood plasma from the alveoli, the greater the oxygen uptake by the hemoglobin. But, the extent of this relationship varies with the PO_2. Hemoglobin combines with oxygen rapidly as PO_2 increases from 10 to 60 mm Hg. At a PO_2 of 60 mm Hg, 90% of the total hemoglobin is combined with oxygen. From 60 to 100 mm Hg, oxyhemoglobin slightly increases to about 98% saturation. Because oxyhemoglobin remains fairly high even at relatively low PO_2, the tissue cells can receive adequate amounts of oxygen to sustain life and to maintain function. Consequently, in work at high altitudes, where the PO_2 may drop drastically to 60 mm Hg from 100 mm Hg at sea level, the oxygen content of hemoglobin remains fairly high at 90%.

Effects of Temperature and Acidity on Hemoglobin Saturation

The hemoglobin-oxygen dissociation curve in Figure 6–14 is based on normal resting conditions where the PCO_2 of the arterial blood is 40 mm Hg, blood temperature is 98.6°F (37°C), and pH is 7.40. However, during work or exercise, when body temperature increases and pH drops, the affinity of hemoglobin for oxygen decreases. Consequently, the hemoglobin-oxygen dissociation curve assumes a different slope (Fig. 6–15). At the cellular level the rise in blood temperature and the increase in blood acidity (pH drop) during exercise result in a greater release of oxygen from hemoglobin at the capillary level.

When blood temperature increases to 102.2°F (39°C) and pH drops to 7.20, hemoglobin may retain only about 17% of its oxygen at the capillary level. In resting condi-

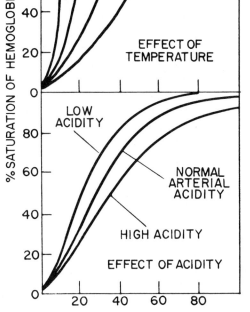

Fig. 6–15. Hemoglobin-oxygen dissociation curves as affected by acidity and blood temperature. (From Vander, A.J., Sherman, J.H., and Luciano, D.S.: Human Physiology—The Mechanisms of Body Function. New York, McGraw-Hill, Inc., 1975. Used with permission of McGraw-Hill Book Co.)

tions, hemoglobin may retain about 33% of its oxygen. Because hemoglobin retains less oxygen at the capillary level during exercise, more oxygen becomes available to the working muscles. This is an advantage in endurance exercises or in athletic events.

But, this advantage is limited with further increases in heat and carbon dioxide. When the pH drops to 7.0 and muscle temperature increases to 104°F (40°C), as occurs in maximum work, the carrying capacity for oxygen by the arterial blood decreases because there is less affinity for oxygen by hemoglobin. However, under most work conditions where effort is submaximal, increased carbon dioxide and temperature enhance oxygen utilization by the working muscles.

Role of Myoglobin in Work

Myoglobin is an iron-containing protein found in skeletal muscle cells and, like hemoglobin, has an affinity for oxygen. In fact, the affinity of myoglobin for oxygen is greater than that of hemoglobin. This is shown by the oxygen dissociation curves for hemoglobin and myoglobin (Fig. 6–16). Whereas the affinity of hemoglobin for oxygen is greatly reduced from a PO_2 of about 40 mm Hg and below, the affinity in myoglobin occurs at a lower pressure of about 20 mm Hg. Consequently, myoglobin releases its oxygen only in fairly heavy exercise when PO_2 drops to 20 mm Hg or less. Often, during mild or moderate exercise, the drop in PO_2 is not sufficient for myoglobin to give up its oxygen. During heavy exercise, when extra oxygen is available from myoglobin, the myoglobin recharges with oxygen if the muscle can relax intermittently. However, if work is continued so that little rest is provided, the importance of myoglobin in pro-

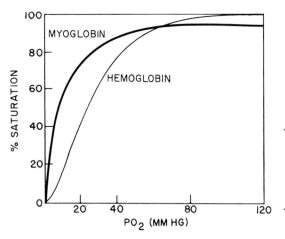

Fig. 6–16.   Oxygen dissociation curves for hemoglobin and myoglobin. (From Vander, A.J., Sherman, J.H., and Luciano, D.S.: Human Physiology—The Mechanisms of Body Function. New York, McGraw-Hill, Inc., 1975. Used with permission of McGraw-Hill Book Co.)

viding additional oxygen to the cells is limited to the early stages of work, or until all its oxygen has been dissociated.

CONTROL OF RESPIRATION

The inspiratory muscles (diaphragm and external intercostals) and expiratory muscles (internal intercostals) are supplied with motor nerves whose cell bodies lie in the medulla at the lower portion of the brain stem near the cardiac and vasomotor regions. Relatively well-defined areas in the medulla contain the inspiratory and the expiratory regions from which impulses are sent to motor neurons going to the respiratory muscles. The centers coordinate function so that, when inspiration occurs, the expiratory center is inhibited. At the end of inspiration at rest, the relaxing inspiratory muscles cause passive expiration. During exercise, when expiration is not passive, the expiratory muscles forcefully contract to expel air rapidly. Breathing is cyclical because of the alternating excitation and inhibition of the respiratory centers. Depth of inspiration depends on the number of motor units firing and their frequency of discharge, whereas respiratory rate depends on the length of time elapsing between firings.

The afferent receptors that influence the respiratory region in the medulla so that the rate and depth of breathing match the metabolic needs of the body are summarized in Figure 6–17. These receptors are located centrally in the medulla of the brain and peripherally in the respiratory muscles, the arteries near the heart, and the skeletal joints. The stimuli that activate the receptors are chemical, such as carbon dioxide, oxygen, and hydrogen ions (H^+), and mechanical, such as the pressure that occurs in a contracting muscle and in a moving joint.

Control of Ventilation by Oxygen, Carbon Dioxide, and Hydrogen Ions

Two different groups of afferent receptors respond to these gases. One group is located at the bifurcation of the carotid arteries and

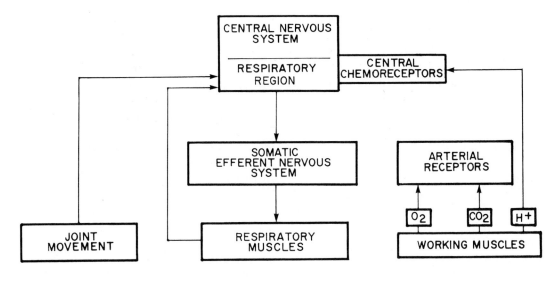

Fig. 6–17. Afferent receptors and stimuli in controlling ventilation.

in the arch of the aorta, close to the baroreceptors that respond to changes in blood pressure. These receptors are called carotid and aortic bodies (see Fig. 5–9), and they are stimulated by oxygen and carbon dioxide. Low arterial PO_2 acts as the primary stimulus to the receptors, although excess carbon dioxide also has an effect. When plasma oxygen is low, or carbon dioxide is high, afferent fibers carry this information from the afferent receptors to the respiratory region in the medulla. From there, the motor neurons to the breathing muscles are stimulated to increase tidal volume and, if plasma oxygen is very low, respiratory rate.

Because these receptors respond only to plasma PO_2 and not to total oxygen in the blood, most of which is combined with hemoglobin, there is no respiratory stimulation from low oxyhemoglobin. In anemia (a physical condition characterized by low quantities of iron in the blood and, in turn, in hemoglobin) ventilation is not increased even though oxyhemoglobin is also in short supply. Ventilation increases only when plasma PO_2 is low. A reduction in oxyhemoglobin by tobacco smoking also does not affect ventilation if PO_2 is normal. Of course, during exercise when aerobic metabolism is greatly involved, low oxyhemoglobin reduces work capacity.

In addition to the afferent receptors responding to oxygen and carbon dioxide in the arteries, other receptors in the brain stem are stimulated by gases. These receptors, however, are influenced only by carbon dioxide and hydrogen ions, not by oxygen. The importance of these afferent receptors in controlling ventilation compared with the control provided by the aortic and carotid bodies can be demonstrated by the differing effects that carbon dioxide and oxygen have on respiration. An increase in alveolar PCO_2 of only 5 mm Hg results in a 100% increase in ventilation. However, breathing 100% oxygen, which is almost a 5-fold increase in the normal amount of oxygen in the atmosphere (20.93%), decreases ventilation by about 10 to 20%. The importance of PCO_2 in respiration is shown by the effects of hyperventilation. When an individual breathes as rapidly and deeply as possible for a minute or so and then breathes normally, the rate of ventilation is greatly reduced, and may even stop for a short time. This effect occurs because the rapid breathing has blown off most of the carbon dioxide in the lungs at a faster rate than it is produced. As a result, the decreased PCO_2 inhibits respiration. Eventually, when the carbon dioxide formed from metabolism gradually builds up PCO_2, breathing resumes at its normal rate. If breathing is curtailed for a prolonged time after hyperventilation, the drop in PO_2 may initiate a faster respiratory rate even before PCO_2 is completely back to normal. This occurs because the carotid and aortic bodies are stimulated by the extremely low PO_2.

The strong influence of PCO_2 in controlling ventilation is also shown by the effects of holding the breath. In a short time, the increase in PCO_2 is so powerful that it overcomes the voluntary inhibition of the respiratory center. In some sporting events that require short bursts of energy followed by rest, such as competitive swimming, holding the breath is not harmful and may be advantageous. But, in underwater swimming for distance, holding the breath after hyperventilation may lower the PO_2 to such an extent that fainting and drowning can result.

Respiratory rate is not influenced by the effects of carbon dioxide itself, but by the concentration of hydrogen ions in the cerebrospinal fluid bathing the nervous tissue in the central nervous system. A high concentration of hydrogen ions stimulates the respiratory centers in the brain stem to increase breathing, whereas a low concentration inhibits the centers. Hydrogen ions are formed from the chemical breakdown of carbon dioxide; however, intermediate, chemical steps are also involved. Carbon dioxide produced in the tissue cells passes out of the cells in a dissolved state. A small amount (8%) remains physically dissolved in the blood plasma and the red blood cells. A large portion of the carbon dioxide (67%) combines with water and changes into carbonic acid (H_2CO_3) and then into bicarbonate (HCO_3^-) and hydrogen ions (H^+).

$$CO_2 + H_2O \rightarrow H_2CO_3 \rightarrow HCO_3^- + H^+$$

The chemical reactions occur primarily in the red blood cells because the reactions require large quantities of a specific enzyme (carbonic anhydrase) that is located in these cells. The hydrogen ions diffuse readily from the blood into the cerebrospinal fluid where their concentration is noted by the respiratory region. The bicarbonate (HCO_3^-) produced with the hydrogen ions (H^+) from the breakdown of carbon dioxide is stored in the blood plasma. The remaining carbon dioxide produced by the tissues (25%) combines directly with hemoglobin (Hb) in the red blood cells to form $HbCO_2$.

When the venous blood reaches the lung capillaries, the relatively smaller PCO_2 in the alveoli than in the blood results in the combining of the bicarbonate in the blood plasma with the hydrogen ions to form carbon dioxide ($HCO_3^- + H^+ \rightarrow H_2CO_3 \rightarrow CO_2 + H_2O$). The carbon dioxide combined with the hemoglobin ($HbCO_2$) is also released. The excess carbon dioxide is then diffused into the alveoli where it is blown off in expiration.

When excess carbon dioxide is not expired by the lungs, which happens during heavy exercise when anaerobic metabolism increases lactic acid, the excess hydrogen ions produce an increase in acidity of the blood. The term used to express the acidity of a solution and its alkalinity is pH. It may be expressed as the power of the hydrogen ion. The range of pH in the body needed to maintain a condition conducive to life is between 7.30 and 7.50 during rest. In strenuous exercise, when lactic acid and hydrogen ions increase, the acidity of the blood may be greatly elevated, as expressed by a pH of 6.80. But, a low pH in exercise is only temporary because, during rest or reduced activity, the body's mechanisms to reduce acidity (elevate pH) start working.

The respiratory mechanism is one way of regulating pH so that a normal level is maintained. An increase in respiratory rate removes more carbon dioxide and, thereby, reduces the concentration of hydrogen ions and elevates pH. The reverse is true when respiratory rate decreases; pH decreases as hydrogen ions increase the acidity of tissues. When the pH is 7.20, ventilation increases about 4 times; but, at pH levels above 7.41, ventilation decreases.

The other two mechanisms of the body that regulate the pH level are: (1) the chemicals in the body fluids, called buffers, which maintain a desired level of hydrogen ions; and (2) the kidneys, which maintain the proper balance of hydrogen ions by the excretion of urine.

These control mechanisms can be better understood when the concept of acid-base balance is known. First, an acid is a chemical compound, such as hydrochloric acid (HCl) or sulphuric acid (H_2SO_4), that gives up hydrogen ions (H^+) in solution. For example,

$$HCl \rightarrow H^+ + Cl^-$$

$$H_2SO_4 \rightarrow H^+ + SO_4^-$$

A base is a chemical compound, such as sodium hydroxide (NaOH) or potassium hydroxide (KOH), that gives up hydroxyl ions (OH^-). For example,

$$NaOH \rightarrow Na^+ + OH^-$$

$$KOH \rightarrow K^+ + OH^-$$

The number of H^+ ions compared with the number of OH^- ions determines whether a solution is acidic or basic. If H^+ ions exceed OH^- ions, the solution is acidic, and vice versa. Directly associated with more H^+ ions, of course, is lower pH, whereas more OH^- ions indicate a higher pH.

Chemical buffers act on acids and bases to diminish their effects in a solution so that a normal level of hydrogen-ion concentration can be maintained. When an acid is added to a solution, such as lactic acid during anaerobic metabolism, the acidity of the solution is reduced by the combining of lactic acid (LA) with the buffer, sodium bicarbonate ($NaHCO_3$), a weak acid. The formula is

The combination of H^+ ions from a strong acid, such as LA, with a salt ($NaHCO_3$) results in a weaker acid and an elevation in pH. When carbon dioxide (CO_2) and the subsequent formation of carbonic acid (H_2CO_3) become excessive in exercise so that pH decreases (indicating higher acidity), bicarbonate (HCO_3^-) acts as a buffer again to reduce acidity as follows:

$$H^+ + HCO_3^- \leftrightharpoons H_2CO_3 \leftrightharpoons CO_2 + H_2O$$

When the formula shifts to the left during strenuous exercise so that the increases in carbon dioxide finally result in more hydrogen ions, there is a shift back to the right by the buffering action of bicarbonate (HCO_3^-) if the excess H^+ cannot be removed via CO_2, ventilation, and the other mechanism controlling pH, the kidney. The importance of bicarbonate as a buffer is indicated by its effect on pH. As bicarbonate ions increase, pH increases. A decrease in this buffer, especially with an increase in dissolved carbon dioxide, decreases pH. The kidney affects pH because it regulates the concentration of hydrogen ions primarily by increasing or decreasing the concentration of bicarbonate ions (HCO_3^-). The kidney does this by storing bicarbonate ions and using them as needed to combine with H^+ ions to form carbonic acid (H_2CO_3) and, thereby, help to retain H^+ ions in the body, or by eliminating them in urination.

Control of Ventilation by Physical Activity

At the beginning of exercise, movement of the skeletal muscles and joints causes a rapid stimulation of the respiratory centers. Pulmonary ventilation increases almost instantly upon initiation of movement. Afterward, PO_2 and PCO_2 contribute to the control of ventilation via the chemical receptors in the arteries and the concentration of H^+ ions in the cerebrospinal fluid. As exercise

$$LA \rightarrow H^+ + LACTATE^- + NaHCO_3 \rightarrow NaLA + H_2CO_3$$

Strong acid + Bicarbonate $\longrightarrow$ Salt + Weak acid proceeds, both joint movement and chemical stimuli regulate pulmonary ventilation.

There are many stretch receptors in the lungs and many muscle spindles in the respiratory muscles. Stretch receptors are located in the pleurae, bronchi, bronchioles, and alveoli of the lungs; spindles are located in the muscles of the diaphragm, the internal and external intercostals, the scaleni, the sternocleidomastoids, and the abdominals. The organs of Ruffini and pacinian endorgans, which are receptors located in the tissues surrounding skeletal joints, also stimulate the respiratory center. Joint movement is the stimulus for these sensory organs. Muscle spindles in the respiratory muscles are activated in two ways: (1) stretching of the skeletal muscles that contain the spindles, and (2) direct stimulation of the spindles by the gamma efferents (Fig. 3–18). During inspiration and expiration, the stretching of muscles stimulates the spindles. At the same time, the spindles are stretched by the gamma motor nerves. The nerve pathways are the same in both mechanisms of stimulation. They follow the spindle afferents to the spinal cord, where they connect to the motor neurons going to the skeletal muscles of respiration. At rest, stretching the spindles in the inspiratory muscles results in a reflex contraction of these muscles and in inhibition of the expiratory muscles. At the end of inspiration, the inspiratory muscles relax, causing the passive exhalation of air by the recoiling of the elastic tissues that were stretched during inspiration. But, during heavy exercise, when the respiratory frequency increases to meet the oxygen needs of the working muscles, the expiratory muscles contract to force air out of the lungs. The expiratory muscles are facilitated to contract by the stretch imposed on their muscle spindles during inspiration. Facilitation refers to the reinforcement of nervous activity so that relatively low frequencies of afferent nerve impulses, when summated with other low impulses, ease the elicitation of a response in an affector neuron. In other words,

stretching the spindles in the expiratory muscles "prepares" or "makes ready" the easier transmission of impulses across the synapses in the spinal cord to the effector nerves of the expiratory muscles.

Effects of Temperature on Ventilation

An elevation of body temperature results in respiratory stimulation. Apparently, the rise in temperature of the fluids bathing the respiratory and cardiovascular regions in the brain stem makes the regions more sensitive to chemical stimuli. Consequently, their response to stimuli may be more exaggerated than when temperatures are lower. The body's ability to lower the acidity of the fluids may also be reduced because of the higher temperatures. This situation is further complicated when the activity of H^+ ions is enhanced, tending to increase the acidity of the cerebrospinal fluid. Even the peripheral chemoreceptors in the arteries may be more responsive to stimuli because of a rise in blood temperature. More secondary effects on ventilation may be indicated by the responses made by the cardiovascular regions to increase core temperatures. The shunting of more blood to the periphery to cool the body by sweating reduces the blood flow to the heart and circulatory system. To maintain cardiac output, heart rate must increase. Stimuli acting on the cardiovascular centers provide input information to the respiratory region, which then coordinates all regions.

Chemical and Neural Factors in Controlling Ventilation in Exercise

During strenuous exercise, arterial PO_2 may drop to between 85 and 90 mm Hg as compared to a normal resting value of between 95 and 100 mm Hg. Arterial PCO_2 may drop to 35 mm Hg or less compared to a resting level of 40 mm Hg, and the concentration of hydrogen ions increases somewhat because of the accumulation of lactic acid. These chemical changes in PO_2, PCO_2, and acidity do not fully explain the increase in ventilation from 6 l./min. at rest to 150 l./min. or more during strenuous exercise. Nor do they explain the rapid increase in ventilation at the beginning of exercise or the abrupt decrease after exercise. Because pulmonary ventilation increases 20-fold or more during exercise, even though the chemical factors of arterial PO_2, PCO_2, and hydrogen ion remain slightly changed, the stimulation for breathing must come largely from neural factors that are stimulated by joint activity. Apparently, chemical factors actually regulate respiratory volume by providing negative feedback via the respiratory regions. When exercise is severe, the increased carbon dioxide and acidity of the blood (low pH) provide feedback to stimulate the gamma, and alpha effector nerves to the respiratory muscles, via the respiratory regions and other areas in the brain stem, to increase pulmonary volume. A drop in PCO_2 and acidity reduces excitation of the gamma and alpha nerves.

The importance of various factors in contributing to the increase of ventilation was estimated by Lambertsen.[28] This estimation was done after examining the factors related to ventilation and the afferent impulses from the great veins, the heart, and the pulmonary circulation. The ventilatory factors are PCO_2, hydrogen ion, pH, PO_2, and temperature as they influence metabolism and joint movement. Only three of these factors were considered to be directly associated with hyperventilation in exercise: increase in core temperature of the body, increase in hydrogen ions of the circulating blood, and increase in movement of the skeletal joints. The metabolic factors of increased temperature and hydrogen ions were estimated to account for at least one third of the ventilatory response in exercise, whereas about half of this response was attributed to the neural mechanisms activated by body movement. Fifteen percent of the total respiratory response to muscular exercise was unaccountable. This estimation was based on a "steady state" of exercise involving aerobic metabolism. In more strenuous work, when the end products of anaerobic metabolism prevail, the relative importance of these factors may change. Although the exact contribution of each factor in controlling or regulating ventilation during exercise is not known, it is a fact that continued and prolonged exercise, in time, improves the efficiency of external and internal respiration.

ATMOSPHERIC PRESSURES AND PERFORMANCE

Barometric air pressure is highest at sea level (760 mm Hg) and decreases with altitude (see Fig. 6–10.) The drop in air pressure is owing to the reduced density of the air as altitude increases. With less air pressure, the gases comprising the atmospheric air also have proportionately less pressure, even though their relative concentrations are the same at all altitudes. At the barometric pressure of 760 mm Hg at sea level, the PO_2 is 159 mm Hg; but, at an altitude of 5,000 ft. (1,524 m.) above sea level, the PO_2 is about 123 mm Hg. The drop in PO_2 in the alveoli at higher altitudes causes a lowered oxygen pressure gradient, which reduces the difference between the alveolar PO_2 and blood PO_2. Consequently, less oxygen diffuses into the blood and, in turn, less oxygen is available to the muscles. This is not a problem under resting conditions but, in heavy work, the quantity of oxygen may not be sufficient for prolonged and continuous aerobic work. At high altitudes, such as 19,000 ft. (5,793 m.), the oxygen saturation of the arterial blood is only 67% compared with an almost 100% saturation at sea level.

In athletic events involving all-out efforts, performance at high altitudes is impaired when success depends primarily on the ability of the respiratory and cardiovascular systems to supply oxygen to the working tissues. The extent of the impairment depends on the duration of the activity and on the altitude at which the work is performed. Generally, the larger the involvement of aerobic processes, the greater the performance decrement at high altitudes.

Endurance Performance in High Altitudes

The diminished oxygen pressure at high altitudes adversely affects performance in events that involve aerobic metabolism. The relationship between distances run and performance decrement at altitudes of 7,340 ft. (2,238 m.) and 5,350 ft. (1,634 m.) are shown in Figure 6–18. Note that impairment occurs at 5,350 ft. when distances run are 1,500 m. and longer, whereas at an altitude of 7,340 ft., impairment occurs when distances run

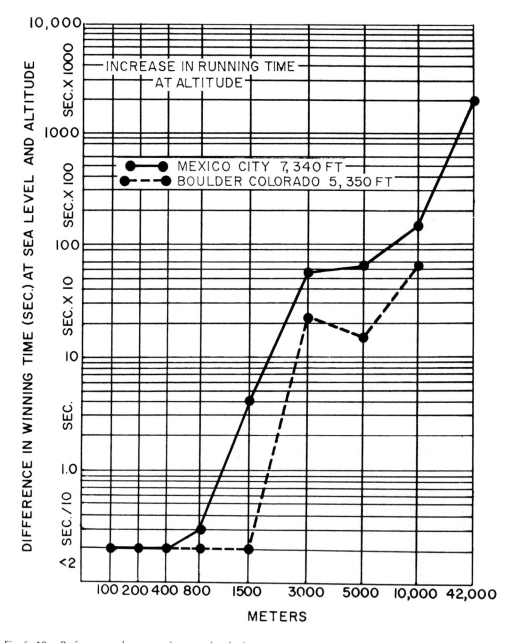

Fig. 6–18.   Performance decrement from sea level when running at various distances at altitudes of 7,340 ft. and 5,350 ft. Data are based on Olympic running times in Mexico City (7,340 ft.) and times in Boulder, Colorado (5,350 ft.) (From Jokl, E., and Jokl, P. (eds.): Exercise and Altitude. S. Karger AG, Basel, 1968.)

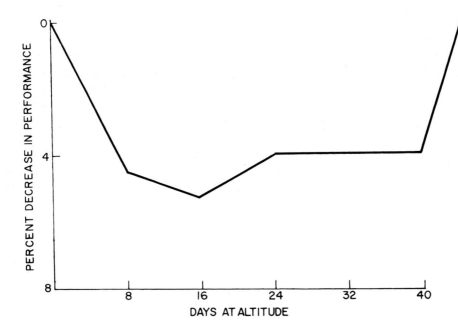
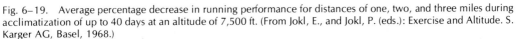

Fig. 6–19.   Average percentage decrease in running performance for distances of one, two, and three miles during acclimatization of up to 40 days at an altitude of 7,500 ft. (From Jokl, E., and Jokl, P. (eds.): Exercise and Altitude. S. Karger AG, Basel, 1968.)

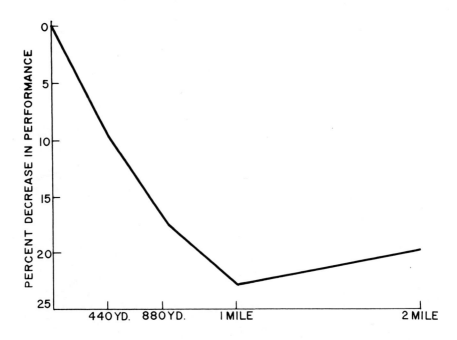

Fig. 6–20.   Percent decreases in performance from sea level after 40 to 57 days of acclimatization at 13,100 ft. (Data from Buskirk, E., et al.: Maximal performance at altitude and on return from altitude in conditioned runners. J. Appl. Physiol., 23:259, 1967.)

are 800 m. and longer. These results are based on athletes who trained at high altitudes before a competition and were largely acclimated to a lower PO_2 in the atmosphere. Similar decrements were found during a period of acclimatization when individuals ran for 1 mile (1,610 m.), 2 miles (3,220 m.), and 3 miles (4,830 m.) at an altitude of 7,500 ft. (2,287 m.). After 8, 16, 24, 32, and 40 days,[29] the decrements were averaged over the 3 distances and related to the days of acclimatization (Fig. 6–19). Performance dropped and then remained relatively constant at about 5 to 6% for the 40 days. At an extremely high altitude of 13,100 ft. (3,994 m.) and after 40 to 57 days of acclimatization, performance decreased even more than at lower altitudes (Fig. 6–20).[30] In fact, at distances of 1 mile and 2 miles, the decrements were about 23% and 18%, respectively.

Physiologic Basis for Performance Decrement at High Altitudes

The ability to perform in aerobic activities depends first on the availability of oxygen to the working muscles. Because PO_2 is lesser at high altitudes than at sea level and, consequently, less oxygen reaches the muscle in work, one can understand how performance is impaired. But, as altitude increases, the degree of aerobic impairment is not proportionate to the drop in PO_2. If it were, running times would be about 40% longer at 13,000 ft. (3,963 m.) than at sea level. However, the running times were about 20% longer (Fig. 6–21). Although the PO_2 reduces at a much greater rate than the loss in work capacity in aerobic metabolism, the actual amount of oxygen reaching the working muscles does not correspond to the proportionate drop in atmospheric PO_2. The reduction in PO_2 at the mitochondrial level of the tissue cells may only fall from 10 mm Hg to 5 mm Hg. The small drop in PO_2 at the cellular level is important because a PO_2 even slightly less than 5 mm Hg would not provide optimal conditions for the activity of oxidative enzymes in the cells. The physiologic responses occurring during work in high altitudes depend on the amount of previous exposure to low atmospheric PO_2. As a con-

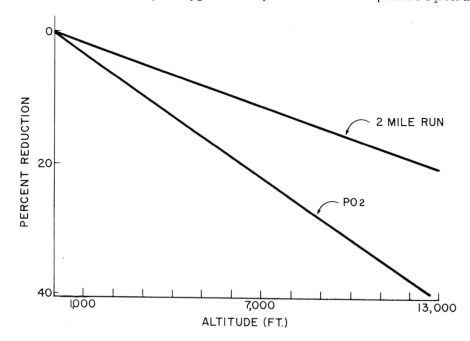

Fig. 6–21.   Percent reduction in PO_2 and performance in running two miles at altitudes ranging from sea level to 13,000 ft. (see Figs. 6–10 and 6–18).

sequence of frequent training at high altitudes, certain physiologic adaptations occur to improve working capacity at high altitudes. The process of adaptation is called acclimatization, and the adaptations are referred to as chronic effects of acclimatization. When an unacclimated individual is exposed to a high altitude, the physiologic effects of his work are referred to as acute effects because they are brought about by an acute exposure to high altitude.

Acute Exposure to High Altitudes and Work Capacity

The physiologic responses during work in high altitudes vary somewhat depending on the extent to which an individual has been previously exposed to lowered PO_2 (hypoxia). Nevertheless, these responses primarily maintain the proper PO_2 at the cellular level. The factors that keep a relatively constant PO_2 at the tissue level during an acute exposure to high altitude by an unacclimated individual are: (1) increased pulmonary ventilation, and (2) increased cardiac output.

Pulmonary ventilation is elevated at high altitudes and may exceed values at sea level for the same work level by 33% at 6,500 ft. (1,982 m.) and by 50% at 9,800 ft. (2,988 m.) (Fig. 6–22). The stimulus for increasing ventilation comes from the low arterial PO_2 in the blood plasma, which acts on the chemoreceptors in the aortic and carotid bodies.[30a] Afferent impulses are sent from the bodies to the respiratory region and, in turn, activate motor nerves to the respiratory muscles. The relaxation and contraction of these muscles are enhanced by the increased firing of impulses over the motor nerves.

Reduced air resistance found in the airway passages of the lungs in less dense, high altitudes also contributes to greater ventilation. Maximum ventilation is considerably greater at high altitudes than at sea level[31,32] and may rise from about 105 l./min. at sea level to 160 l./min. at 9,800 ft. (2,988 m.).[33]

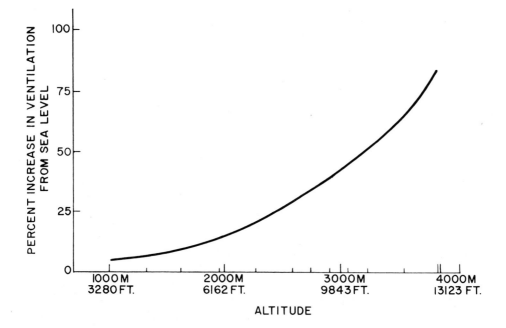

Fig. 6–22. Pulmonary ventilation at various altitudes while working at approximately 67% of maximum oxygen consumption at sea level. (Data from Åstrand, P.O.: The respiratory activity in man exposed to prolonged hypoxia. Acta Physiol. Scand., *30*:343, 1954.)

Increased cardiac output, another important factor in maintaining an adequate PO_2 at the cellular level when moving from sea level to high altitude, occurs even when working at the same relative work load.[34] Cardiac output is increased primarily because heart rate increases whereas stroke volume is not appreciably changed or may drop slightly. Although cardiac output increases at high altitudes, the greater flow of oxygenated blood may not be sufficient to compensate for the low atmospheric PO_2, especially as work intensity increases. But at low submaximal work, the increased cardiac output may provide sufficient oxygen to the muscle cells to permit sustained activity. In maximum work at high altitudes, however, oxygen uptake by the cells drops because cardiac output is maximum (as are heart rate and stroke volume). In fact $\dot{V}O_2$ max at a high altitude may only be 72% $\dot{V}O_2$ max at sea level even though cardiac output is maximum. The main reason for the difference in $\dot{V}O_2$ max is the lowered PO_2 in the capillary blood supplying the tissues when working at high altitude.[34a] Cardiac output, although maximum during maximum work in acute exposure to low PO_2, does not respond the same way once acclimatization has occurred. After acclimatization of several months at an altitude of 19,024 ft. (5,800 m.), cardiac output may be reduced by 30% compared to its value at sea level.[35]

Chronic Exposure to High Altitude and Work Capacity

The adaptations that occur from exposure to high altitudes during training are related to the amount of exposure. Short-term adaptations to acclimatization occur over a period of days, weeks, and months; long-term adaptations take years. The adaptations involve: (1) a sustained increase in pulmonary ventilation, (2) an adjustment in the pH level of blood and other fluids, (3) an improvement in the capacity of arterial blood to carry oxygen, and (4) a modification in cardiac output, especially during maximum work.

A chronic response to high altitude is a noticeable increase in pulmonary ventilation after only four weeks. This increase may exceed the value at sea level by 40 to 100%, depending on the amount of work being done.[2] Ventilation remains elevated in high altitudes because of the continued reflex action of the chemoreceptors in the aortic and carotid bodies, which are stimulated by low arterial PO_2. Pulmonary ventilation drops after several years of living at a high altitude, but remains higher than ventilation at sea level. After long-term acclimatization, pulmonary ventilation may be about 24% higher than at sea level in rest and about 12% higher than at sea level in exercise at 14,900 ft. (4,543 m.).[36]

With the elevation in pulmonary ventilation there is a reduction in PCO_2 in the alveolar air as the amount of carbon dioxide blown off is greater than the amount produced. In an acclimated individual living at 15,000 ft. (4,573 m.), alveolar PCO_2 may be maintained at about 28 mm Hg, or even less at higher altitudes, compared to the usual PCO_2 of 40 mm Hg at sea level. A lower plasma PCO_2 of 28 mm Hg does not inhibit ventilatory rate at sea level because of other adaptations of acclimatization. The H^+ ion concentration in the body fluids, which largely controls ventilation, is maintained at a normal level even though pulmonary ventilation is enhanced at high altitudes and tends to lower PCO_2 and H^+ ions. A normal level of H^+ ions is maintained after acclimatization, in spite of a low PCO_2, by the elimination of more bicarbonate (HCO_3^-) in the urine. The reduction in bicarbonate reduces blood alkalinity and, consequently, increases the acidity of the blood (lower pH level). The higher acidity continues to exert a stimulating effect on the respiratory centers in the brain stem.

Changes in the ability of arterial blood to carry more oxygen occur as a consequence of acclimatization. If the PO_2 in the atmosphere alone decided how much oxygen could be carried in arterial blood, there would be about 94% saturation of hemoglobin with oxygen at an altitude of 15,000 ft. (4,573 m.) and about 89% saturation at 20,000 ft. (6,098 m.). But, other factors increase arterial oxygen to a level similar to that found at sea level.[37] These additional factors are a result of acclimatization.

In long-term acclimatization, total hemoglobin increases.[38] As a result, oxygen content of arterial blood is approximately the same at 15,000 ft. (4,573m.) as at sea level before acclimatization.[30] The increase in the production of erythrocytes, or red cells, which may amount to 25% at an altitude of 14,900 ft. (4,543 m.) results in a corresponding increase in hemoglobin.[37] However, even though arterial blood may contain the same quantity of oxygen at high altitude as at sea level, less oxygen reaches the tissues at high altitudes. The reason for this is the decreased oxygen pressure gradient between blood and tissues at high altitude. Consequently, less oxygen moves from the hemoglobin to the tissue cells.

In the early stages of acclimatization, the response in cardiac output is similar to that obtained in acute exposure, i.e., cardiac output does not diminish at high altitudes during submaximal work or maximal work.[39] But, as acclimatization occurs, cardiac output decreases in maximal work. The main reason for less cardiac output after prolonged stays at high altitude seems to be reduced stroke volume,[35,40–42] but a reduced heart rate also contributes.[35,39,42,43] In fact, after only 10 days to 2 weeks at altitudes from 10,240 ft. (3,122 m.) to 14,038 ft. (4,280 m.), stroke volume reduces by as much as 20% during maximal work.[42] The physiologic basis for variations in cardiac output, stroke volume, and heart rate at different altitudes is not completely known. However, the reduction in heart rate is not believed to be a result of oxygen deficit at high altitudes.[44]

The physiologic adaptations, which are a result of acclimatization, minimize the adverse effects of low atmospheric PO_2 on the working tissues. The total effect of these adaptations is shown by the pressure gradient for oxygen at the mitochondrial or cellular level. As a result of acclimatization, the pressure gradient only drops from a PO_2 of 10 mm Hg at sea level to a PO_2 of 5 mm Hg at high altitude. In addition, adaptations take place at the cellular level that increase the utilization of oxygen by enzymatic changes.[45] Also, there is evidence that more capillaries are formed within muscle tissue as a response to work in high altitudes.[46,47] Consequently, the distance between the capillaries and the muscle fibers reduces, thereby expediting more blood flow.

Training at High Altitude and Performance at Sea Level

The stress placed on the working muscles and the cardiovascular-respiratory systems in work at high altitude is similar in some ways to the stress encountered while training at sea level. Both involve, in varying degrees, an oxygen deficit or hypoxia. The training effects at both sea level and high altitude indicate that the same organic systems are involved. Training at all altitudes results in increases in hemoglobin, red-blood-cell count, total blood volume, and mitochondria, and in improved changes in cellular enzymes. As a result, maximum oxygen uptake is also improved. The added stress of hypoxia in training, which is afforded by training at high altitude, may add significantly to the training effect encountered at sea level. This possibility has been examined in several studies, but with contradictory results.[48–50] When nonathletes were trained at altitudes of 7,400 ft. (2,256 m.) to 11,300 ft. (3,445 m.) in one study[50] and at an altitude of 7,500 ft. (2,287 m.) in another study,[51] performances improved significantly at sea level when oxygen consumption was the criterion in the first study and running times in 880-yd (805 m.), 1-mile (1,610 m.), and 2-mile (3,220 m.) runs were the criteria in the second study. However, after the third and fifteenth days after a return to sea level from altitude, performance in the 1- and 2-mile runs was poorer.[51] Another study involved athletes training at

7,500 ft. (2,286 m.) and their subsequent performances 35 to 42 days after returning to sea level. No appreciable improvement occurred in running 1 (1,610 m.), 2 (3,220 m.) or 3 miles (4,830 m.)[52] at sea level.

The reasons for these conflicting results can only be speculated. In the two studies where nonathletes improved performance at sea level after training at high altitudes,[50,51] it is possible that the same improvements, or greater, could have been achieved if training were at sea level. In the case of the studies using athletes[30,52] who either did not improve or had a performance decrement after training at high altitudes, the inability to reach a maximal stroke volume and/or to train at the same intensity in high altitudes may have had a deleterious effect on oxygen consumption and performance. Whatever the reasons, they should not obviate the need to train at high altitudes, especially when preparing for a future sport event in a high altitude.

Because complete acclimatization takes years to accomplish and still does not allow the same work capacity as at sea level, it is difficult to determine exactly now many days are necessary to achieve acclimatization in preparation for an impending athletic event. Nevertheless, events held in altitudes above 5,000 ft. (1,524 m.) and requiring more than 2 to 3 min. of continuous work should be prepared for by training at the specific altitude at which the contest will be held. The number of days needed to achieve acclimatization depends on the altitude. Generally, most of the immediate physiologic adaptations of acclimatization to altitudes of 15,000 ft. (4,573 m.) and below occur in 21 days. Fewer days may be sufficient to acclimatize at lower altitudes. For competition at 10,000 ft. (3,049 m.), 7 to 10 days may be sufficient. There is no indication that better trained individuals require less time to acclimate than do others.[53] Consequently, the benefits of acclimatization should be similar for all individuals provided the days of training and the relative intensity of workouts are approximately the same.

OXYGEN SUPPLEMENTS AND PERFORMANCE

If a decrease in the PO_2 at high altitudes is associated with a decrement in performance in events involving primarily aerobic metabolism, one may logically assume that an increase of PO_2 in the inspired air would improve aerobic endurance. With increased oxygen pressure in the alveoli, more oxygen would be absorbed by the blood and greater amounts would be made available to the working muscles. But, whether or not higher oxygen saturation of the blood results in increased utilization of oxygen at the cellular level to such an extent that aerobic endurance is improved depends on when the increased PO_2 is administered. Oxygen administered before work affects endurance differently than does oxygen administered during work. Studies have been performed to determine the effects of increased inspired oxygen on work and also on recovery from work. In these studies, oxygen to the lungs was enhanced by either inhaling more oxygen at normal atmospheric pressure, breathing normal amounts of oxygen but under greater atmospheric pressure, or using hyperoxygenated air under high pressure.

Oxygen Administration Before Exercise

When oxygen is administered before exercise, performance appears to improve slightly. Several research studies have shown that, when oxygen is inhaled just before work, the ability to run 250 yd. (229 m.) and 880 yd. (805 m.) is enhanced.[54] When work involves holding the breath, improvement occurs in running short distances[55] and in running in place.[55] However, unless oxygen is administered for 1 to 2 min. or less before exercise, little advantage, if any, is achieved.[55] In most athletic events, it is not possible to breathe excess amounts of oxygen just before competition. Consequently, any benefits from oxygen inhalation are negligible.

Oxygen Administration During Exercise

Increasing the availability of oxygen at the cellular level during exercise by increasing alveolar PO$_2$ above that found at sea level permits more work to be done.[56,56a] The improvement in work capacity as a consequence of greater PO$_2$ is reflected in other physiologic responses, such as oxygen consumption, pulmonary ventilation, and lactate. Increases in oxygen consumption[57,58] and decreases in ventilation[57,58] and lactate[59,60] have resulted with greater alveolar PO$_2$. The reason for better work performance is primarily larger quantities of oxygen absorbed by the entire musculature. This increase is shown when the same amount of work is performed at sea level and at conditions with higher PO$_2$. Under higher PO$_2$, the muscles of the limbs and respiration can function more aerobically and can perform with less stress on the heart and circulatory system. For the same reason, more aerobic work can be done when the PO$_2$ is increased during work. However, the application of this information is limited for improving performance in sports. The impracticability of administering oxygen during a long run or during a game of football is obvious. Even if it were possible, the sanctioning organizations in athletic sports would not approve such a procedure.

Oxygen During Work Recovery

Breathing air that contains a PO$_2$ higher than that at sea level is common among some athletes, especially professional football players. But, a more rapid recovery as a consequence is questionable. Studies show that no differences are evident in heart rate[61-63] or oxygen debt[61,64] following the administration of oxygen after exercise. Apparently, the large reduction in metabolism after exercise compared to the large intake of oxygen in recovery under the usual atmospheric conditions encountered in sport competition provides a situation that encourages optimal, or near optimal, quantities of oxygen to be absorbed by the worked muscles. Perhaps future research will add more information supporting the use of oxygen supplements during recovery; however, the available evidence provides little support for this practice.

PRINCIPLES FOR TRAINING

1. Cigarette smoking increases the amount of oxygen needed by the respiratory muscles to maintain pulmonary ventilation during exercise.[16-18] Smoking has varying effects on oxygen cost of breathing during exercise, depending on how soon before exercise it occurs. Smoking one cigarette immediately before exercise can result in a two- to three-fold increase in airway resistance. Even when a chronic smoker abstains for 24 hours before a race, the cost of ventilation may be 50% higher than that of nonsmokers. In activities of a continuous nature, such as running or cycling for five minutes or more, or when movement is less sustained at a given rate but more sporadic and prolonged, such as in soccer and basketball, smoking may have deleterious effects on the endurance aspects of performance.

2. When preparing to race for 2 to 3 min. or longer at altitudes above 5,000 ft. (1,524 m.), training should also take place at an altitude above 5,000 ft. The length of training to achieve most of the acclimatization depends on the altitude. Generally, training for 7 to 10 days at 10,000 ft. (3,049 m.) and 21 days at 15,000 ft. (4,573 m.),[29] is sufficient. However, performance will still be poorer than at sea level.

3. Training at high altitudes of 7,500 ft. (2,287 m.) to 13,000 ft. (3,963 m.) may not improve endurance performances at sea level among conditioned individuals at running distances of 440 yd., 880 yd., 1 mile, 2 miles, or 3 miles.[30,52] Although nonathletes show improvement at sea level after training at high altitudes,[50,51] it is not known how much of the training effects, if any, are the result of high altitude and how much are caused by work stress alone.

4. The administration of extra amounts of

oxygen (increased PO$_2$) 1 to 2 min. before exercise enhances performance in races lasting about 1 to 3 min.[54,55] Although aerobic endurance is also enhanced by breathing more oxygen while exercising,[56,56a] such a procedure is not practical in athletic competition. Increased oxygen breathing apparently does little to improve recovery rate.[56a,61–63]

REFERENCES

1. Campbell, E.J.M.: An electromyographic study of the role of the abdominal muscles in breathing. J. Physiol., *117:*222, 1952.
2. Åstrand, P.O., and Rodahl, K.: Textbook of Work Physiology. New York, McGraw-Hill Book Co., 1977.
3. Åstrand, P.O.: Experimental studies of physical working capacity in relation to sex and age. Copenhagen, E. Munksgard, 1952.
4. Lyons, H.A., and Tanner, R.W.: Total lung volume and its subdivisions in children: normal standards. J. Appl. Physiol., *17:*601, 1962.
5. Robinson, S.: Experimental studies of physical fitness in relation to age. Arbeitsphysiol., *10:*251, 1938.
6. Åstrand, I.: Aerobic work capacity in men and women with special reference to age. Acta Physiol. Scand., *49:*169, 1960.
7. Milic-Emili, G., Petit, J.M., and Deroanne, R.: The effects of respiratory rate on the mechanical work of breathing during muscular exercise. Int. Z. Angewandte Physiol. einschliesslich Arbeitsphysiol., *18:*330, 1960.
8. Milic-Emili, G., and Petit, J.M.: Mechanical efficiency of breathing. J. Appl. Physiol., *15:*359, 1960.
9. Shephard, R.J., and Bar-Or, O.: Alveolar ventilation in near-maximum exercise. Med. Sci. Sports, *2:*83, 1970.
10. Bachman, J.C., and Horvath, S.M.: Pulmonary function changes which accompany athletic conditioning programs. Res. Q., *39:*235, 1968.
11. Saltin, B., and Åstrand, P.O.: Maximal oxygen uptake in athletes. J. Appl. Physiol., *23:*353, 1967.
12. Nocker, J., and Bohlau, V.: Abhangigkeit der leistungsfahigkeit vom alter und geschlecht. Münchener Medizinische Wochenschrift, *97:*1517, 1955.
13. Norris, A.H., et al.: Pulmonary function studies: age differences in lung volume and bellows function. J. Gerontol., *11:*379, 1956.
14. Rizzato, G., and Marazzini, L.: Thoracoabdominal mechanics in elderly men. J. Appl. Physiol., *28:*457, 1970.
15. Turner, J.M., Mead, J., and Wohl, M.E.: Elasticity of human lungs in relation to age. J. Appl. Physiol., *25:*664, 1968.
15a. Burger, M.: Zur pathophysiologie der geschlechter. Münchener Medizinischer Wochenschrift., *97:*981, 1955.
15b. MacNab, R.B.J., Conger, P.R., and Taylor, P.S.: Differences in maximal and submaximal work capacity in men and women. J. Appl. Physiol., *27:*644, 1969.
15c. Cumming, D.: Correlation of athletic performance with pulmonary function in 13 to 17 year old boys and girls. Med. Sci. Sports. *1:*140, 1969.
15d. Wilmore, J.H., and Sigerseth, P.O.: Physical work capacity of young girls, 7 to 13 years of age. J. Appl. Physiol., *22:*923, 1967.
16. Comroe, J.J., Jr.: The lung. Sci. Am., *214*(2):56, 1966.
17. Rode, A., and Shepard, R.: The influence of cigarette smoking upon the oxygen cost of breathing in near-maximal exercise. Med. Sci. Sports, *3:*51, 1971.
18. Shephard, R.J.: The oxygen cost of breathing during vigorous exercise. Q. J. Exp. Physiol., *51:* 336, 1966.
19. Holmgren, A., and Åstrand, C.O.: DL and the dimensions and functional capacity of the O$_2$ transport system on humans. J. Appl. Physiol., *21:*1463, 1966.
20. Kaufmann, D., et al.: Pulmonary function of marathon runners. Med. Sci. Sports, *6:*114, 1974.
21. Maksud, M., et al.: Pulmonary function measurements of Olympic speed skaters from the U. S. Med. Sci. Sports, *3:*66, 1971.
22. Newman, F., Smalley, B.F., and Thomson, J.L.: Effect of exercise, body and lung size on CO diffusion in athletes and non-athletes. J. Appl. Physiol., *17:*649, 1962.
23. Bannister, R.G., et al.: Pulmonary diffusing capacity on exercise in athletes and non-athletic subjects. J. Physiol., *152:*66, 1960.
24. Reddan, W., et al.: Pulmonary function in endurance athletes. Fed. Proc., *22:*396, 1963.
25. Reuschlein, P., et al.: Effect of physical training on the pulmonary diffusing capacity during submaximal work. J. Appl. Physiol., *24:*152, 1968.
26. Saltin, B., et al.: Response to submaximal and maximal exercise after bedrest and training. Circulation [Suppl. 7], *38:*1, 1968.
27. Bretschneider, H.J.: Oxygen requirement and supply of the myocardium. Verh. Dtsch. Ges. Kreislaufforsch., *27:*32, 1961.
28. Lambertsen, C.J.: Interactions of physical, chemical, and nervous factors in respiratory control. *In* Medical Physiology. 12th Edition. Vol. I. Edited by V. B. Mountcastle. St. Louis, The C. V. Mosby Co., 1968.
29. Jokl, E., and Jokl, P. (eds.): Exercise and Altitude. New York, S. Karger, 1968.
30. Buskirk, E., et al.: Maximal performance at altitude and on return from altitude in conditioned runners. J. Appl. Physiol., *23:*259, 1967.
30a. Heymans, J.F., and Heymans, C.: Sur les modifications directes et sur la regulation reflexe de l'activite du centre respiratoire de la tete isolee du chien. Arch. Internat. Pharmacodyn. Therap., *33:*272, 1927.
31. Miles, S.: The effect of changes in barometric pressure on maximum breathing capacity. J. Physiol., *137:*85, 1957.
32. Ulvedal, F., et al.: Ventilatory capacity during pro-

longed exposure to simulated altitude without hypoxia. J. Appl. Physiol., *18:*904, 1963.

33. Åstrand, P.O.: The respiratory activity in man exposed to prolonged hypoxia. Acta Physiol. Scand., *30:*343, 1954.

34. Steinberg, J., Ekblom, B., and Messin, R.: Hemodynamic response to work at simulated altitude. J. Appl. Physiol., *21:*1589, 1966.

34a. Rahn, H.: Introduction to the study of man at high altitudes: conductance of O_2 from the environment to the tissues. *In* Life at High Altitudes. Scientific Publ. 140, Pan-American Health Organization, WHO, Washington, D.C., September, 1966.

35. Pugh, L.G., et al.: Muscular exercise at great altitudes. J. Appl. Physiol., *19:*431, 1964.

36. Pugh, L.G.C.E.: Physiological and medical aspects of the Himalayan scientific and mountaineering expedition, 1960–61. Br. Med. J., *2:*621, 1962.

37. Hurtado, A., et al.: Mechanisms of natural acclimatization. Studies on the native resident of Morococha, Peru, at an altitude of 14,900 feet. Technical Documentary Report No. Sam-TDR-56-1, Washington, D.C., 1956, USAF School of Aerospace Medicine.

38. Surks, M.I., Chinn, K.S., and Matoush, L.O.: Alterations in body composition in man after acute exposure to high altitude. J. Appl. Physiol., *21:*1741, 1966.

39. Åstrand, P.O., and Åstrand, I.: Heart rate during muscular work in man exposed to prolonged hypoxia. J. Appl. Physiol., *13:*75, 1958.

40. Alexander, J.K., et al.: Reduction of stroke volume during exercise in man following ascent to 3,100 m. altitude. J. Appl. Physiol., *23:*849, 1967.

41. Hartley, L.H., et al.: Subnormal cardiac output at rest and during exercise in residents at 3,100 m. altitude. J. Appl. Physiol., *23:*839, 1967.

42. Saltin, B., et al.: Maximal oxygen uptake and cardiac output after two weeks at 4,300 meters. J. Appl. Physiol., *25:*400, 1968.

43. Vogel, J.G., Hansen, J.E., and Harris, C.W.: Cardiovascular responses in man during exhaustive work at sea level and high altitude. J. Appl. Physiol., *23:*531, 1967.

44. Blomqvist, G., and Stenberg, J.: The ECG response to submaximal and maximal exercise during acute hypoxia. *In* The Frank Lead Exercise Electrocardiogram. Edited by G. Blomqvist. Acta Med. Scand., *178* [Suppl. 440]:82, 1965.

45. Barbashova, J.I.: Cellular level of adaptation. *In* Handbook of Physiology, Adaptation to the Environment. Edited by D. B. Dill. Washington, D.C., American Physiological Society, 1964.

46. Cassin, S., Gilbert, R.D., Johnson, E.M.: Capillary development during exposure to chronic hypoxia. Report SAM-TR-66-16, USAF School of Aviation Medicine, Randolph Field, Tex., 1966.

47. Vannotti, A.: The adaptation of the cell to effort, altitude and to pathological oxygen deficiency. Schweiz. Med. Wochenschr., *76:*899, 1946.

48. Consolazio, C.F.: Submaximal and maximal performance at high altitude. *In* The International Symposium on the Effects of Altitude on Physical Performance. Edited by R. F. Goddard. Chicago, The Athletic Institute, 1967.

49. Grover, R.F., and Reeves, J.T.: Exercise performance of athletes at sea level and 3,100 meters altitude. *In* The International Symposium on the Effects of Altitude on Physical Performance. Edited by R. F. Goddard. Chicago, The Athletic Institute, 1967.

50. Roskamm, H., et al.: Effects of a standardized ergometer training program at three different altitudes. J. Appl. Physiol., *27:*840, 1969.

51. Faulkner, J., Daniels, J., and Balke, B.: Effects of training at moderate altitude on physical performance capacity. J. Appl. Physiol., *23:*85, 1967.

52. Faulkner, J., et al.: Maximum aerobic capacity and running performance at altitude. J. Appl. Physiol., *24:*685, 1968.

53. Billings, C.: Cost of submaximal and maximal work during chronic exposure at 3,800 m. J. Appl. Physiol., *30:*406, 1971.

54. Hill, L., and MacKenzie, J.: The influence of oxygen on athletes. J. Physiol., *38:*28, 1909.

55. Karpovich, P.V.: The effect of oxygen inhalation on swimming performance. Res. Q., *5:*24, 1934.

56. Bannister, R.G., and Cunningham, D.J.C.: The effects on the respiration and performance during exercise of adding oxygen to the inspired air. J. Physiol., *125:*118, 1954.

56a. Cunningham, D.A.: Effects of breathing high concentrations of oxygen on treadmill performance. Res. Q., *37:*491, 1966.

57. Welch, H.G., et al.: Effects of breathing O_2 enriched gas mixtures on metabolic rate during exercise. Med. Sci. Sports, *6:*26, 1974.

58. Wilson, G.D., and Welch, L.G.H.: Effects of hyperoxic gas mixtures on exercise tolerance in man. Med. Sci. Sports, *7:*48, 1975.

59. Hickam, J.B., et al.: Respiratory regulation during exercise in unconditioned subjects. J. Clin. Invest., *30:*503, 1951.

60. Hughes, R.L., et al.: Effect of inspired O_2 on cardiopulmonary and metabolic responses to exercise in man. J. Appl. Physiol., *24:*336, 1968.

61. Bjorgum, R.K., and Sharkey, B.J.: Inhalation of oxygen as an aid to recovery after exertion. Res. Q., *37:*462, 1966.

62. Hagerman, F.C., et al.: The effects of breathing 100 percent oxygen during rest, heavy work, and recovery. Res. Q., *39:*965, 1968.

63. Miller, A.T.: The influence of oxygen administration on cardiovascular function during exercise and recovery. J. Appl. Physiol., *5:*165, 1952.

64. Elbel, E.R., Ormond, D., and Close, D.: Some effect of breathing O_2 before and after exercise. J. Appl. Physiol., *16:*48, 1961.

Assessment of Physical Performances as Expressions of Physiologic Functions

CHAPTER 7

Previous chapters were concerned with physiologic function and the structural changes of various tissues and organ systems as a result of exercise and work. Organ and systemic functions were presented at various levels of rest and work. When these functions are viewed from another perspective, such as physical performance and its component parts, all the physiologic mechanisms activated in exercise become of interest as they interact with each other. The nature of the performance and the varying stresses placed on the organs determine where the training effects occur. For example, in an exercise such as long-distance running, the specific component of physical performance primarily stressed and the component that provides an explanation for success or failure in the run is cardiovascular endurance. Another activity, such as weight lifting, involves primarily the performance component of muscle strength. Again, the level of performance depends largely on the functional capacity of the tissues involved. In this case, the ability to perform is determined by the force capacity of skeletal muscle tissue. These two activities place the greatest stress on different systems or tissue, but they both obviously involve the same physiologic mechanisms. Muscle force is needed to run, and cardiovascular function is needed to lift weights.

This chapter views physical performance as involving the interacting effects of all the physiologic mechanisms presented in previous chapters. First, the reader focuses on the uniqueness of a particular physical performance and, second, on the physiologic mechanisms involved in that activity. To understand more precisely the relationship between the two, the reader must know the component parts or aspects making up all possible physical performances. Some of these components are muscle strength, muscle power, and muscular and cardiovascular endurance. When a component can be defined in a "pure" sense, with as little overlapping of other components as possible, the physiologic systems and tissues directly associated with the component can be better understood from an exercise or work point of view. Often in sports or industry, where individuals are assessed on physical performance to either establish norms, evaluate work capacity, or screen athletes or job applicants, the criterion is actual job performance. On occasion, in sports and especially in industry, actual job performance cannot be assessed. If 200 sport candidates or prospective employees must be screened, a problem obviously exists because of the administrative difficulty in testing large groups of people on the criterion of actual job performance. To solve this problem, testing personnel use alternate tasks that can be more easily administered to large numbers of people. But, each test must measure one or more of the components considered important for performing the job successfully. If it does not, the test is invalid. The relationship between the physical components required in the job and the physiologic systems evoked by each component should be known. Thus, a test that stresses the same physiologic systems with the same intensity as do the actual job tasks is valid for screening purposes. This is one example of how knowledge of the relationship between physical performance and the physiologic mechanisms involved may be applied.

COMPONENTS OF PHYSICAL PERFORMANCE

The components of physical performance can be observed in a variety of different activities, both in sports and in occupations. All the movements of man that involve relatively large muscle mass and require an expenditure of energy significantly greater than that expended at rest can be expressed by descriptive action verbs, such as running, jumping, throwing, lifting, pushing, pulling, and carrying. An additional term is used when the duration of performance is a concern. This term is endurance, and it reflects physiologic fatigue. The ability to perform movements of high repetitions over a prolonged time period largely depends on endurance. The following section isolates the various performance components by offering a model based on empiric data and research.

Identifying the Components of Physical Performance

Numerous research studies have been done to ascertain the components comprising physical performance. Most of these studies have identified the same or similar components, although the terms selected to describe these components are not always the same. One component considered essential for evaluating performance is strength because it is required to some degree by

every movement. Research studies have dissected strength into subcomponents; each component is unique in terms of primary physical expression. Some of the terms used to describe the different kinds of strength are explosive, power, dynamic, and static strength. Each kind of strength is expressed differently in physical performance. Other components identified in research studies as essential in physical performances are flexibility, agility, speed, balance, coordination, and endurance. Each of these has been further dissected in attempts to identify its subcomponents. Researchers use a statistical technique to decide which components are basic to physical performance. Such a technique involves correlational test data. Generally, test scores relate to each other because they have something in common. The quality that makes them common is called a factor in statistical terminology and a component in performance parlance. The same statistical technique is used to further examine each component and to determine whether additional delineation can add to the understanding of a component.

STRENGTH. The subcomponents of strength are examined separately. They all are related to each other because the force capacity of muscle in slow movements is indicative (not perfectly) of force in quick movements, whether body weight alone or an external object is moved.

Explosive strength or power is seen in quick movements when body weight is propelled either upward or forward. It is characterized by one short burst of energy and is seen in such tests as the standing long jump, vertical jump, and short runs. Other power expressions are shown in activities that apply an explosive force to an external object even though the quick movement of a large or small segment of body mass can be associated with the move. Such tests as shot put and medicine-ball throw are examples of this kind of strength. When a heavy shot is putted by moving the entire body several feet forward just prior to the release of the shot, the distance putted depends on two "power abilities." The first occurs in the rapid movement of body mass, and the second occurs in the application of an explosive force to the shot.

Another form of strength is observed when a force is applied to an external object that does not move appreciably as a result. An isometric contraction is usually involved in this kind of test. A good score does not depend on the explosiveness of muscles, but on maximum force capacity. The measurement of strength in this way is called static strength. A similar expression of strength occurs when the muscles exert maximum force to an external object that moves. But, this kind of strength differs from static strength because the muscles contract concentrically rather than isometrically and because a score is the amount of weight lifted one time rather than the amount of force applied to an immovable object. The term given to identify this kind of strength is dynamic strength. The word dynamic denotes movement.

When only body weight is lifted repeatedly, but with significant difficulty for each repetition, strength is measured by number of repetitions. The strength component is only involved if muscle force is relatively high for each movement. Exercises that elicit this kind of strength are chinning, dipping on parallel bars, push-ups, and rope climbing. Activities such as side-straddle-hop and toe touch do not fall into this category because their performance does not require much muscle force for each repetition.

FLEXIBILITY. The ability to move the trunk and limbs throughout a range of motion is associated with large muscle movement and performance capacity. This ability is termed flexibility, and it is concerned with stretching of the muscles and tissues around skeletal joints. There are basically two kinds of flexibility: one involves a substantial amount of movement, and the other involves only a minimum amount of movement.[1] Certain skills in gymnastics and in swimming require the limbs to move rapidly

and through a large range of movement. This kind of flexibility is called dynamic flexibility because the movement itself is an essential aspect. At other times, muscles may contract isometrically to maintain a certain bodily posture, such as during leg splits or certain stationary stunts in gymnastics. Although concentric contractions place the limbs in the desired, stretched positions, the actual range of motion maintained depends on the stretch capacity of the tissues and on the isometric forces acting on the concerned joints. Flexibility involving these characteristics is referred to as static flexibility.

SPEED. Moving quickly is a basic requirement for achieving success in many sports. A successful sprinter or offensive back requires quick movements of the legs. But, qualities other than speed are associated with these particular movements. Coordination of limb movements of the upper body, lower body, and trunk are essential. Running speed and body control cannot reach full fruition without good coordination. Speed, as a component of physical performance, has been difficult to isolate in research because of its relationship to other qualities of performance, such as strength, agility, coordination, and endurance. In the laboratory, speed of the limbs can be measured with high accuracy. The scores are less likely to become contaminated with other qualities than are the running times in the 40-yd. dash. But, even in the laboratory, speed of the upper limbs is not a good indicator of leg speed or vice versa. This fact adds to the difficulty in measuring speed per se by field tests of running and agility.

AGILITY. Some of the problems with speed measurement have also been encountered with agility. The strong emphasis of speed in this component has led some researchers to name agility "speed-of-change-of-direction." Certainly, the ability to move quickly from one point to another while stopping abruptly along the way or skirting around objects requires speed. But, when the agility qualities of dodging, and stopping and starting quickly are added to speed, such as in the tests of shuttle run and dodge run, separation of the two components becomes difficult. Another term frequently used in place of agility to describe the qualities required to move quickly between objects is "coordination." Although coordination is involved in agility, it does not emphasize, in common usage of the term, the component of speed. In addition, coordination in performance is more difficult than agility or speed to identify from field tests of physical prowess.

BALANCE. The body must be balanced to walk a tight rope or to maintain a handstand. But, these two activities require different kinds of balance. In one, an individual is constantly moving to cover a prescribed distance. The other performance is done in the same place, and movement is minimal. When moving the entire body from one point to another on a base of support that is relatively small, as in walking a tight rope or balance beam, the balance required is called dynamic balance. If the body is required to assume a fixed position of equilibrium, the balance required is static balance. These two forms of balance are only slightly related. However, they both measure qualities that are different from those measured by agility and speed tests. Although running quickly between objects certainly requires some qualities of dynamic balance, balance has not been statistically isolated as an important factor in agility or speed performances.[2] As a result, balance alone is not a predictor of physical fitness or physical performance.

ENDURANCE. The ability to endure muscular work is a universally accepted component of physical performance. In practice, most physical fitness tests include a distance run to measure aerobic capacity and a test (usually sit-ups) to measure muscular endurance. Some test items measure varying degrees of muscular endurance, such as chinning and push-ups. But, these tests are usually selected to assess strength. Even when sit-ups is a test item and an individual cannot do more than about 20 repetitions, the component mostly stressed is strength. Nevertheless, there is a common agreement that both muscular endurance and aerobic endurance are important components of performance.

The various components presented were gleaned from the research literature.[2-4] Actually, each component has been investigated in more detail than is implied by this discussion. Researchers do not agree as to which components are involved in all the physical performances common to sports, physical fitness testing, and heavy industrial occupations. The interacting functions of physiologic systems contribute to this difficulty. For example, the vestibular apparatus is largely concerned with maintaining balance of the limbs and is greatly involved in agility and balance tests. However, when its functions are joined to muscle force, the proprioceptors, and all the other physiologic functions that come into play, its ability to accomplish balance cannot be clearly discerned. Because the body functions as a whole, the researcher can identify components only by determining which physiologic mechanisms are primarily involved in performing a task. When ability depends mostly on muscle force, the component of primary concern is strength. If performance in running long distances depends mainly on the efficiency with which oxygen is delivered to, and utilized by, the working muscles, the primary component involved is aerobic endurance. A model using this approach has been developed to identify the components of physical performance.

MODEL OF PHYSICAL PERFORMANCE

All human movement, which takes a variety of forms, involves at one time or another one or more of the components just discussed. Specific intensities of muscle contractions that often involve varying amounts of muscle mass are associated with each component. An arm exercise in weight training, for example, involves contractions of high force. In an activity such as jogging, the leg and hip muscles contract with considerably less force. These activities also differ in the amount of muscle mass used and in the duration of contractions. Ten repetitions of a weight-training lift take about 20 to 25 sec. to complete, whereas jogging can continue for minutes on end. Weight training is obviously an activity that involves the component of absolute strength whereas jogging involves the component of aerobic endurance. In addition, each component elicits its own specific physiologic functions. With this in mind, a model of physical performance is presented that unites, in a logical manner, such expressions of human movement as muscle force, duration, and muscle mass, with the physiologic systems that are evoked by these responses. The model is presented in schematic fashion in Figure 7–1.

Practically all human movement can be explained by, and identified within, this model. The approach taken in developing the model began with the intensity of contraction. An activity with high muscle force, represented on the left in Figure 7–1, involves primarily either strength, if movement is relatively slow, or power, if speed is high. If strength is involved, the high force of muscle contraction comes either from lifting a heavy external load, such as a barbell, or from lifting body weight. Strength used to lift a maximum external load is considered absolute strength. The strength used to lift body weight, for less than 25 repetitions using maximum effort, is relative strength. In a fast, explosive movement in which power is evident, a muscle contracts rapidly when either moving an external load or moving body weight. If moving an external load, the component is called absolute power; if moving body weight, the component is called relative power.

The rationale for dividing strength and power into components that are designated as absolute and relative was supported by Fleishman.[2] The ability to move a heavy external load (absolute strength) or a lighter external load with acceleration (absolute power) is not indicative of the ability to move body weight repetitively (relative strength) or quickly (relative power). In fact, young adult males with higher-than-average absolute strength and power often have lower-than-average relative strength and power (see Fig. 1–25).[2]

Low muscle forces in human movement during maximum performance is associated with endurance. The right side of Figure 7–1 contains the breakdown emanating from low muscle force. The kind of endurance,

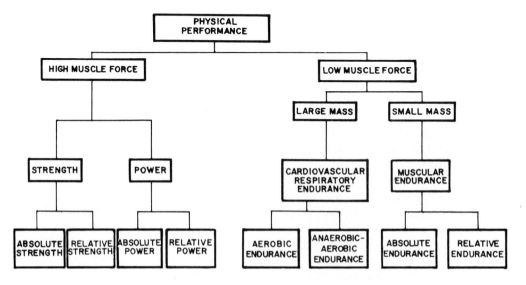

Fig. 7–1.   A model of physical performance.

whether cardiovascular or muscular, depends on the amount of muscle mass involved in an activity. When a relatively large mass is represented, the limitations in performance lie largely within the cardiovascular system. On the other hand, when small muscle mass is contracting and work is maximum, the ensuing high repetitions are a result of factors residing primarily within the muscle itself. In this case, muscular endurance is evident.

Work stressing the cardiovascular system, brought about by activity of large muscle mass, may elicit primarily either aerobic metabolism or anaerobic metabolism. When aerobic metabolism is elicited, the intensity of muscle contractions is relatively small. However, when the contractions are so intense that blood flow is greatly impeded, anaerobic metabolism may dominate. The balance between aerobic and anaerobic metabolism as the two main sources for the formation of ATP was shown in Table 2–3. Note how work intensity, indicated by running times, is related to this balance. To identify cardiovascular endurance in terms of the involvement of aerobic metabolism, one must consider two different performance components. These components are aerobic endurance and anaerobic-aerobic endurance. Activities that stress the cardiovascular system for three minutes or longer in maximum work are expressions of the aerobic component. Activities of less than three minutes and closer to two minutes manifest the anaerobic-aerobic component.

The extreme right of Figure 7–1 depicts the factor of muscular endurance. This factor involves work done with relatively small muscle mass for more than 25 repetitions. In human movement, muscular endurance is elicited in basically two ways: by work done with an external load and by work done using body weight as the load. In either way, the muscles may be stressed similarly. Two components were chosen to describe muscular endurance under the two load conditions. Work with an external load expresses

absolute muscular endurance. But, when body weight is the load, relative muscular endurance is manifested. The division of muscular endurance into two separate components provides a more logical basis for measuring this quality in physical performance. This will be made clearer in the section on assessing physical performance.

The eight basic components of physical performance are defined in Table 7–1. The physiologic mechanisms primarily activated when these components are involved in a performance follow.

PHYSIOLOGIC MECHANISMS EVOKED BY THE PHYSICAL PERFORMANCE COMPONENTS

In a particular sport or occupation, there may be primarily only one component involved or there may be many components operating in some kind of sequence. Some sports, such as football, involve a variety of tasks when an athlete must push against heavy opponents, run around them, or run over them. Each task requires a different component. In such sports as track or swimming, performance is limited to fewer components, such as aerobic and anaerobic endurance. But, regardless of the sport and the particular components it requires, the physiologic mechanisms associated with the activity operate as a team. Although muscle force is involved largely in tackling an opponent in football, the heart and circulation must also work to provide the muscles with oxygenated blood. At the same time, the lungs are discarding carbon dioxide and taking in oxygen. Related to these functions is the autonomic nervous system, which coordinates many of the physiologic activities. Other physiologic systems and organs are equally supportive of the task of tackling and thereby add to the complexity of the teamwork. The physical stress may be on the heart and circulation at one moment; at other moments, stress may be on muscular endurance; and, at other times, the stress may fall on muscle force. But, wherever physiologic stress is found, the physical per-

Table 7–1.

Physical Performance Components: Their Definitions and Measurements

Component	Operational Definition	Measurement
Absolute strength	Strength in moving a heavy object other than body weight or applying force to an immovable object.	Maximum force applied to an external object, such as a barbell, in movement (concentric contraction) or a dynamometer (isometric contraction).
Relative strength	Strength in moving body weight or strength per pound of body weight.	Chins, dips, push-ups, rope climb, or any measure where maximum number of repetitions with body weight is less than about 25.
Absolute power	Strength or force in moving an external weight quickly and explosively.	Medicine ball put, lifting an external load rapidly, and leg power test are examples.
Relative power	Strength or force in moving body weight quickly and explosively. (Sometimes referred to as speed when running in one direction, or agility and coordination when running around obstacles.)	Standing broad jump, vertical jump, shuttle run, dodge run, 50-yd. dash, softball throw, and 10-yd. dash are examples.
Aerobic endurance	Endurance in moving large muscle groups repeatedly for 3 min. or more, but preferably for over 5 min. The limitations in performance are primarily in the oxygen delivery system and at the cellular level.	All-out running, swimming, or cycling for more than 3 min.
Anaerobic-aerobic endurance	Endurance in moving large muscle groups repeatedly for at least 1 min., but not for more than 2 min. The limitations in performance lie within the muscles' short-term energy supply and the oxygen delivery system.	All-out running, swimming, or cycling for 1 to 3 min.
Relative muscular endurance	Endurance is repeatedly lifting body weight or a light load that is a proportion of maximum strength, by concentric contractions, or sustaining these loads by an isometric contraction. The limitations in performance reside primarily within the muscle itself.	Performance tests that permit more than 25 repetitions using body weight or an external load that is the same relative load for everyone. Sit-ups and leg raises are examples of appropriate tests. Also, maintaining a sustained isometric contraction for more than about 60 sec., such as in a bent arm chin, is an effective measurement.
Absolute muscular endurance	Endurance in repeatedly lifting an external weight or in sustaining it by an isometric contraction.	Performance tests that permit more than 25 repetitions with loads that are the same for all testees.

formance associated with the stress can be expressed in terms of the components. Likewise, the expression of a component in physical performance can be identified with specific physiologic stresses and mechanisms.

Strength and Physiologic Response

A muscle may contract maximally in a work task involving either absolute or relative strength. A muscle cannot distinguish lifting a heavy barbell once (1-RM) from lifting body weight once using maximum effort. Thus, the physiologic response is the same in both situations. Often, in work and in sports, when both strength components are evident, an individual will lift a submaximal load repeatedly. Working on a production assembly line may require heavy loads to be removed or placed on a conveyor belt or gymnastics may require body weight to be lifted repeatedly. In both activities, the components of muscular endurance play a larger role as the duration of work increases. But, the primary component may still be strength. Endurance also enters into performances when strength is measured by the number of repetitions with which a load is lifted. Strength tests of this kind include chinning and push-ups. When repetitions are less than 25, muscle force is still the primary component, but endurance is also a concern. Muscular endurance, although contributing somewhat to strength performances when duration or repetition is a factor, is discussed later with the endurance components.

The primary source of energy in high forces of muscular contractions is the ATP-CP stored within the muscle cells. Eliciting energy for high muscle forces does not depend on a steady supply of oxygen to the muscles. The anaerobic source of energy, however, is depleted in about 10 sec. when maximum force is evoked (see Table 2–3). Consequently, force capacity drops noticeably after this period.

Because of the high forces in contraction and their rapid elicitation in strength per-

formances, more white, fast-twitch fibers than red, slow-twitch fibers are involved. More rapid splitting of ATP-CP for energy, larger motor neurons, and greater conduction velocities are primarily responsible for the shorter contraction times in white fibers than in red fibers. But, by the same token, the more rapid depletion of ATP in the white fibers leads to a similarly quick reduction in glycogen stores and to an increase in lactic acid. Thus, high muscle forces cannot be sustained for long periods. The large quantities of lactic acid that build up in the muscles lead to a rapid onset of fatigue and diminished performance. Also contributing to the greater fatigability of white fibers are the relatively fewer capillaries supplying them and the fewer mitochondria in their cells. Less oxygenated blood flow and fewer manufacturing ''plants'' for the production of ATP in white fibers lead to less endurance in white fiber muscle cells than in the red fibers.

The extent of muscle force is related to the number of motor units firing at one time and to the frequency of their firing. Consequently, afferent input from the working muscles, which has a positive influence on motor unit involvement, contributes significantly to strength. Before applying a force, an individual gets ''set.'' As a result, gamma bias increases. Gamma neurons are facilitated to be excited on shorter notice when action begins. And, even before action begins, gamma influence on muscle spindles results in greater muscle force just prior to a maximum effort. In addition, the synergistic effect of other muscles not directly involved in moving the load enhances force capacity of the primary muscles. These synergists facilitate and make easier the activation of motor neurons to the working muscles. But, to prevent excessive force and to avoid injury, the Golgi tendon organs may come into action to inhibit contractile tension. If so, strength is less likely to reach its maximal capacity. Associated with a contraction of the working muscles is the action of reciprocal inhibition, which affects the antagonistic muscle. The opposing muscle relaxes further so that the agonists can move with less restriction and more strength.

The cardiovascular and respiratory responses to work of maximum contractions are a result of the overall effects of skeletal muscles on blood flow.[5-8] Total peripheral resistance increases greatly as the contracting muscles squeeze on the blood vessels. Respiration either is greatly curtailed or may cease during the effort. During repetitive movements, breathing may be only partially impaired. However, when only one maximum effort is required, breathing often stops temporarily. The drop in venous return to the heart may be great enough to reduce blood flow and oxygen to the brain. This Valsalva maneuver leads to dizziness and, at times, to fainting. The reduction in venous return may decrease cardiac output if the proportional drop in stroke volume is greater than the relative increase in heart rate. But, cardiac output does not affect performance because it does not contribute to the amount of muscle force achieved in one maximum effort. However, if strength is measured by repetitive movements that alternately contract and relax the muscles, such as in chinning or push-ups, cardiac output plays a larger supportive role and contributes more to the performance. In this case, venous return is less affected, and cardiac output increases with stroke volume and heart rate. Some of the changes in cardiovascular and respiratory responses during strength activities that involve repetitions are caused by the effects of the sympathetic nervous system. The accelerating effect on heart rate and respiratory rate and the vasoconstriction effect in the nonworking tissues by sympathetic stimulation are some of the changes that enhance performance.

Power and Physiologic Response

The exertion of a maximum force in a quick movement is characteristic of both absolute and relative power. Although the resistance load propelled is an external load in one component and body weight in the other, the muscles providing the force respond the same way physiologically. Force of contraction is not as great in power movements as it is in activities where strength per se is emphasized. This was shown in Figure 1–19 where the relationship between velocity of muscle shortening and muscle force is illustrated. Nevertheless, in power movements, muscle force is usually significantly larger than in endurance activities where muscles must work for long periods of time.

The physiologic responses in power movements are similar in many ways to those occurring in primarily strength efforts. Some differences between the two are associated with the time interval over which forces are applied. In activities of all-out effort when only one tremendous contraction is involved, such as in lifting a maximum load when measuring strength, or when only one explosive jump is involved, such as in power, maximum strength takes longer to achieve than maximum power does. As a result, the longer and greater tension developed in the muscles during a maximum strength performance depletes the ATP-CP energy stores at a faster rate than in a power movement. Both require stored ATP-CP as the primary energy source, however. In addition, both involve the white fibers to a much greater degree than the red fibers because high force and rapid contractions fire these fast-twitch fibers. But, by the same token, the rapid depletion of ATP-CP stores in the muscles does not permit maximum strength or power to continue over a long time span.

Neural control of movement in power activities is qualitatively the same as in strength activities. However, the rapidity of power moves requires quicker responses by the afferent receptors and the integration and interpretation of their input in the central nervous system. In a series of fast movements involving a specific sequential pattern of muscular contractions, the body as a whole and/or the limbs are displaced from one position to another. These rapid alterations in body posture call for appropriate neural input and output so that balance is maintained and limbs do not exceed their joint ranges. Balance is achieved by effector responses to input from the proprioceptors in the muscles, joints, skin, and vestibular apparatus. Movement activates these afferent receptors, and their impulses are conveyed to the central nervous system for interpretation. Involved in integrating and interpreting this input are the cerebellum, cerebral cortex, and other neural tissues in the brain. The motor response prevents the limbs and entire body from moving beyond a balanced posture. The cerebellum prevents "overshoot," and the vestibular apparatus and neck receptors help to keep the center of gravity above the base of support. Hyperextension of the limbs is prevented by the coordinating relationship between the muscle spindles and the Golgi tendon organs. Muscle force is greater at the beginning of a power move than at any other joint angle because the muscle is usually at its longest length and the spindles are maximally stimulated. At the same time, the antagonistic muscles are especially placid from the effects of reciprocal inhibition. But, near the end of the joint range, the Golgi tendons of the agonists are stimulated, thus relaxing the muscle and contracting the antagonist to prevent undue tension at the skeletal joint. For example, when putting a shot, the triceps muscle contracts to extend the arm. However, at the completion of extension, the triceps relax as the biceps contract to prevent hyperextension.

The responses made by the heart, blood vessels, and respiratory system are similar to what occurs when strength is the primary component involved. That is, heart rate may or may not increase at the moment of maximum effort because of the short time required in one explosive movement. However, soon after, heart rate is elevated to meet the increased metabolic needs of the previously worked muscles. When a power event is repetitive, such as a short running dash, heart rate increases during the run. The contraction of skeletal muscle in power activities provides a resistance to blood flow and an increase in blood pressure. Usually, ventilation is temporarily suspended because the breath is often held. Immediately afterward, blood pressure may stay elevated briefly while metabolic needs are met.

Endurance and Physiologic Response

To work continuously, a muscle must have a high energy supply and the capacity to produce ATP. Because most of the ATP is produced in the presence of oxygen, or aerobically, adequate blood flow is essential for optimal endurance. If oxygenated blood is plentiful during work, the limitations in performance depend on the amount of glucose and stored glycogen in the muscles. When energy stores run out, fatigue sets in and movement is impaired. In other kinds of endurance work, the ability to perform is not limited by the stored energy in the muscles, but by an inadequate blood flow. Unless large quantities of oxygen are available to muscles, the potential energy stores cannot be tapped. Insufficient blood flow or quantity of available fuel can be the limiting factor in endurance. The primary cause of either is related to the intensity of muscle force. There is a direct and an inverse relationship between blood flow and force of a muscle contraction.[9,10,10a] Large numbers of muscle fibers contracting at once increase force; however, an increase in contracting fibers decreases the blood to the fibers. Associated with greater contractions is an increased shifting from aerobic metabolism to anaerobic metabolism. Smaller contraction forces and increased blood flow allow the production of ATP primarily by aerobic metabolism.

When relatively small muscle mass is working, the cardiovascular system can easily provide large quantities of blood. Whether it reaches the muscle fibers is another matter and depends on the extent to which blood flow is impeded. But, as more muscle mass is involved and oxygen needs increase, greater importance is attached to the ability of cardiovascular function to provide large quantities of blood. The distinction between cardiovascular endurance and muscular endurance is based on the degree to which the heart and circulation are stressed in work. Ordinarily, performances involving large muscle mass with low muscle forces increase the demands placed on the oxygen delivery system in work of long duration. When small muscle mass is worked and relatively little stress is placed on the heart and circulation, muscular endurance is the primary component involved. The limitations in performance when muscular endurance is primarily emphasized lie within the muscle fibers themselves and not within the oxygen delivery system of the heart and circulation. However, in cardiovascular endurance, the limitations are found in both the delivery system and the muscles.

The physiologic responses in both absolute and relative muscular endurance are the same. Their limitations in endurance are determined by the contraction forces of the muscle. The ATP-CP stores in the muscles are depleted rapidly in work or exercise when the forces are high. In fact, in a maximum sustained effort, they are depleted in about 10 sec. If work is less intense and some blood flow is possible, ATP energy is produced both anaerobically and aerobically. Usually in sport activities, where work is near maximum or maximum, the limiting factor of performance is the muscle's capacity to provide ATP by anaerobic metabolism and, at the same time, to neutralize the acidity in the muscles caused by lactic acid buildup.

MEASUREMENT OF THE PHYSICAL PERFORMANCE COMPONENTS

Each component of physical performance, when elicited in work or exercise, is associated with a specific kind of muscle contraction. A strength component is related to high muscular contractions; a power component to fast contractions; and an endurance component to sustained or repeated contractions. These kinds of muscle responses are evoked when either body weight or an external weight is the resistance load. In addition to the specific kind of muscle contraction elicited by the different components, a different amount of muscle mass is also involved in some of the components. To elicit the aerobic component, large muscle mass must contract repeatedly. The muscular endurance component, however, is often elicited with relatively small muscle mass. Table 7–2 indicates the extent to which force, contractile velocity, repetitive contractions, and muscle mass are involved in each component and the nature of the resistance load, whether it is body weight or an external load. From this table, tests to measure each component can be ascertained.

Tests That Measure Absolute Strength

Refer to the absolute strength component in Table 7–2. The columns associated with absolute strength identify the unique characteristics of this component in terms of muscle response, muscle mass involved, and resistance load against which the muscles contract. Column 1 indicates that high muscle force is a characteristic of this component. Therefore, to achieve a high contraction force, either a heavy weight must be lifted once or a maximum force must be applied to an immovable object. The resistance load is external (col. 5) in any case. Because only one maximum effort is required, both repetitions (col. 3) and velocity of contraction are low (col. 2). Muscle mass measured for absolute strength is unlimited. Therefore, all subcolumns in column 4 are checked. A common measure of absolute strength is the amount of weight lifted once (1-RM) using a barbell or Universal Gym. When strength is measured by an isometric contraction, a back and leg dynamometer or a tensiometer is frequently used (see Figs. 1–34, 1–35). These instruments can be used to measure strength of athletes, industrial workers, and students in physical education classes. But, when large numbers of individuals must be

Table. 7–2.
Physical Performance Components and the Associated Muscle Responses, Muscle Mass Involvement, and Load Lifted

Component	Muscle Force			Contraction Velocity			Repetitions			Muscle Mass			Resistance Load	
	High	Moderate	Low	High	Moderate	Low	High	Moderate	Low	High	Moderate	Low	Body Wt.	External Load
Absolute strength	X					X			X	X	X	X		X
Relative strength	X					X			X	X	X	X	X	
Absolute power		X		X					X	X	X	X		X
Relative power		X		X					X	X	X	X	X	
Aerobic endurance			X			X	X			X			X	
Anaerobic-aerobic endurance		X			X	X	X			X			X	X
Absolute endurance		X	X		X	X	X				X	X		X
Relative endurance		X	X		X	X	X				X	X	X	X (% of max.)

tested and time is a factor, a situation commonly found in the schools, other tests are often used to measure strength. The fairly high relationship between maximum strength and number of times or repetitions a heavy load can be lifted permits an estimate of 1-RM strength. The statistical relationship between maximum strength of the elbow flexors and number of repetitions with which 65 lb. can be curled among college males is high (R = .90), as was shown in Figure 1–30.[11] This relationship is understandable because individuals with high levels of strength have a greater capacity for lifting a given load repeatedly than do those of lower strength, even though muscular endurance may also be involved to some degree in the performance. But, as the load becomes lighter and the ability to perform depends more and more on muscular endurance, some individuals of less strength can out-perform stronger individuals because of the much greater role played by endurance than by strength. This is brought out clearly by the low (but statistically significant) relationship between maximum strength and number of repetitions with 25 lb. (R = .39) (see Fig. 1–30).

To accurately predict maximum absolute strength from number of times a load is lifted, an individual must lift a relatively heavy load that does not permit more than 25 repetitions. With this load, the relationship between strength and repetitions is high (R = .90), as was shown in Figure 1–30. Table 7–3 can be used to predict maximum strength from number of repetitions and load lifted provided repetitions do not exceed 25. For example, 80 lb. is lifted 10 times (10-RM or the load with which 10 repetitions can be performed using maximum effort). To predict maximum strength or 1-RM, first locate the number 10 in the first column. Second, divide the 80 lb. by .80, the number in the second column and same row. The quotient, 100 lb., is the estimated maximum strength or 1-RM. If 80 lb. is lifted 5 times, divide 80 lb. by .90 to arrive at a 1-RM of 89 lb. (rounded off). The error in predicting the

Table 7–3.

Predicting Maximum Absolute Strength (1-RM) from Maximum Number of Repetitions When Repetitions are 26 or Less*

Maximum number of Repetitions	Divisor
2	.96
3	.94
4	.92
5	.90
6	.88
7	.86
8	.84
9	.82
10	.80
11	.78
12	.76
13	.74
14	.72
15	.70
16	.68
17	.66
18	.64
19	.62
20	.60
21	.58
22	.56
23	.54
24	.52
25	.50

*To predict the 1-RM, divide the load by the divisor in the row corresponding to the number of repetitions with which the load was lifted.

1-RM by this procedure is usually less than 5%.[12]

Absolute strength may also be predicted by using body weight as the resistance load with which repetitions are performed. Again, repetitions must not be higher than about 25.[13] There are two tests of this kind: maximum chin and dip. From the number of chins or dips and from body weight, the 1-RM can be predicted by using Table 7–3. Either of these tests are not only excellent predictors of strength of the arm and shoulder muscles but also are fair predictors of the strength of other muscles (see Table 1–6). When both are predicted and their values are combined in an equation, they predict total strength for college males with high accuracy (R = .90) (total strength = 1.05 1-RM chin + .74 1-RM dip + 322).[12] Total strength in this prediction is the sum of the 1-RM values of 7 weight-training lifts involving all the large muscle groups of the body. The lifts were: curl, upright rowing, overhead press, bench press, dead lift, squat, and sit-up.

Tests that Measure Relative Strength

The muscle response for relative strength is much the same as for absolute strength in terms of muscle force (col. 1), contraction velocity (col. 2), and muscle mass (col. 4) in Table 7–2. There is some difference in the repetitions area (col. 3) because repetitions may go up to 25 whereas in absolute strength only one repetition is involved. The most distinct difference between the two kinds of strength is in the resistance load (col. 5). Relative strength is measured by the number of times body weight is lifted whereas absolute strength involves the application of a single force to an external load. This difference between the two strengths accounts for the higher contraction force in absolute strength. But, nevertheless, the contraction force in relative strength is still high, provided repetitions do not exceed about 25. A test that allows higher repetitions measures strength and muscular endurance to a large extent. And, as repetitions increase, the test becomes farther removed as a measure of strength. Some common tests of relative strength are push-ups, chins, and rope climb. But, even these tests may not be good measures of strength among individuals who either cannot do one repetition or who easily perform over 25 repetitions. Often, young children and most females of all ages cannot perform one push-up or dip. In these cases, the tests do not measure relative strength. Occasionally, some individuals exceed 25 repetitions in these tests. Consequently, the quality of strength becomes less of a factor in performance. (Generally, however, the stronger individuals are those that exceed the 25-repetition limit.)

Tests that Measure Absolute Power

The most common characteristic of power is high contraction velocity (see Table 7–2, col. 2). As a result, muscle force is moderate because of the inverse relationship between force and velocity of muscle shortening. (see Fig. 1–19). Because only one explosive move is usually involved, the repetitions are low (col. 3). Any amount of muscle mass may be moved (col. 4), but the resistance load is primarily external to the body. Of course, the total resistance load is not limited to an outside load because limbs are always moved when muscles shorten. But, when the external load is substantial in weight, such as an 8-lb. medicine ball or 16-lb. shot, the component of absolute power plays a prominent role in successful performance.

As expected, generally high absolute power is associated with high absolute strength. The ability to apply a large force to a heavy barbell increases the ability to propel a lighter weight farther. As a result, power athletes often train for absolute strength so that power will increase. Field tests that measure absolute power should confine body movements to the muscles actually pushing against the external object. Otherwise, relative power may become a significant factor. For example, in the shot-put, an athlete moves his body across a circle before putting the shot. The distance of the toss reflects both the initial movements associated with relative power and the final movements involving the component of absolute power. For "pure" absolute power to be measured, the relative power aspect must be minimized. One way to accomplish this in the shot-put is to eliminate the move across the circle and to confine the test to the final move. In this way, the distance putted better reflects absolute power. Other kinds of tests to measure absolute power involve tossing an 8-lb. medicine ball with two hands while in a sitting or standing position.

Tests that Measure Relative Power

The major difference between these tests and those measuring absolute power is the load propelled. Body weight is the main resistance load (Table 7–2, col. 5). Otherwise, muscle force is still moderate (col. 1), contraction velocity is high (col. 2), repetitions are generally low (col. 3), and muscle mass is of variable amounts (col. 4). Many tests measure relative power. Quick movements of the total body are characteristic of such tests as the 50-yd. dash, vertical jump, standing long jump, shuttle run, and softball throw. Although the actual movements differ among these tests, the basic component common to each, and the underlying quality primarily contributing to the performance, is relative power. Some laboratory tests measure power by the use of electronic equipment. In one such test, the Margaria power test,[14] an individual stands in front of a staircase. When ready, he runs up the stairs as rapidly as possible, taking three steps at a time. An electronic clock starts when the foot touches the third step and stops when the foot touches the ninth step. The power expressed by the movement is a product of the individual's body weight and the vertical distance, divided by the time (hundredths of a second). The formula is

$$P = \frac{W \times D}{t}$$

where P=power, W=body weight, D=vertical distance, and t= time.

The Kalamen-Margaria test also measures leg power by the electronic devices and is practically the same as the Margaria test.[15] However, in this test, an individual begins the move 6 m. in front of a staircase instead of directly in front of the first step. The two tests are the same in all other ways.

Just as absolute strength and absolute power are related, so are relative strength and relative power. Individuals of high strength per pound of body weight ordinarily can project themselves with speed, agility, and coordination better than those of less strength. Again, as with absolute power, individuals training to increase relative power usually incorporate weight training as an essential form of exercise. Other than by improving sport skills, the only way an individual can increase the capacity to run faster or jump higher and farther is to improve the contractile force of muscle.

Tests that Measure Aerobic Endurance

For ATP energy to be created aerobically during work, blood flow to the exercised muscles must not be hindered significantly. With a free flow of oxygenated blood and a steady production of ATP, work can be carried out for long periods, provided that the glycogen stores in the muscle are plentiful. Aerobic endurance or endurance accomplished with adequate supplies of oxygen, is associated with muscular contractions of low intensity. The oxygen required for the work matches closely the energy needs of the muscles. Higher muscle contractions unbalance the relationship between oxygen availability and energy requirements. When this happens, more and more of the energy is produced anaerobically.

The intensity of a muscle contraction is directly related to the degree of ATP production either aerobically or anaerobically; and both are related to work duration. Aerobic metabolism is associated with work of relatively long duration, whereas anaerobic metabolism is associated with work of shorter duration. The involvement of each in maximum work of different durations is shown in Table 7–4. Note that, as exercise duration increases, more of the energy produced comes from aerobic metabolism. Of course, longer work times are accomplished with low forces of muscle contraction and (see Table 7–2, col. 1), therefore, low contraction velocity (col. 2). Because work is continuous and prolonged, high repetitions are evident (col. 3). With the great activation in aerobic endurance of the heart and cir-

Table 7–4.

Relative Contribution of Anaerobic and Aerobic Metabolism at Various Maximum Run Times, and Approximate Distances Run at Each Time for Young Adult Males and Females

Maximum Run Time (min.)	Relative Contribution of Energy Production*		Running Distance**	
	Anaerobic	Aerobic	Male	Female
1	60	40	380 yd.	250 yd.
2	40	60	600 yd.	430 yd.
3	33	67	850 yd.	600 yd.
4	27	73	1,025 yd.	840 yd.
5	20	80	1,275 yd.	1,025 yd.
6	16	84	1,450 yd.	1,210 yd.
7	14	86	1,600 yd.	1,350 yd.
8	12	88	1,760 yd.	1,510 yd.
9	11	89	1,910 yd.	1,650 yd.
10	9	91	2,060 yd.	1,810 yd.

*These values are based on several research studies[18–20] as reported by Gollnick.[21]
**Estimated by interpolation and extrapolation for young adults.[22]

culatory systems and of the respiratory functions, a large amount of muscle mass must be involved (col. 4). The resistance load against which the muscles contract during aerobic work may be limited to body weight, such as in running or swimming, or to an external load, such as a bicycle ergometer or rowing machine (col. 5).

One of the best ways to test for aerobic capacity is by measuring $\dot{V}O_2$ max. This procedure is performed by gradually increasing a work load on a bicycle or treadmill until an additional work increment does not elicit more oxygen consumption. Numerous laboratory methods are used to measure oxygen consumption. A representative sample of these methods is described in Table 7–5. In addition to work loads provided by a treadmill and bicycle ergometer, maximum oxygen consumption

Table 7–5.

Some Methods Used on the Treadmill and Bicycle Ergometer in Determining Maximum Oxygen Consumption

Method	Type of Work	Testing Procedure
Åstrand and Saltin[17]	Leg work on bicycle ergometer at 50 rpm	10 minute warm-up at 55% $\dot{V}O_2$ max followed by work to exhaustion in 2 to 8 minutes
Åstrand and Saltin[17]	Graded treadmill running	Run at 7 mph to exhaustion on successive days. Elevate treadmill by 2.5% each day. $\dot{V}O_2$ max is determined when exhaustive run is less than 2.75 minutes.
Costill and Fox[23]	Graded treadmill running	7 minute warm-up at 7.44 mph, 0% grade. 4 minute work at 8.9 mph at 0% grade followed by 4% grade. Successive increases of 2% after every 2 minutes until exhaustion.
Katch, Girandola, and Katch[24]	Leg work on bicycle ergometer at 60 rpm	Work begins at 2.5 kp (measure of force) and increases by 0.5 kp every 2 minutes until exhaustion.

can be assessed by swimming,[16] cross-country skiing,[17] or working both the arms and legs simultaneously.[10a]

Although laboratory assessments of aerobic capacity are highly valid, they may be impractical when large groups of individuals must be tested in field conditions. In addition, the expense of laboratory equipment is prohibitive in many schools. Nevertheless, aerobic capacity is often measured with high accuracy from field tests involving running. This was shown by the highly significant relationships found between oxygen consumption (ml./kg./min.), considered the best measure of aerobic capacity, and some field test of endurance.[22] Forty-four adult males, whose ages ranged from 17 to 30 years, participated in a study to determine the physiologic factors common to both laboratory and field tests of working capacity. Field tests that measured aerobic and anaerobic endurance, each in varying degrees, were related to $\dot{V}O_2$ max (ml./min.) (Table 7–6). The highest correlation coefficients were between $\dot{V}O_2$ max and the tests that strongly measured aerobic capacity such as the 1-mile, 12-min.-run, and 600-yd. tests. Smaller coefficients found with the field tests of 300-yd., 50-yd., and 10-yd. runs indicate a greater involvement of anaerobic metabolism in performance.

Table 7–6.

Correlation Coefficients Between Maximum Oxygen Consumption and Various Running Field Tests

Test	Maximum Oxygen Consumption (ml./kg./min.)
12-min. run (distance)	.90
1 mile	−.74*
600 yard	−.78*
300 yard	−.52*
50 yard	−.29*
10 yard	−.23*

*Negative signs indicate relationships between scores where higher scores on one variable are associated with lower scores on another variable.[24]

These relationships are understandable because the duration of maximum work, which is highest in the 12-min. run test and lowest in the 10-yd. dash test, indicates the extent to which aerobic and anaerobic metabolism are involved. This was clearly shown in Table 7–4 where maximum run times (work duration) were associated with anaerobic-aerobic energy production and estimated running distances for young adult males and females. Based on these figures, a test of aerobic endurance should elicit maximum effort for 3 min. or more, preferably over 5 min. For young adult males, this time period corresponds to running distances between 850 and 1,275 yd.; for females, 600 to 1,025 yd. During these runs, most of the ATP produced comes from aerobic metabolism. These figures also apply to other activities, such as cycling, swimming, or rope jumping, provided that work is continuous and maximum for 3 or more minutes.

Tests that Measure Anaerobic-Aerobic Endurance

The greater intensity of muscle force (Table 7–2, col. 1) and the correspondingly faster velocity of muscle shortening (col. 2) in anaerobic-aerobic endurance compared to aerobic endurance are the two most important distinctions between these two endurance components. The shifting from primarily aerobic metabolism to more anaerobic metabolism and the associated limitations in ATP production reduce work time significantly. At a maximum run time of 10 min., only about 9% of the energy is produced anaerobically; at a more intense run of 1 min., anaerobically produced energy increases to about 60% (see Table 7–4).

If running tests are used to assess this component, the distances that require 1 to 2 min. to run will elicit both anaerobic and aerobic metabolism to approximately the same extent. Of course, the distances required to achieve a 1 to 2 min. run depend on several factors that are related to work capacity. Age and sex differences result in varying endurance performances. Distances run in 1 to 2 min. are longer for young adults than for young children. Even among young adults, differences exist with males exceeding females on the average. Because of these factors, running distance to measure anaerobic-aerobic endurance depends on age and sex. Table 7–4 shows the distances run by young adult males and females at the various maximum run times. This information can be used to develop a running test that can elicit any percentage combination of anaerobic and aerobic endurance. If an individual wants to measure primarily aerobic endurance, but also a limited degree of anaerobic endurance, the average running time of 4 min. would be achieved at distances of 1,045 yd. for males and 840 yd. for females. At 4 min., about 27% of the ATP comes from anaerobic metabolism and 73% comes from aerobic metabolism.

The duration of 1 to 2 min. for measuring anaerobic-aerobic endurance also applies to cycling, rope skipping, and swimming as long as the work duration and intensity are the same.

Tests that Measure Absolute Muscular Endurance

Both aerobic and anaerobic metabolism are involved in muscular endurance, but the extent of their involvement depends on the energy requirements per contraction. During high intensity work, anaerobic metabolism dominates; in work of low intensity, aerobic metabolism is emphasized. In higher intensity contractions, impairment of circulation to the working muscles and the correspondingly decreased oxygen availability lead to more anaerobic involvement for energy. The intensity of muscle force need only be a little more than 15% of maximum strength for anaerobic metabolism to play a highly significant role in energy formation.[25]

Muscular endurance, whether absolute or relative, is evidenced by low or moderate muscle force (see Table 7–2, col. 1) and contraction velocity (col. 2). Repetitions are high (col. 3), a characteristic of all endurance performances. Muscle mass is generally low or moderate (col. 4), and the resistance load is external (col. 5).

Tests to measure absolute endurance require applying a force to an external load that is the same for everyone. As long as the load is over 15% of maximum strength for everyone, scores are comparable among all test subjects. Smaller loads may be lifted indefinitely and, therefore, would not be appropriate for measuring muscular endurance. Because the load is the same for everyone, the test subjects with the highest absolute strength can generally perform more repetitions and, thus, have more muscular endurance than do the weaker individuals. But the importance of strength in endurance depends on the load lifted. The heavier the load, the better the performance of the stronger individuals. Even with a light load, stronger persons tend to perform better, but to a lesser degree. This was shown in Figure 1–30 where the relationship between maximum strength and absolute endurance became less as the load lifted became lighter (the r decreased from .90 to .36).

Tests that Measure Relative Muscular Endurance

The energy sources for relative endurance are the same as for absolute endurance and depend on the intensity of each repetitive contraction. The two components differ in the load used to measure relative endurance. Although absolute endurance is measured with the same load for everyone, relative endurance is measured with a load that either is a proportion of maximum strength or is body weight. When the load is the same proportion of maximum, but light enough to permit more than 25 repetitions, work intensity for each repetitive movement is about the same for all test subjects. Any differences among individuals would then be attributable to cellular adaptability to work stress. If an individual with a maximum lift of 200 lb. can lift 100 lb., 30 times, he has the same relative endurance as a person with maximum strength of 150 lb. who can lift 75 lb., 30 times. Most studies have shown that stronger individuals cannot sustain an isometric contraction as long as weaker individuals can,[26-28] nor can they perform as many repetitions when work is done with concentric contractions.[11,29]

Relative endurance can also be measured by the number of times body weight is lifted in whole or in part, provided that the repetitions exceed 25. Less than 25 repetitions measure primarily relative strength. Individuals of high relative strength tend to perform well on the component of endurance. This result is understandable because less effort is needed per repetition when strength per pound of body weight is high. Consequently, more repetitions can be done. Some field tests of relative endurance are sit-ups, leg raises, and push-ups.

The physical performance components, their definitions, and the field tests that measure them are summarized in Table 7–1. It should be reiterated that only seldom does just one component operate in work or exercise. Often, many components are involved; some are involved to a high degree whereas others are involved only slightly. Usually, the highly involved components primarily determine the quality or quantity of a performance. If an important component essential for high-level performance in a sport or occupation is possessed to a high degree, success is more likely.

RELATIONSHIP OF BODY SIZE AND STRUCTURE TO PHYSICAL PERFORMANCE COMPONENTS AND ATHLETIC SPORTS

Athletes at high levels of performance in their particular sports possess physical characteristics that favor their success. In the field events of shot-putting, discus throwing, and hammer throwing, the participants are large and muscular; in distance running, the athletes are generally small; and in gymnastics, the athletes are short and muscular. Although sports training affects, to some degree, the muscularity and excess adipose tissue in athletes, some basic body structures are optimally suited for some

sports and not for others. The massive football lineman would not be successful as a gymnast; nor would the smaller gymnast succeed as a defensive tackle. If an individual has a body size that contributes to success in specific performance components, he will likely succeed in the sports that require those components for high-level ability. An individual with a large and muscular skeletal frame will likely possess a high level of absolute strength and power, a component important for successfully performing as a shot-putter. Understanding the relationship between body size and athletic performance begins first with knowing which physical components are especially affected by body size.

Body Size and Performance of the Physical Components

Correlation coefficients between body size and scores from tests that measure various performance components indicate

Table 7–7.

Relationships Between Body Size and Tests That Measure the Components of Physical Performance*

Test	Height	Weight	Primary Component
deep knee bend	−.33	−.22	
rope climb	−.43	−.48	relative
dips	−.41	−.32	strength
bent-arm hang	−.32	−.48	
pull-ups	−.42	−.45	
push-ups	−.33	−.25	
medicine ball put			
standing	.17	.39	absolute
sitting	.18	.32	power
hand grip	.25	.49	absolute
arm pull	.23	.39	strength
trunk pull	.32	.42	
50-yard run	−.24	−.32	relative
shuttle run	−.31	−.38	power

*Based on 201 males of average age 18.25 years; height, 70 inches; and body weight, 150.6 pounds; from Fleishman.[2] Coefficients of .20 are significant at the .05 level.

whether body weight and height contribute to a component score. Table 7–7 shows the relationships between body size and the component tests to which it is associated. The negative coefficients between body size and the tests that measure the components of relative strength and relative power indicate that a tall and heavy person has poor performances on these components. But, on the components of absolute strength and power, the opposite occurs. A large stature contributes to performance in activities of absolute strength and power.

Although most of these relationships are statistically significant, they are, nevertheless, too low to accurately predict performance. Certainly, every heavy person does not have a high level of absolute strength, nor does every light person have low strength. The same reasoning holds true for the other components when they are related to body size. However, on the average, an individual of large body size has more absolute strength and power than does an individual of small stature. The same reasoning applies for the average small individual, who has more relative strength and power than a larger individual.

The explanation for these differences in performance as they relate to body size is centered around strength per pound of body weight. The relationship between relative strength (strength/lb.) and absolute strength is inverse (Fig. 1–25). Although absolute strength increases with body weight, strength per pound decreases. As a result, heavier people can exert a larger quantity of muscle mass to an external object. But, in tasks where body weight must be lifted or propelled quickly, the larger strength per unit body weight allows for better performance by the smaller person.

Lighter body weight and, in turn, greater strength per pound are advantages for the components of aerobic endurance, anaerobic-aerobic endurance, and relative endurance when body weight is the resistance load. More strength per unit weight makes carrying the body easier. Consequently, oxygen cost

per pound is also less. So, in a long-distance race, the athlete with more strength per pound can maintain the faster pace. Even in shorter races, where running times are 1 to 2 min., and anaerobic-aerobic endurance is the primary component involved, the individual with more strength per pound should be able to run faster. More strength per pound is also an advantage in relative endurance when body weight is lifted. Movements can be repeated more often and contractions sustained longer in supporting body weight. Push-ups and sit-ups are two expressions of relative muscular endurance when repetitions exceed about 25.

For the component of absolute endurance, where an external load is lifted, large muscle mass and, concomitantly, high absolute strength are advantages. This component favors the large individual who can repeatedly raise and lower a weight with less effort than can an individual of small muscle mass. As a result, the work capacity and endurance of the stronger individual exceeds that of the smaller individual.

The importance of body size in the performance of the components is summarized in Table 7–8. Remember that there are exceptions to the rule; some heavy individuals have high strength per pound of body weight

Table 7–8.

Importance of Body Weight in the Physical Performance Components Among Young Adult Males

Component	Body Weight	
	high	low
Absolute strength	X	
Relative strength		X
Absolute power	X	
Relative power		X
Aerobic endurance		X
Anaerobic-aerobic endurance		X
Absolute muscular endurance	X	
Relative muscular endurance with body weight		X

whereas some small individuals have low strength per pound of body weight.

Body Size, Skeletal Structure, and Performance in Athletics

In some sports, body size obviously affects performance. The relation between body size and athletic performance is shown in Table 7–9. Although there are numerous exceptions to these relationships, they nevertheless indicate the high significance of body size to performance. Some of these exceptions are owing to different anthropometrical relationships between various parts of the skeleton, even among those of similar body size. This is brought out by the unique skeletal structures of certain athletes. High jumpers generally are tall and light, but also tend to have relatively long legs and short upper bodies. This arrangement is an advantage because the trunk, which must be lifted over a bar, is lighter in weight because of the shorter upper body. But, the higher center of gravity of the jumper makes him poorly designed for contact sports where maintaining balance on the ground is highly important. With a higher weight center, an athlete is more likely to lose balance when struck by an opponent. Also, in such sports as soccer and judo, long-legged individuals may find the execution of abrupt changes in direction difficult.

The ratio of the length of the lower leg to the thigh, called the crual index, is related to performance. Individuals with a high index (proportionately longer lower leg than upper leg) tend to have an advantage in jumping. Almost all jumping animals have a high crual index.[30] The length of the heel bone (calcaneus) may also contribute to differences in performance. If the bone is long, there is a greater mechanical advantage for jumping and running. Longer limbs are an advantage in throwing. The range of motion through which the hand passes allows a pitcher to impart acceleration to the ball. In tests of power, where objects are either thrown or pushed, arm length is an important factor in performance. All these anthropometric factors play a part in explaining athletic performance.

EVALUATION OF PHYSICAL PERFORMANCE

Physical performance is expressed by a variety of physical tasks that are used to assess physical fitness, athletic ability, or work capacity in industry. In the physical assessment of performance, basic steps that apply to all situations must be followed, whether the purpose is to determine physical fitness or to develop a screening test for job applicants. Once the purpose is known, one must identify the physical components primarily involved in the performance to be assessed. The next step is the selection of tests that measure these components. Finally, the tests are administered and the scores evaluated. This approach is used in the assessment of physical fitness, athletic ability, or work potential in industry.

Physical Fitness Testing

To assess physical fitness, one must identify the physical components considered most essential for achieving a high level of fitness. Of course, physical fitness must be defined before the important components can be identified. Physical fitness is considered here as an ability possessed in varying degrees by everyone. Specifically, physical fitness is defined as the ability to perform tasks that involve the components of strength, power, and endurance. Thus, by varying the tasks (but not the components), a different battery of test items can be used to measure physical fitness specifically for different age levels or sports. The components of strength, power, and endurance are considered basic because they are involved in the characteristic movements of man in work and play. These movements are running, jumping, lifting, and throwing.

Thus, the first step in the assessment process, defining physical fitness and identifying the components, has been accom-

Table 7–9.

Relation Between Body Size and Athletic Performance*

Body Height	Body Weight	Sport	
		Men	Women
Tall	Heavy	Heavyweight boxing Football end Football tackle Heavyweight wrestling	Field hockey goalie Soccer goalie Lacrosse
Tall	Medium	Discus thrower, javelin thrower Basketball center Baseball pitcher	Modern dance Softball pitcher Volleyball
Tall	Light	High jumper, hurdler Tennis Middle-distance runner Fencing Cross-country runner	Tennis Basketball Softball, first base
Medium	Light	Distance runner Badminton Baseball second baseman Lightweight boxer	Fencing Badminton Softball infielder
Short	Light	Soccer forward Tumbling Figure skater Jockey	Tap dancing Tumbling Soccer forward
Short	Medium	Gymnastic apparatus Handball Springboard diver Water polo guard	Diving Skiing Figure skater
Short	Heavy	Baseball catcher Ice hockey defense Weight lifter	Softball catcher Backfield-soccer Backfield-hockey
Medium	Heavy	Shot putter Football fullback Football guard, tackle, or center	Speedball Archery Bowling
Medium	Medium	Distance swimming Golf Bowling	Swimming Field hockey forward Golf Synchronized swimmers

*(From Morehouse, L. E., and Rasch, P. J.: Sports Medicine for Trainers. 2nd Edition. Philadelphia, W. B. Saunders Co., 1964.)

plished. The second step is the selection of test items that measure these components. But, before this selection can be done, one must also define the group of individuals or population that will be tested. A group is usually defined by such characteristics as age, sex, and group affiliation. The group is identified so that the most appropriate test items can be selected. For example, push-ups is an inappropriate test for young children because a significant number cannot perform them. The last characteristic of the group, called group affiliation, refers to a physical education class, athletic team, or a group of individuals trying to make an athletic team. The test items used to measure physical fitness will differ according to a particular group. In a physical education class, the teacher is concerned about measuring physical fitness with items that involve a variety of muscles and movements. This may not be the case with a coach who is interested in screening individuals trying out for a football team. A coach may select items that measure more specifically the tasks in football, such as sprint running and leg power in pushing a sled, and other items that measure upper body strength.

To assess physical fitness in a physical education class, with the main components being strength, power, and endurance, test items are selected to measure absolute and relative strength, absolute and relative power, and aerobic and anaerobic-aerobic endurance. Test items used to measure these components for young adult males are presented in Table 7–1. At least one test item is selected to measure each component. Tests that measure primarily the component of muscular endurance are seldom chosen to measure physical fitness. The significant relationship between strength and muscular endurance guarantees to some extent that the strength items will assess muscular endurance. Muscular endurance is also omitted as an essential component to minimize the number of test items. In a school setting, physical fitness should be assessed with as few items as possible because of the time

factor. Sometimes, however, muscular endurance is measured directly for some individuals who find the test items of relative strength easy to perform (individuals who can do more than 25 repetitions). One test item that measures muscular endurance for most is the all-out sit-up. This item becomes more a test of relative strength if a 1-min. time limit is used.[29]

If time for administering the test items is critical, only the aerobic or the anaerobic component can be measured. The relatively high relationship between these two components indicates that a good score on one probably results in a good score on the other (r = .78).[31]

IMPORTANCE OF PHYSICAL PERFORMANCE COMPONENTS IN SPORTS

The assessment of athletic performance focuses on the primary components that are essential for success. Athletic skill is not a consideration here. Athletic potential is assessed with the assumption that, if an individual possesses the necessary components to a significant level, the basic ingredients upon which to build skill are present. But, if the basic components are insufficient, no amount of skill can replace them. With this in mind, the primary components of several athletic sports are indicated in Table 7–10. A further breakdown within some sports is made because certain playing positions or events depend more on some components than on others for success.

FOOTBALL. In the sport of American football, the playing positions of interior lineman and running back emphasize different components. The interior lineman must move heavy opponents to either make or prevent a tackle. Consequently, high relative power is needed to get to the opponent quickly and, once there, high absolute power and strength are needed for the restraining aspect of the task. Although the offensive back and the interior lineman require the same components, the emphasis is a little different. The running back depends

Table 7–10.
Most Important Components Underlying Performance in Various Sports

Sport	Absolute Strength	Relative Strength	Absolute Power	Relative Power	Aerobic Endurance	Anaerobic-Aerobic Endurance	Muscular Endurance
Football							
offensive back	X		X	X		X	
defensive back	X		X	X		X	
interior lineman	X		X	X		X	
wide receiver				X		X	
tight end	X		X	X		X	
line backer	X		X	X		X	
quarterback				X		X	
Baseball			X	X		X	X
Basketball				X	X	X	
Soccer				X	X	X	
Field Hockey				X	X	X	
Wrestling	X	X	X	X	X	X	X
Fencing				X		X	X
Track-Running Events							
100 m.				X		X	
200 m.				X		X	
400 m.						X	
800 m.						X	
1 mile (1500 m.)					X		
2 mile					X		
5,000 m.					X		
10,000 m.					X		
Marathon					X		
Track-Field Events							
shot-put			X	X			
discus			X	X			
hammer-throw			X	X			
pole vault				X			
high jump				X			
long jump				X			

more on high relative power to elude tacklers, but, once contact is made, high absolute strength and power are important for "breaking" tackles. The most important component for the defensive back is relative power, which provides the speed and body control that keeps him from being outmaneuvered. Certainly other components, such as absolute strength and power and anaerobic-aerobic endurance, are involved when making a tackle. But, without an exceptional quality of relative power, the position cannot be played well. In addition, because of the many repeated and relatively long runs required from a defensive back, anaerobic-aerobic endurance is especially important. Primarily, wide receivers catch passes. Therefore, they must possess high relative power, which is reflected in running speed and "faking out" an opponent. The varied roles played by line backers, where heavy opponents must be pushed out of the way to make tackles and pass coverage involves quick movement of the entire body, require a high degree of additional components, such as absolute strength and power and relative power. Because the area of the playing field covered by a linebacker is extensive, an especially high level of anaerobic-aerobic endurance is also essential. Like the wide receiver, the tight end must have good relative power for catching passes; however, he must also block heavy linemen on running plays, which requires a high degree of absolute strength and power. Of course, anaerobic-aerobic endurance is important at all positions because of the repeated short, all-out bursts of energy required. Each play from the line of scrimmage usually lasts for several seconds with about a 15 to 20 sec. rest between plays. However, because each team consists of an offensive squad and a defensive squad, there are adequate rest periods for most players.

The significance of body size in the various playing positions reflects the importance of the different components to which body weight is related. Because high absolute strength and power are essential to blocking and tackling in the interior of the line, the strongest athletes are required in those positions. And, because large body mass is associated with high absolute strength, one can understand why the heaviest players are found at those positions. But, when the most important component is relative power, which is basic to running speed and total body coordination and is a quality highly important for a defensive back, smaller individuals often perform best. The higher strength and power per body weight in smaller football athletes makes them better adapted for playing as defensive backs. The same is true for offensive backs because they must elude tacklers. But, because offensive backs are called on more frequently to block or "break tackles," absolute strength and power play a larger role in their performance than in that of defensive backs. Consequently, running backs are generally heavier in body weight and, thereby, have more absolute strength and power. Although there are exceptions to the rule in terms of body size and playing position, there are fewer exceptions at the highest levels of performance in professional football.

BASEBALL. The basic activities in baseball are running, hitting, and throwing. Because running is fast and, of necessity, short in duration, the endurance component is anaerobic-aerobic endurance. Because running is relatively infrequent, and the times between runs quite lengthy, recovery from fatigue is usually assured. However, if a player hits for extra bases, he must have enough endurance to avoid being tagged out. Running endurance is not frequently exhibited, but, when it is, winning or losing may be in the balance. Relative power is probably more important than anaerobic-aerobic endurance in running. Beating out a hit or stealing a base requires running speed. In defensive play in the outfield or infield, players must be able to move their entire bodies rapidly and in a coordinated fashion. Relative power is important at such times.

Hitting and throwing involve applying a

force to external objects with high velocity and acceleration. The nature of the moves and the resistance loads involved point to absolute power as an important component for both tasks. The acceleration imparted to the bat when contact is made with the ball directly influences the distance the ball travels. Generally, players with the greatest muscle mass hit the most home runs because stronger players can impart greater acceleration to a bat. This also applies to throwing, but to a lesser degree. That is, stronger, and often larger, individuals tend to throw fast. In professional baseball, pitchers tend to be of substantial body size, indicating the association between absolute power and muscle mass. Because the ball is thrown repeatedly by a pitcher, the muscular endurance factor plays a larger role in the performance of this position than it does for others, especially in the muscles of the arm and shoulders. The metabolic emphasis is anaerobic because of the short and explosive nature of the muscular contractions. The ability of the body to replenish the ATP-CP in the throwing muscles between pitches determines, to a large extent, the consistency with which a pitcher can throw a ball with high acceleration.

BASKETBALL. A basketball player must perform a variety of tasks in a game. Some of the movements involve primarily relative power, as shown by a fast break; anaerobic-aerobic endurance, as shown by repeated, fast runs up and down the court; and aerobic endurance, as shown by movements that are not necessarily explosive, but are continuous and highly repetitive. Dribbling the ball while moving rapidly, jumping in the air while shooting or recovering rebounds, faking out an opponent, and chasing a loose ball are moves that involve relative power. And, when they are repeated frequently, endurance enters the picture. Components of lesser importance (although not indicated for basketball in Table 7–10) are absolute and relative strength, which operate when "fighting" over a rebound or loose ball. Although these two components are generally less important for success in playing

basketball, they are essential for some individuals with exceptionally low levels of strength. A tall player may not be able to take advantage of height if body weight is not in proportion to weight, or strength is not in proportion to height. As a result, going up for a rebound makes this player more vulnerable to the effects of excessive body contact by opponents.

SOCCER AND FIELD HOCKEY. These sports are considered together because they involve the same components in varying degrees. The continuous nature of the activities, alternating between short explosive bursts of effort, more drawn-out but reasonably intense runs, and less intense work, elicit the full gamut of endurance responses: anaerobic, anaerobic-aerobic, and aerobic endurances, respectively. Chasing the ball or puck as an offensive or defensive maneuver, or getting into playing position quickly in anticipation of an opponent's move, requires relative power to a high degree. The speed and coordinated aspects of these moves are critical for optimum performance. Relative power is probably a little more important than endurance for the goalie. Short, quick movements in preventing the opposing team from scoring are common responses of a goalie and involve mostly relative power. Of course, if most of the playing time is spent at one end of the field, endurance becomes more of a factor for the goalie at that end.

WRESTLING. This sport requires all the essential components for optimum performance. Movement of the body on a continuous basis, sometimes relatively slowly and sometimes quite quickly, brings into play all the components of endurance. Muscular endurance is associated with the high intensities of contractions (when the strength components are evident) and their prolonged involvement. Here, the inability to continue work at a high level is owing to factors residing primarily within the muscles and not within the oxygen transporting mechanisms. But, while muscular endurance is operating, other muscles are functioning at various levels of anaerobic and aerobic metabolism, thus taxing the heart and circulatory system as well. Fast movements of the body when applying wrestling holds show relative power. Once an opponent is engaged and his body weight is tossed about, absolute power becomes an important component. Because all these components are operating at more or less the same time, one can easily understand why wrestling is so physiologically demanding.

FENCING. The sporadic bursts of quick energy observed when lunging toward or retreating from an opponent indicate an emphasis on relative power of the legs, hips, and upper-body muscles. When these movements are repeated often enough, both anaerobic-aerobic endurance and muscular endurance are involved. The weight of the weapon is light enough so that absolute strength of the arm and shoulder muscles is not a great factor in performance. However, the ability to recuperate between a series of repeated bouts is largely dependent on the same physiologic mechanisms and tissues underlying endurance in many other sports.

TRACK-RUNNING EVENTS. The intensity of muscle force with each step in running determines whether the energy cost can be met primarily aerobically or anaerobically. If the forces are high, as in the sprint events, ATP is used more rapidly than it can be supplied by aerobic metabolism. In the 100-m. run, almost all the energy is supplied anaerobically by the stored ATP-CP in the muscles. Consequently, for the outstanding and conditioned sprinter, running time reflects primarily relative power rather than endurance. However in the 200-m. run, although the ATP-CP stores still play the largest role, the anaerobic-aerobic component contributes, in some degree to the performance. In the middle distances, where muscle force is less than in the races of shorter distances, more of the energy can be produced aerobically, but a high component of anaerobic metabolism is still involved. Consequently, the anaerobic-aerobic component is involved. As the distances in-

crease and each step is taken with less muscle force, aerobic metabolism provides most of the energy. So, in races of 1 mile or 1,500 m. and more, the most important component is aerobic endurance. Of course, its importance becomes absolute in races of 30 min. or more (see Table 7–4).

TRACK-FIELD EVENTS. The explosive nature of the field events in track is evidence for the importance of the power component. In such events as shot-put, discus, and hammer throw, where body weight is moved rapidly as a force is applied to an external object, both the relative and absolute power components are involved. But, in the high jump and long jump, where body weight is propelled upward and forward, relative power is the primary component in performance. Pole vaulting requires much relative power to rapidly raise the body toward the pole, but relative strength also contributes largely to the lift over the bar. A high level of relative strength, or strength per pound, permits a higher lift of the body and better performance.

IMPLICATIONS FOR ATHLETIC TRAINING

The first step in developing training programs to improve athletic performance is to identify the most important components for success in a sport. The next step is to incorporate exercises in the program that stress the physiologic mechanisms and tissues specifically involved when these components are elicited. To accomplish this, the particular actions of the skeletal joints when performing in the sport should be known. With this information, the muscles producing these actions can be identified. Generally, the best way to train the muscles is by the same movements required in the sport. If this is not possible, then other movements involving the same muscles are employed in training. The specific method of training these muscles depends on the components that need developing: strength, power, or endurance. But, the training principle that applies to all the components is the overload principle. For improvement to occur from training, the muscles and physiologic systems must be continually stressed to varying degrees on a long-term basis. The particular form or mode of overloading used, however, determines the specific component trained. For example, heavy loads as a form of overload training, such as in weight training, improve the components of strength whereas high repetitions as a form increase the endurance components.

Absolute and Relative Strength

Performance in the strength components can be enhanced by training that increases the force capacity of muscle. To accomplish this, overloading is done with heavy loads and, therefore, with relatively few repetitions (10 or less). There are actually four ways of overloading to increase strength: by repetitions, exercise load, sets, and training days per week. When overloading is provided by repetitions, the athlete begins a program with a heavy load that can be lifted for a specific number of repetitions, e.g., six. He strives to lift this weight more times in training and, as a result, there is an overloading effect. When 10 repetitions are possible, more weight is added to the exercise load. Increasing the training load is the second method of overloading. For best results, the loads added are 5% or less of the previous training load. The third form of overloading involves the number of times or sets an exercise is repeated. Usually, these three forms of overloading—repetitions, exercise load, and sets—are all employed. It is customary to establish a specific number of sets, usually three, during the earlier stages of training. When each of three sets can be performed for a predetermined number of repetitions, such as 10, additional weight is lifted at the next training session. Later in training, more sets may be added to further increase the overloading effect. However, more than five sets may result in overtraining; consequently, adding sets as a form of overloading is less frequently used than are repetitions and exercise load. The fourth method of overloading is by increasing the number of training days a week, but this has its limitations. The necessary rest day between training sessions only allows three or four weekly sessions at most. If training begins with three weekly sessions, only one session could be added. However, if the same muscles are not exercised every day, strength training can occur five or six days a week. In this way, the muscles are still able to recuperate between training sessions.

Absolute and Relative Power

Power is improved when the force capacity of a muscle is increased in a fast movement, such as when body weight or an external object of relatively light weight is moved. Maximum forces are not achieved in power movements because of the inverse relationship between force and velocity of shortening. Slow movements, associated with lifting heavy weights, elicit high contractile tensions, whereas light loads, when moved as rapidly as possible, are done with considerably less muscle force. But, the best way to improve muscle force in power events is by training for maximum strength using the overloading methods previously described for the strength components. The training effects in power, however, may not be as dramatic as the increases in maximum strength. There is not a high relationship between maximum strength and running speed or speed in throwing a baseball. Consequently, increasing strength may not always increase power. This possibility is illustrated in Figure 7–2 for a hypothetic case before and after strength training. Movement was controlled so that force alone could be measured at a variety of velocities. When these forces were measured before and after training, two different slopes evolved. Note that, as movement velocities increased, there was a relatively smaller increase in force. And, at the fastest velocity, no differences in force were shown before and after strength training. Movement speed in running may not always improve from strength training, especially at the fastest movement. However, when heavy external

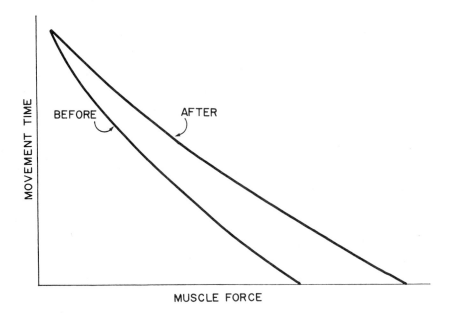

Fig. 7–2.   Changes in muscle force at various movement velocities before and after weight training. A hypothetic athlete.

weights and body weight are both moved, such as in shot-putting or hammer throwing, there is a better chance that strength training will improve power and performance.

Anaerobic and Aerobic Endurance

These endurance components operate in a variety of athletic sports. Although the physiologic stresses on the heart and circulation are similar in various sports, there are large differences between them in the specific muscles used and the movements made. Running involves movements and muscles that are somewhat different from those used in rowing or wrestling. Nevertheless, the principles of training, as they apply to the two endurance components, are much the same.

The intensity of work and its duration determine which component is most affected. Table 7–4 indicates the various work intensities and the primary energy sources associated with them. To develop anaerobic-aerobic endurance, work durations between 1 and 2 min. are best; for aerobic endurance, work of more than 3 min. (preferably 5 min.)

is most effective. The overload principle in endurance training is applied in a variety of ways.

Interval Training. This is a system of conditioning in which work is done in regularly repeated bouts with rest periods between. Overloading is provided by rate and distance of the work, number of times the work is repeated, length of rest periods between work bouts, and number of training sessions per week. If the primary concern is to improve anaerobic-aerobic endurance, the distance run in interval training should take about 1 to 2 min. For a young adult male, the distance would be about 440 yards. If the primary concern is to improve aerobic endurance, the distance run would be 880 yards or more. Rest periods between runs may be from 0.5 to 3 times the running times. It is common to work about six bouts each training session and to train at least three times weekly. However, the competitive runner invariably trains for more bouts and weekly sessions.

Continuous Movement Training. Programs of continuous movement are carried out for durations exceeding 5 min. and, therefore, develop primarily aerobic endurance. These programs vary in terms of movement rate and distances covered. If slow running is the activity, distances covered are in miles. Jogging falls in this category and usually is associated with slow, continuous running. Therefore, distances run exceed one mile.

Muscular Endurance

There are basically two ways to overload the muscles to increase muscular endurance. One is by strength training, which involves heavy weight, and the other is by high repetitive movements. Absolute muscular endurance is increased particularly by strength training. As a consequence of an improvement in force capacity, more work can be done. An athlete before training, who bench presses 150 lb., may perform 40 repetitions with 60 lb. After training, when his maximum bench press is 175 lb., the 60-lb. weight can be lifted probably more than 50 times. The other way to overload is by practicing high repetitions with a relatively light load. Whereas strength training usually increases muscle mass and, as a result, force capacity, high repetitive training affects more the structural and chemical makeup of the muscle fibers to enhance their ability to utilize oxygen and produce energy. Perhaps a more effective program to increase endurance would involve a combination of both strength training and high repetitive movements. Instead of lifting the same weight for 50 times, a heavy weight is lifted for 10 times, each of five sets with no rest between sets. But, for each succeeding set after the first, the weight is dropped by about 20%. In this way, the effort per repetition is high to increase strength, but, because the movements are continuous for high repetitions, the endurance aspects of the muscle fibers are also enhanced.

Although the specific principles of overload training to improve strength, power, and endurance are easily understood, the variety of methods used by coaches to apply these principles may be confusing. Part of the problem is the inability of the observer to identify the common components affected by a variety of seemingly unrelated training programs. An educated eye is often necessary to see the commonality of components among different sport movements. Although an understanding of the physiologic mechanisms primarily involved in each of the components is essential for analyzing training programs and their effects, if the components cannot easily be identified, then the physiologic effects of training may not be known. Therefore, to function optimally as a practitioner in sports or athletic training, both physiologic responses and performance components must be understood as inseparable partners.

REFERENCES

1. Harris, M.: A factor analytic study of flexibility. Res. Q., *40*:62, 1969.
2. Fleishman, E.A.: The Structure and Measurement of Physical Fitness. Englewood Cliffs, Prentice-Hall, Inc., 1964.
3. Baumgartner, T.A., and Zuidema, M.A.: Factor analysis of physical fitness tests. Res. Q., *43*:443, 1972
4. Jackson, A.S.: Factor analysis of selected muscular strength and motor performance tests. Res. Q., *42*:164, 1971.
5. Åstrand, I., Guharay, A., and Wahren, J.: Circulatory responses to arm exercise with different arm positions. J. Appl. Physiol., *25*:528, 1968.
6. Bevegard, S., Freyschuss, U., and Strandell, T.: Circulatory adaptation to arm and leg exercise in supine and sitting position. J. Appl. Physiol., 21:37, 1966.
7. deVries, H.A., and Adams, G.M.: Total muscle mass activation vs. relative loading of individual muscle determinants of exercise response in older men. Med. Sci. Sports, *4*:146, 1972.
8. Freyschuss, U., and Strandell, T.: Circulatory adaptation to one-and-two leg exercise in supine position. J. Appl. Physiol., *25*:511, 1968.
9. Lind, A. R., and McNicol, G.W.: Muscular factors which determine the cardiovascular responses to sustained and rhythmic exercise. Can. Med. Assoc. J., *96*:706, 1967.
10. Lind, A.R., and McNicol, G.W.: Cardiovascular responses to holding and carrying weights by hand and by shoulder harness. J. Appl. Physiol., *25*:261, 1968.
10a. Åstrand, P.O., et al.: Intra-arterial blood pressure during exercise with different muscle groups. J. Appl. Physiol., *20*:253, 1965.
11. Berger, R.A.: Relationship between strength and absolute muscular endurance with various resis-

tance loads. Unpublished study. Biokinetics Research Laboratory, Temple University, 1970.

12. Berger, R.A.: Prediction of total dynamic strength from chinning and dipping strength. J. Assoc. Phys. Ment. Rehabil., *19*:18, 1965.

13. Berger, R.A.: Determination of a method to predict 1-RM chin and dip from repetitive chins. Res. Q., *38*:330, 1967.

14. Margaria, R., Aghemo, P., and Rovelli, E.: Measurement of muscular power (anaerobic) in man. J. Appl. Physiol., *21*:1662, 1966.

15. Kalamen, J.: Measurement of Maximum Muscular Power in Man. Doctoral Dissertation, The Ohio State University, 1968.

16. Magel, J.R., and Faulkner, J.A.: Maximum oxygen uptakes of college swimmers. J. Appl. Physiol., *22*:929, 1967.

17. Åstrand, P.O., and Saltin, B.: Maximal oxygen uptake and heart rate in various types of muscular activity. J. Appl. Physiol., *16*:977, 1961.

18. Saltin, B., and Hermansen, L.: Glycogen stores and prolonged severe exercise. *In* Nutrition and Physical Activity. Edited by G. Blix. Upsala, Almqvist and Wiksell, 1967.

19. Saltin, B., and Karlsson, J.: Muscle glycogen utilization during work of different intensities. *In* Muscle Metabolism During Exercise. Edited by B. Pernow and B. Saltin. New York, Plenum Press, 1971.

20. Saltin, B.: Metabolic fundamentals in exercise. Med. Sci, Sports, *5*:137, 1973.

21. Gollnick, P.D., and Hermansen, L.: Biochemical adaptations to exercise: anaerobic metabolism. *In* Exercise and Sport Sciences Reviews. Edited by J.H. Wilmore, New York, Academic Press, 1973.

22. AAHPER Young Fitness Test Manual. Washington, D.C., American Association for Health, Physical Education, and Recreation, 1965.

23. Costill, D.L., and Fox, E.L.: Energetics of marathon running, Med. Sci. Sports, *1*:81, 1969.

24. Katch, F.S., Girandola, R.N., and Katch, V.L.: The relationship of body weight on maximum oxygen uptake and heavy-work endurance capacity on the bicycle ergometer. Med. Sci. Sports, *3*:101, 1971.

25. Rohmert, W.: Die beiziehung zwischen kraft und ausd uer bei statischer muskelarbeit, schriftenreihe arbeitsmedizin, sozialmedizin, arbeitshygiene. Band *22*:118, A.W. Gentner Verlag, Stuttgart, 1968.

26. Martens, R., and Sharkey, B.J.: Relationship of phasic and static strength and endurance. Res. Q., *37*:435, 1966.

27. Tuttle, W.W., Janney, C.D., and Thompson, C.W.: Relation of maximum grip strength to grip strength endurance. J. Appl. Physiol., *2*:663, 1950.

28. Tuttle, W.W., Janney, C.D., and Salzano, J.V.: Relation of maximum back and leg strength to back and leg strength endurance. Res. Q., *26*:96, 1955.

29. Berger, R.A.: Relationship between dynamic strength and dynamic endurance. Res. Q., *41*:115, 1970.

30. Davenport, C.B.: The crual index. Am. J. Phys. Anthropol., *17*:333, 1933.

31. Burke, E.J.: A Factor Analytic Investigation into the Validity of Selected Field Tests of Physical Working Capacity. Doctoral dissertation. Temple University, 1973.

Index